FUNDAMENTALS OF NURSING
for
General Nursing and Midwifery

FUNDAMENTALS OF NURSING
for
General Nursing and Midwifery
(Including First Aid)

| Third Edition |

SN Nanjunde Gowda MSc (N) PhD
Professor and Ex-Principal
Anil Baghi College of Nursing
Ferozepur, Punjab, India

Jyothi Nanjunde Gowda MSc (N)
Ex-Vice-Principal
Anil Baghi College of Nursing
Ferozepur, Punjab, India

Forewords
Nagarajaiah
BN Muninarayanappa

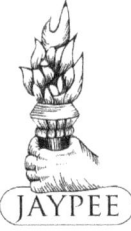

JAYPEE BROTHERS MEDICAL PUBLISHERS
The Health Sciences Publisher
New Delhi | London

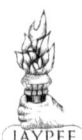

Jaypee Brothers Medical Publishers (P) Ltd

Headquarters

Jaypee Brothers Medical Publishers (P) Ltd
EMCA House, 23/23-B
Ansari Road, Daryaganj
New Delhi 110 002, India
Landline: +91-11-23272143, +91-11-23272703
+91-11-23282021, +91-11-23245672
Email: jaypee@jaypeebrothers.com

Overseas Office

J.P. Medical Ltd
83 Victoria Street, London
SW1H 0HW (UK)
Phone: +44 20 3170 8910
Email: info@jpmedpub.com

Corporate Office

Jaypee Brothers Medical Publishers (P) Ltd
4838/24, Ansari Road, Daryaganj
New Delhi 110 002, India
Phone: +91-11-43574357
Fax: +91-11-43574314
Email: jaypee@jaypeebrothers.com

EU GPSR Authorised Representative

Logos Europe, 9 rue Nicolas Poussin
17000, La Rochelle, France
Phone: +33 (0) 6 67 93 73 78
E-mail: Contact@logoseurope.eu

Website: www.jaypeebrothers.com
Website: www.jaypeedigital.com

© 2024, Jaypee Brothers Medical Publishers

The views and opinions expressed in this book are solely those of the original contributor(s)/author(s) and do not necessarily represent those of editor(s) and publisher of the book.

All rights reserved. No part of this publication may be reproduced, stored or transmitted in any form or by any means, electronic, mechanical, photocopying, recording or otherwise, without the prior permission in writing of the publishers.

All brand names and product names used in this book are trade names, service marks, trademarks or registered trademarks of their respective owners. The publisher is not associated with any product or vendor mentioned in this book.

Medical knowledge and practice change constantly. This book is designed to provide accurate, authoritative information about the subject matter in question. However, readers are advised to check the most current information available on procedures included and check information from the manufacturer of each product to be administered, to verify the recommended dose, formula, method and duration of administration, adverse effects and contraindications. It is the responsibility of the practitioner to take all appropriate safety precautions. Neither the publisher nor the author(s)/editor(s) assume any liability for any injury and/or damage to persons or property arising from or related to use of material in this book.

This book is sold on the understanding that the publisher is not engaged in providing professional medical services. If such advice or services are required, the services of a competent medical professional should be sought.

Every effort has been made where necessary to contact holders of copyright to obtain permission to reproduce copyright material. If any have been inadvertently overlooked, the publisher will be pleased to make the necessary arrangements at the first opportunity.

Inquiries for bulk sales may be soliciated at: jaypee@jaypeebrothers.com

Fundamentals of Nursing for General Nursing and Midwifery

First Edition: 2006
Second Edition: 2010
Third Edition: **2024**

ISBN: 978-93-5465-978-2

The more credit you give away,

The more will come back to you.

The more you help others,

The more they will want to help you.

Brain Tracy

Advisors

Devi Nanjappan
Principal
Nagarathnamma College of Nursing
Bengaluru, Karnataka, India

BV Kathyani
Principal
National Institute of Mental Health and Neuro Sciences
Bengaluru, Karnataka, India

Foreword to the Third Edition

The challenge of preparing new generations of nurses who are effective in the clinical community has become increasingly more complex. The target outlined in the nursing practice required knowledge and skill that are truly rooted in the science of nursing. The scope and depth of knowledge required by students and faculty alike demand educational resources that are interesting. Textbooks that meet this standard are rare and precious. Fortunately, some of the textbooks meet the standard, and hence students and teachers are able to select such precious textbooks.

The authors have taken out time to upgrade Foundation of Nursing for the 3rd edition, according to latest syllabus. I am happy to note that this title started one decade back and has been utilized by many educational institutions in India and other countries. The 3rd edition of this textbook promotes nursing as an evolving art and science directed to human health and well-being.

The authors created students experience in mind. The student-friendly writing style ensures that the students will retain information with responsible caring practice. The students will master the cognitive and technical skills they will need to effectively nurse the patient in their care.

I recommend this book to be used for the General Nursing Midwifery program and should be on the bookshelf of every student, teacher, and practicing nurse today.

Nagarajaiah MSc (N) PhD
Former Additional Professor
National Institute of Mental Health and Neuro Sciences
Bengaluru, Karnataka, India

Foreword to the First Edition

The Indian Nursing Council (INC) is a national statutory body to establish a uniform standard of nursing education for the nurses in the country. The INC has revised the syllabus for the Diploma in General Nursing and Midwifery Training program. In this context, I appreciate the authors of the Fundamentals of Nursing for General Nursing and Midwifery, for bringing out the book as per the syllabus in order to help the students for their easy understanding.

Fundamentals of Nursing for General Nursing and Midwifery is based on revised syllabus. The authors have used their clinical skills and teaching expertise to bring out the contemporary and innovative thoughts practiced in Indian hospitals and nursing institutes.

This book could also be called as insight for students, and it is in very simple English. To write this type of book, one needs dedication and devotion of time and energy which authors have proved by covering all the units in one volume. I am confident that this book will be able to prepare the nurses to provide qualitative nursing care in the hospital and community.

I recommend this book to be used for general nursing students and should be in the bookshelf of every student and teacher of today. I congratulate the authors for bringing together the most important ideas from the old and new nursing principles under one cover as Fundamentals of Nursing for General Nursing and Midwifery.

BN Muninarayanappa
Registrar
Karnataka Nursing Council
Karnataka, India

Preface to the Third Edition

The nursing profession always depends on change and challenges. Nursing requires broad knowledge, skill, and ability to apply it to their patients while providing care. The role of a nurse includes safeguarding nursing practice and demonstrating its contribution to the health care of our nation.

The third edition of Foundation of Nursing is revised to prepare today's students for the challenges of tomorrow. This edition is designed for both students and teachers. The comprehensive coverage provides fundamental concepts, skills, and procedures for firm foundation in nursing. The language used is student-friendly. This edition includes a number of key current practice issues and prepares the students and teachers to address the unique healthcare needs of patients.

Key features
Coverage of all fundamentals of nursing content:
- **Safety guidelines in nursing unit** provides incident involving and safety precaution
- **Nursing process** provides historical perspective and steps for benefit and format for nursing care
- **Physical examination** provides technique and preparation to perform physical examination
- **Hygienic needs, assessing vital signs, and medication administration** provides knowledge base for nurses
- **Diagnostic measure** provides specific guidelines for nursing role in preparation, during procedure, and aftercare nurse's role
- **Managing emergencies** improves the role of a nurse in addressing cardiopulmonary resuscitation (CPR) and other emergencies
- **Infection control** provides chain of infection, mode of spread and hospital-acquired infection and prevention.

SN Nanjunde Gowda
Jyothi Nanjunde Gowda

Preface to the First Edition

Though the numbers of books written by Western authors are available, they focus on care related to Western, sociocultural milieu. Studies have highlighted the importance of environmental and cultural aspects of patient while providing care. Hence books written by Indian authors are very useful to students and beginning practitioners in nursing to understand the importance of sociocultural milieu of patients which specifically focuses on need based nursing care and leads to greater satisfaction of patients.

The format of this book has been well organized into eight units, with pictures, tables, checklists and so on. In the beginning of each unit, objectives have been specified of what is expected by the readers after completion of each unit or chapters which are found to be very useful particularly for beginners so that they know what they are expected to learn and understand from each unit.

To ensure that this edition reflects current practice and future trends in fundamental of nursing the reviewers have taken keen interest to review. They are from all specialties of nursing including hospital and community practice, education and research. Their knowledge, experiences and skills have made this edition a valuable practical instructional guide to all categories of students and nurse practitioners.

Those who read this book as a student, as a novice nurse, an expert practitioner, a preceptor or teacher, the book will provide the wealth of knowledge and skills derived from many sources from professional nursing practice, from research and from the experience of countless patients and clients.

Finally, what is noteworthy in this book is the organization of contents around the core aspects of fundamental practice of care required by patients which manifest the oneness of knowing-being-doing and oneness of art, science and technology of caring and healing practice adapted based on Indian context.

SN Nanjunde Gowda
Jyothi Nanjunde Gowda

Acknowledgments

The preparation of this book and the continued third edition resulted from the combined effort of many talented professionals. As an author, I acknowledge their support and professionalism. I am very proud to be associated with such fine individuals. My special thanks go to the nursing teachers and students who supported me and professional members who offered suggestions for completing this edition.

My warm appreciation and thanks go to Jaypee Brothers Medical Publishers (P) Ltd., New Delhi, India, who helped and guided me, Shri Jitendar P Vij (Group Chairman), Mr Ankit Vij (Managing Director), Mr MS Mani (Group President), Dr Madhu Choudhary (Director-Educational Publishing), Ms Pooja Bhandari [Director-Production (Books and Journals)], Ms Sunita Katla (Executive Assistant to Group Chairman and Publishing Manager), Mr Ajay Kumar Sharma [DGM–Production (Books and Journals)], Ms Seema Dogra (Cover Visualizer), Ms Neelam Kakriya (Proofreader), Mr Dinesh Bhardwaj (Typesetter), Mr Manoj Pahuja (Graphic Designer), and their team members for sharing our vision for foundation of nursing and giving me the chance to turn this vision into reality.

I would like to extend my heartfelt gratitude and special appreciation to Ms Jitika Royal (Content Strategist), for her unwavering support and dedication during the book revision process. Her invaluable contributions have made this endeavor truly remarkable, and I will forever cherish her guidance and encouragement.

I would also like to express my sincere thanks to all the dedicated editorial team members who have played a crucial role in shaping this project. Your hard work and commitment have been instrumental in its success.

In addition, I would like to acknowledge the exceptional contributions of two outstanding individuals, Ms Samina Khan (Executive Assistant to the Director of Educational Publishing) and Mr Rajesh Sharma (Production Coordinator). Their support and cooperation have been instrumental in bringing this project to fruition, and I am deeply grateful for their efforts.

My sincere thought is that if the nursing teachers, students, and other healthcare personnel apply the scientific principles which are described in this book, they will be getting immense satisfaction. I sincerely welcome constructive criticism from readers that will help me to enrich my knowledge to contribute more to the profession.

Above all, I am thankful to **ALMIGHTY GOD** for bestowing his bountiful grace for the success of this book.

Contents

1. **Introduction to Nursing**   1
   - Nursing Concept   1
   - Nursing: Definition   2
   - Scope of Nursing   3
   - Nature of Nursing   3
   - Functions of Nurse   4
   - History of Nursing   5
   - The Emergence of Professional Nursing   9
   - Ethics in Nursing, Roles and Responsibilities of a Nurse   13
   - **Types of Healthcare Agencies/Services**   **18**
   - Types of Healthcare Agencies   18
   - Major Hospital Health Services Departments   19
   - Nursing Unit   22
   - Rehabilitation Center   22
   - Healthcare Teams   23
   - Modern Approaches to Nursing Care   23
   - Health and Disease   23
   - Definition of Health   23
   - Determinants of Health   24
   - Dimensions of Health   25
   - Maslow's Hierarchy of Needs   25
   - Health Illness Continuum   26
   - Factors Influencing Health   26
   - Causes and Risk Factors for Developing Illness   27
   - Effect of Hospitalization   28

2. **Nursing Care of the Patient**   29
   - Emotional Needs of Patients   33
   - Common Emotional Responses to Illness and Nursing Implications   34
   - **Admission, Transfer, and Discharge Procedures**   **35**
   - Hospital Admission and Discharge   35
   - Room Preparation   36
   - Admission of Patient to an Emergency Department   37
   - Internal Transfer of Patients   39
   - Discharge from the Hospital   39
   - **Basic Nursing Skills**   **40**
   - Communication   40
   - Factors Influencing the Communication Process   44
   - Nurse-Patient Relationship   50
   - Recording and Reporting   51
   - Types of Client Records   52
   - Methods/Systems of Documentation/Recording   54
   - Reporting   55
   - Nursing Process   56
   - Historical Prospective of Nursing   56
   - Steps in the Nursing Process   57
   - Benefits of the Nursing Process   57
   - A Framework for Accountability   57
   - Process of Assessment   57
   - Nursing Diagnosis   59
   - Planning   61

3. **Meeting the Basic Needs of a Patient**   70
   - Comfort, Rest, and Sleep   71
   - Body Mechanics   73
   - Range of Motions   73
   - Beds and Bed Making   81
   - Elimination Needs   95
   - Nutritional Needs   109
   - Psychological and Spiritual Needs   120
   - Care of Terminally ill and Dying Patient   120

4. **Assessment of Patient/Client**   125
   - Health Assessment   125
   - Physical Examination and Assessment   126
   - Specific Areas of Examination   129
   - Physiological Assessment   137
   - Pulse   143
   - Respiration   145
   - Blood Pressure   148
   - Collection of Specimen   151
   - Venipuncture (Venous Blood)   152
   - Specimen Collection   159
   - Cervical Scrape   159
   - Ear Swab   159
   - Eye Swab   160
   - Collecting a Stool Specimen   160
   - Nasal Swab   162
   - Penile Swab   162
   - Rectal Swab   163
   - Semen   163
   - Throat Swab   164
   - Urine   164
   - Vaginal Swab   165
   - Wound Swab   165
   - Psychological Assessment   166

5. Infection Control — 170
- Nature of Infection — 170
- Hospital Acquired Infection (Nosocomial Infection) — 173
- Introductory Concept of Asepsis, Medical, and Surgical Asepsis — 175
- Medical Asepsis — 178
- Surgical Asepsis (Sterile Technique) — 180
- Aims of Standard Precautions Against Hospital-Acquired Infection — 181
- Biomedical Waste Management — 182

6. Therapeutic Nursing Care — 183
- Patients with Upper Respiratory Airway Infection — 183
- Patients with Pulmonary Diseases — 185
- Care of Patient with Altered Body Temperature — 189
- Care of Patient with Fluid and Electrolytes Imbalance — 190
- Care of Unconscious Patient — 193
- Care of the Patient in Traction — 197
- Care of Patient with Pain — 199
- Planning — 201
- Care of Patients with Body Elimination Deviation — 202

7. Introduction to Clinical Pharmacology — 208
- **Administration of Medication: General Principles, Considerations, Purpose of Medication — 209**
- General Principles — 209
- Purpose of Medication — 209
- Drug Nomenclature — 209
- Drugs Forms — 211
- Routes of Administration of Medication — 211
- Parenteral Administration — 213
- System of Drug Measurement — 221
- Topical Administration, Types, Purpose, Site, Equipment, Procedure — 223
- Ear Irrigation and Instillation of Ear Drops — 226
- Application of Drugs in Other Forms (Tropical Drugs) — 227
- Inhalation — 227
- Meaning of Parenteral Route of Epidural, Intrathecal, Intraosseous, Intraperitoneal, Intrapleural, Intra-arterial — 232
- Important Dates in Nursing — 232
- World Nursing Organization History — 233
- World History of Nursing Journal — 234

8. First Aid — 236
- Definition of First Aid — 237
- Aims of First Aid — 237
- General Principles of First Aid — 237
- Concept of Emergency — 239
- **Procedures and Techniques in First Aid — 239**
- Preparation of First Aid Kit — 239
- Dressing, Bandaging and Splinting — 239
- Cardiopulmonary Resuscitation: External Cardiac Massage — 248
- **First Aid In Emergency — 256**
- Hemorrhage — 256
- Shock — 256
- Drowning — 259
- Injuries to the Bones, Joints, and Muscles — 260
- First Aid for Accident — 264
- First Aid for Burns and Scalds — 265
- First Aid for Poisoning — 267
- First Aid for Food Poisoning and Poisonous Plants — 269
- First Aid for Bleeding — 270
- First Aid for an Insect Bite — 272
- **Community Emergencies — 274**
- Community Emergencies and Community Resources — 274
- Types of Disaster — 275

Index — 279

Syllabus

NURSING FOUNDATIONS

Placement: First Year

Time: 210 hours
Fundamentals of Nursing: 190 hours
First-Aid: 20 hours

FUNDAMENTALS OF NURSING

Course Description

This course is designed to help students develop an ability to meet the basic health need of the patients with regard to nursing care and develop skill in the competencies required for rendering effective patient care.

General Objectives

Upon completion of the course, the students shall be able to:

- Describe the physical, mental and social adjustment required of a sick individual and his family.
- Carry out basic nursing techniques and care with the application of sound scientific principle.
- Explain the concept of comprehensive nursing care.
- Develop skills in assessment, planning, implementation and evaluation of the nursing care rendered to the patients.
- Communicate effectively and establish good interpersonal relationship with the patients, their relatives and other health team members.
- Demonstrate skills in observation, recording and reporting.
- Recognize and utilize opportunities for planning and implementing need-based health teaching programme(s) for individuals, groups, families and communities.

Total Hours: 190

Unit	Learning Objectives	Content	Hours	Method of Teaching	Assessment Methods
I	• Define nursing and explain its nature, meaning, scope, ethics and principles in nursing. • Identify the qualities of a professional nurse health care agencies and its functions. • Describe the holistic approach to nursing and the determinants of health and the effects of illness.	**Introduction to Nursing** • Nursing—concept, meaning, definitions, scope and functions. • History of nursing in India • Nursing as a profession • Nursing professional—qualities and preparation. • Ethics in Nursing—roles and responsibilities of a nurse. • Health care agencies—hospital and community service—types and function of hospitals health team. • Modern approaches to nursing care including holistic nursing care • Health and Disease > Definition of health, determinants of health status. > Basic human needs > Illness and its effects on individual	25	Lecture cum discussions	• Short answer • Objective type • Essay type

Unit	Learning Objectives	Content	Hours	Method of Teaching	Assessment Methods
II	• Describe nursing care of the patient/client in hospital using nursing process. • Demonstrate skill in the admission and discharge process, maintenance of safe environment and records and reports	**Nursing care of the patient** • Patient environment in the hospital: Patients unit • Therapeutic environment ➢ Physical factors—lighting temperature, ventilation, humidity, noise, pestilence. ➢ Safety needs, prevention of environmental hazard ➢ Psychosocial and aesthetic factors. • Patient's adjustment to the Hospital. ➢ Understanding the patient as a person, socio-economic, and cultural background, health status, etc. ➢ Effect of hospitalization on patient and family. ➢ Admission, transfer, discharge procedures • Basic nursing skills ➢ Communication ➢ Nursing interview ➢ Recording and reporting • Nursing process ➢ Meaning and importance ➢ Assessment, nursing diagnosis ➢ Planning, implementation and evaluation ➢ Nursing care plan.	6	• Lecture cum discussions. • Demonstration of maintaining the records and reports • Role play	• Short answer • Objective type • Essay type • Return demonstration
III	• Describe basic needs of the patient • Demonstrate skill in meeting basic care of the patient	**Meeting the Basic Needs of a patient** • Physical needs: ➢ Comfort, rest, sleep and exercise ➢ Importance and its promotion ➢ Body mechanics—moving, lifting, transferring ➢ Position and posture maintenance ➢ Comfort devices ➢ Beds and bed making—Principles of bed making, types and care of bed linen ➢ Safety devices, restraints and splints ➢ Exercises—Active and Passive • Hygienic needs: ➢ Personal and environmental hygiene personal ➢ Nurses note in maintaining personal and environmental hygiene. ➢ Care of eyes, nose, ears, hands and feet. ➢ Care of mouth, skin, hair and genitalia ➢ Care of pressure areas, bed sores. • Elimination needs: ➢ Health and sickness ➢ Problems—constipation and diarrhea, retention and incontinence of urine. ➢ Nurse's role in meeting elimination needs. ➢ Offering bed-pan and urinal ➢ Observing and recording abnormalities. ➢ Preparation and giving of laxative, suppositories, enemas, bowel wash, flatus tube. ➢ Perineal care, care of patient with urinary catheter, diapers. ➢ Maintenance of intake and output records	65	• Lecture cum discussion • Demonstration	• Short answer • Objective type • Essay type • Return demonstration • Assessment using checklist

Unit	Learning Objectives	Content	Hours	Method of Teaching	Assessment Methods

		• Nutritional needs
		  ➢ Diet in health and disease
		  ➢ Factors affecting nutrition in illness
		  ➢ Nurse's role in meeting patients nutritional needs.
		  ➢ Modification of diet in illness.
		  ➢ Diet planning and serving.
		  ➢ Feeding helpless patients including artificial methods of feeding.
		• Psychological and spiritual needs
		  ➢ Importance
		  ➢ Nurse's role—diversional and recreational therapy
		• Care of terminally ill and dying patient
		  ➢ Dying patient's signs and symptoms needs of dying patient and family
		  ➢ Nursing care of dying: Special considerations; advance directives, euthanasia, will, dying declaration, organ donation, etc.
		  ➢ Medicolegal issues
		  ➢ Care of the dead body
		  ➢ Care of unit
		  ➢ Autopsy
		  ➢ Embalming			

IV	Describe the principles of assessment demonstrate skills in assessing the patient	**Assessment of patient/client**
		• Physical assessment
		  ➢ Importance, principles, methods of assessment
		  ➢ Height, weight, posture
		  ➢ Head to toe examination.
		• Physiological assessment
		  ➢ Vital signs, normal, abnormal Characteristics, factors influencing the variations
		  ➢ Observation and collection of specimens- urine, stool, vomitus and sputum.
		• Psychological assessment
		  ➢ Mood, intelligence, emotions—normal and abnormal behavior.
			14	• Lecture cum discussions
				• Demonstration
					• Short answer
					• Objective type
					• Essay type
					• Return demonstration
					• Assessment using checklist

V	• Describe the infection control, methods in the clinical setting.
	• Demonstrate infection control practices
		Infection control
		• Infection control:
		  ➢ Nature of infection
		  ➢ Chain of infection transmission
		  ➢ Defence against infection: natural and acquired
		  ➢ Hospital acquired infection (nosocomial infection)
		• Concept of asepsis:
		  ➢ Medical and surgical asepsis
		  ➢ Isolation precautions, barrier nursing
		  ➢ Handwashing: Simple, hand asepsis, surgical asepsis (scrub)
		  ➢ Isolation: Source and protection
		  ➢ Personal protective equipments types, uses and techniques of wearing and removing
			20	• Lecture cum discussion
				• Demonstration
				• Explain using manual of biomedical waste management of Government of India
				• Demonstration
				• Videos
				• Simulation
				• exercises
					• Short answers
					• Essay type
					• Objective type

Unit	Learning Objectives	Content	Hours	Method of Teaching	Assessment Methods
		➢ Decontamination of unit and equipment ➢ Transportation of infected patient ➢ Standard safety precaution ➢ Transmission based precautions • Biomedical waste management ➢ Importance ➢ Types of hospital wastes ➢ Hazards associated with hospital waste ➢ Decontamination of hospital waste ➢ Segregation and transportation ➢ Disposal			
VI	Describe therapeutic nursing care	**Therapeutic Nursing Care** • Care of patients with respiratory problems/dyspnea ➢ Deep breathing and coughing exercises ➢ O_2 inhalation ➢ Dry and moist inhalation ➢ Oronasal suctioning • Care of patient with altered body temperature—hot and cold applications • Care of patients with fluid and electrolyte imbalance • Care of unconscious patient • Care of the bed-ridden patient (traction, fractures, etc.) • Care of patient with pain • Care of patients with body elimination deviation	30	• Lecture cum discussions • Demonstration	• Short answer • Objective type • Essay type • Return demonstration • Assessment using checklist
VIII	Explain the principles, routes, effects of administration of medications	**Introduction to Clinical Pharmacology** Administration of medication: • General Principles/Considerations ➢ Purposes of medication ➢ Principles: Rights, special considerations, prescriptions, safety in administering medications and medication errors ➢ Drugs forms ➢ Routes of administration ➢ Storage and maintenance of drugs and nurses responsibility ➢ Broad classification of drugs ➢ Therapeutic effect, side effect, toxic effect, allergic reaction, drug tolerance, drug interactions ➢ Factors influencing drug actions ➢ Systems of drug measurement: metric system, household measurements. ➢ Converting measurements units: conversion within one system, between systems, dosage calculations. ➢ Terminologies and abbreviations used in prescription of medications. • Oral drug administration: oral, sublingual, buccal—equipment and procedure. • Parenteral: ➢ General principles ➢ Types of parenteral therapies.	30	• Lecture cum discussions • Demonstration	• Short answer • Objective type • Essay type • Return demonstration • Assessment using checklist

Unit	Learning Objectives	Content	Hours	Method of Teaching	Assessment Methods
		➢ Types of syringes, needles, cannulas and infusion sets ➢ Protection from needlestick injuries, giving medications with a safety syringe. ➢ Routes of parenteral therapies: Purposes, site equipment, procedure and special considerations in giving intradermal, subcutaneous, intramuscular and intravenous medications. ➢ Advanced techniques: epidural, intrathecal, intraosseous, intraperitoneal, intrapleural, intraarterial ➢ Role of nurse • Topical administration: purposes, site, equipment, procedure, special considerations for applications to skin and mucous membrane. • Direct application: ➢ Gargle, throat swab ➢ Insertion of drug into body cavities: nasal pack, suppositories/medicated packing into rectum / vagina ➢ Instillations: ear, eye, nasal, bladder and rectal. ➢ Irrigations: eye, ear, bladder, vaginal and rectal. ➢ Spray: nose and throat • Inhalations: nasal, oral, endotracheal, tracheal (steam, oxygen and medications) – purposes, types, equipment, procedure and special considerations. • Recording and reporting of medications administered.			

FIRST-AID

Course Description

This course is designed to help students develop and understanding of community emergencies and be able to render first-aid services as and when need arises.

General Objectives

Upon completion of this course, the students shall be able to:
* Describe the rules of first aid.
* Demonstrate skills in rendering first aid in case of emergencies.

Total Hours: 20

Unit	Learning Objectives	Content	Hours	Teaching-Learning Activities	Assessment Methods
I	Describe the importance and principle of first aid	**Introduction** • Definition, aims and importance of First Aid • Rules/General principles of First Aid • Concept of emergency	2	Lecture cum discussions	• Short answer • Objective type

Unit	Learning Objectives	Content	Hours	Teaching-Learning Activities	Assessment Methods
II	Demonstrate skill in first aid techniques	**Procedures and Techniques in First Aid** • Preparation of First Aid kit. • Dressing, bandaging and splinting (spiral, reverse spiral, figure of 8 spica, shoulder, hip, ankle, thumb, finger, stump, single and double eye, single and double ear, breast, jaw, capelin), triangle bandage uses, abdominal binder and bandage, breast binder, T and many tail bandage, knots reef, clove. • Transportation of the injured • CPR: Mouth to mouth, Sylvester, Schafer, external cardiac massage	8	Lecture cum discussions • Demonstration • Videos • Simulation exercises	Short answer • Objective type • Return demonstration
III	Describe first aid in common emergencies	**First Aid in emergencies** • Asphyxia, drowning, shock • Wounds and bleeding • Injuries to the bones, joints and muscle-fractures, sprains, strains, hanging, falls • Burns and scalds • Poisoning—ingestion, inhalation, bites and stings • Foreign body in eye, ear, nose and throat	6	• Lecture cum discussions • Videos • Demonstration	• Short answer • Objective type • Return demonstration
IV	List various community emergencies and community resources.	**Community Emergencies and Community Resources** • Fire, explosion, floods, earthquakes, famines, etc. • Role of nurses in disaster management • Rehabilitation • Community resources • Police, ambulance services • Voluntary agencies—local, state, national and international	4	• Lecture cum discussions • Videos • Mock drill • Simulation exercise • Videos • Field visit to voluntary agencies.	• Short answer • Objective type • Essay type

"Service to Man is Service to God"

A NURSE'S PRAYER

As I care for my patients today, be there with me, Oh Lord, I pray "Make my word kind, it means so much and in my hands, place your healing touch, let your love shine through, in all that I do so those who are in need, may hear you, feel you, see you in me."

Nursing Code of Professional Conduct

The code indicates that the nurse's primary responsibility is to meet the needs of the people those who require nursing care:

1. Act always in such a manner as to promote and safeguard the interests and the wellbeing of the patients and the clients.
2. Ensure that within your scope of responsibility, you take no action or fail to act in a manner that harms the well-being, condition, or safety of the patient and client.
3. Continuously enhance and update your professional knowledge and competence.
4. Recognize and acknowledge the boundaries of your knowledge and skills, and refrain from accepting responsibilities that you cannot safely and effectively fulfill.
5. Foster open and collaborative relationships with patients, clients, and their families to empower their independence and actively involve them in care planning and delivery.
6. Collaborate effectively with fellow healthcare professionals and other team members, recognizing and valuing their unique contributions within the care team.
7. Show unwavering respect for the dignity of every patient or client, responding to their needs with compassion and care, regardless of their background, beliefs, or health conditions.
8. Promptly report any concerns or conscientious objections to the appropriate authority, recognizing that these may impact your professional practice.
9. Avoid any misuse of your privileged relationship with patients and clients, as well as the access granted to their person, property, residence, or workplace.
10. Safeguard for all confidential information acquired during professional practice concerning patients or clients, disclosing it only with their consent or when mandated by a court order or in cases where disclosure can be justified in the broader public interest.
11. Report to the appropriate authority, taking into account the physical, psychological, and social well-being of the client, any circumstances within the care environment that could compromise the standard of care.

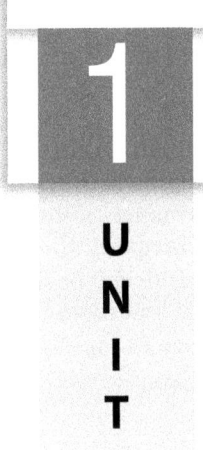

UNIT 1

Introduction to Nursing

LEARNING OBJECTIVES

After completing this unit, learner will be able to:
- Explain nursing concept, meaning, definitions, scope, and functions.
- Discuss history of nursing in India.
- State nursing as a profession.
- Discuss nursing professional-qualities and preparation.
- List ethics in nursing, roles and responsibilities of a nurse.
- Understand health care agencies, hospital and community services, types, and function of hospitals health team.
- Explain modern approaches to nursing care including holistic nursing care.
- Discuss health and disease.
- Explain definition of health and determinants of health status.
- List basic human needs.
- Explain illness and its effect on individual.

INTRODUCTION

Nursing means different to different people today, as it depends on the place you live, the tradition you follow, and the practice of nursing in your society. Most of the people still think of nursing as a concept of caring for the sick or assisting the doctor in his treatment and care of the patient, but nursing is much more than these.

NURSING CONCEPT

Nursing has always been directed at serving the health care needs of the society. Nursing originated with the desire to keep people healthy and to provide comfort, care, and assurance.

Modern nursing involves many kinds of concepts and skills related to health and social sciences and with basic science on contemporary issues. Nursing as a profession, is unique because it addresses humanistically and holistically, the response of client and families to actual and potential health problems.

Nursing profession has become an epicentric concept in the modern world, with the changing life style within the culture and thinking of the people it serves as the guiding force for service and for the peace of the society. At present, the world is experiencing major social and political change reflecting in the struggle of the people as they seek to live out their national, political, and religious aspirations. But sadly, conflict and violence are frequently the hall mark of these struggles as it is evident with the worlds on going wars, uprising massacres terrorism, and extended civic unrest. The untold mission of the people who died or injured in these conflict seems to be growing as the numbers of refugees and forced migrants. If nurses are in fact professionally committed to those important tenets of human rights, then there is an abundant opportunity to act on these commitments. Nurses can work to promote peace and healthful environment. The challenges, of course, are to find ways in which more nurses can make a greater differences at all levels (regional, national, and international).

Nursing is a helping profession and as such it provides services, which contribute to the health and well being of the people. Nursing is a vital consequence to the individual receiving service. It fulfills needs which cannot be met by family (or) other individuals in the community or the person himself. The essential components of professional nursing are **care, cure, and coordination**. It deals with the human beings under stress. Nursing is an art (skill, how to work and observe) and a science (body of knowledge of human behavior). Nursing as an art has been practiced ever since the human world began.

Mothers were the first practitioner of the art of nursing and women have always been found to care their children, the aged, and the ill persons. The skills required were passed informally from one person to another.

NURSING: DEFINITION

Defining nursing is difficult. In prehistory, very little is known about the nurse. One nurse historian writes, from the dawn of civilization, it seems that nurturing has been essential to the preservation of life. Survival of the human race, therefore, is very closely linked to the development of nursing. Nursing should be a caring. Nurse is to be a care giver for patients by managing, physical needs, preventing illness and treating health condition. This is the reason why nursing proper can only be taught by the patient's bed side and the sickroom or word lecturers and books are but valuable accessories.

One of the reasons, why it is difficult to develop clear and concise definitions of nursing is because there is a lack of separation from medicine. The interdependence exists between the two professions, medicine and nursing, and they have developed together throughout the history. However, anyone who has been involved in the profession of nursing, for any period of time will be quick to assure that differences exist. Primarily the differences are focused on the major goal of each profession. In general, medicine is concerned with the diagnosis and treatment (cure when possible) of disease. Nursing is concerned with caring for the person in a variety of health-related situations.

Early Definition of Nursing

Beginning with the simplest definition, a nurse is a person who nourishes, fosters, and protects a person who is prepared to care for the sick, injured, and aged person. In this sense, "nurse" is used as a noun and is derived from the Latin word "nutrix", which means "nursing mother". Another early use of the word "nurse" was associated with the meaning of a woman who suckled a child, usually not her own—a wet nurse. Dictionary definitions of nurse also include such words as "suckles or nourishes", to take care of a child or children "to bring up, rear". With such an origin, it is understandable that people generally have associated nursing with women.

A few early nurses wrote definitions of nursing, but it has been over the past 50 years that most of the developments of written definitions of nurse and/or nursing have occurred, following are some of the important definitions of nursing.

Florence Nightingale's (Founder of Modern Nursing)

Definition of nursing attributed to Nightingale is "The goal of nursing is to put the patient in the best condition for nature to act upon him, primarily by altering the environment" (1859). It signifies the proper use of fresh air, light, warmth, cleanliness, and the proper selection and administration of diet, which is the vital power to the patient.

Virginia Henderson (American Nurse Educator)

In 1996, Virginia Henderson, wrote a definition of nursing, stating that "The unique function of the nurse is to assist the individual, sick or well, in the performance of those activities contributing to health or its recovery (or to peaceful death), that he would perform unaided, if he had the necessary strength, will, or knowledge and to do this in such a way as to help him independence as rapidly as possible" (1966).

American Nurse' Association (1980)

Nursing is the diagnosis and treatment of human responses to actual or potential health problems.

World Health Organization (WHO)

"Nursing as an integral part of the health care system, encompasses the promotion of health, prevention of illness, and care of physically ill, mentally ill, and disabled people of all ages, in all health care and community settings within the broad spectrum of health care, the phenomena of particular concern to nurse are individual, family, and group responses to actual or potential health problems".

These human responses range broadly from health restoring reactions to an individual episode of illness, to the development of policy in promoting the long-term health of a population. Within the total health care environment, nurse share with other health professionals and those in other sectors of public service, the function of planning, implementation, and evaluation, to ensure the adequacy of the health system for promoting health, preventing illness, and caring for ill and disabled people.

Hildegard Peplau (1952)

Nursing is viewed as an interpersonal process involving interaction between the two or more individuals that has as its common goal assisting the individual who is sick or in need of health care.

Betty Neuman (1982)

Nursing responds to individuals, groups, and communities who are in constant interaction with environmental stressors that create disequilibrium. A critical element is the client's ability to react to stress and factors that assist with reconstitution or adaptation.

Sister Callista Roy (1984)

The goal of nursing is the promotion of adaptive responses (those things that positively influences health) that are affected by the person's ability to respond to stimuli. Nursing involves manipulating stimuli to promote adaptive responses.

Martha Rogers (1984)

Nursing is an art and science that is humanistic and humanitarian and directed toward the unitary human and is concerned with the nature and direction of human development.

SCOPE OF NURSING

Nursing practice is defined as the range of roles, functions, responsibilities, and activities in which registered nurses are educated and authorized to perform.

The broad scope of nursing practice reflects all of the roles activities. This includes health promotion, health protection, health maintenance, health restoration, rehabilitation, and palliation. Nursing practice is directed toward the goal of assisting client to achieve and maintain optimal health in order to maximize quality of life across the lifespan.

The scope of practice of an individual nurse is influenced by the nurse's knowledge, practice setting, employer requirements, and client needs.

Advanced Nursing Practice

Advanced nursing practice (ANP) roles have evolved in response to the changing needs of client and society, and trends in the delivery of health care. However, advanced practice nurses constantly challenge and extend the boundaries of nursing practice.

Competencies

Competencies are defined as the integrated knowledge, skills, attitudes, and judgment required to safely and effectively practices nursing. It reflects what is required of the registered nurses to function in specific roles of practice setting.

Classification

Entry to practice nursing

Competencies are identified as the knowledge attitude, judgment, critical thinking, communication, and psychomotor intervention expected of the entry level registered nurses, e.g., wound care, health assessment, and counseling.

Specialty nursing competencies

Identified as activities currently practiced as new emerging interventions that involve a higher level of complexity than the entry level competencies, e.g., removal of chest tube, administering chemotherapy, changing outer tracheotomy tube, etc.

Shared competencies

These are identified as health-related client intervention that is determined to be within the scope of practice, e.g., medication administration, maintenance of airway, etc.

Nursing Practice

Nursing involves an interrelationship of many people concerned with a client's response to potential or actual health problems. Today, there is an emphasis on the whole, people are seen not merely as physical beings but as biopsychosocial beings. Nursing practice involves a complex of knowledge and skills applied to the whole client. Nurses are also involved with support persons and the community as a whole. For this reason, nurses must be aware of how the support persons and community affect the client's well-being and consider the well-being of these support persons and the community.

Health Promotion

Health promotion means helping people to develop resources to maintain or enhance their well-being. The goal of health promotion is to improve people toward their own optimum level of health and well-being or wellness. An example of a nursing action that promotes health is explaining the benefits of an exercise program to a client.

Health Maintenance

Health maintenance means helping people to improve health following health problems or illness. Health maintenance nursing activities are those actions that help clients to maintain their health status. An elderly person in a long-term care facility can be taught and encouraged to exercise to maintain muscle strength and mobility.

Health Restoration

Health restoration means helping people to improve health following health problems or illness. Examples of activities that help restore health are teaching a client to protect an incision and to change a surgical dressing or assisting handicapped individuals to attain the highest level of physical strength of which they are capable.

Care of the Dying

Care of dying means comforting and caring for people of all ages while they are dying. Nurses carrying out these activities work in homes, hospitals, and extended care facilities. Some agencies, called hospices, are specifically designed for this purpose.

NATURE OF NURSING

Scope means the breadth of opportunity to function or range of activity.

The scope of nursing can be characterized by:
- Educational opportunity
- Service opportunity can be divided into—
  - Opportunities in clinical areas and
  - Opportunities in educational institutes

Educational Opportunities at Present

Educational opportunities at present are available to prepare nurses to function at various levels of the health care delivery system in the country.
- Auxiliary Nurse Midwives (ANMs)/Multipurpose health workers (MPHW) (F), 1½ year training program.
- Diploma in General Nursing and Midwives (GNM), 3 years and 6 months program.

- ❖ BSc Nursing Basic, 4 years program.
- ❖ Post certificate and postgraduate courses:
  - ♦ Post certificate BSc nursing, 2 years program
  - ♦ Post certificate diploma in clinical specialties like nursing education and nursing administration. 1 year course available in some states only because nursing education and nursing administration submerged with BSc nursing program.
- ❖ Postgraduate education; MSc nursing education. In 1969, MSc nursing program was started in CMC Vellore, affiliated to Madras University.
- ❖ MPhil program: To strengthen the research capabilities of nurses MPhil program started in October 15, 1986.
- ❖ PhD program for nurses started in few colleges from 1990 onward. Psychiatric nursing PhD program also started in NIMHANS, PhD is offered in Sri Ramachandra Medical College and Research Institute, Perur, Chennai and Vinayaka Mission Institute in Tamil Nadu, RAK College of Nursing New Delhi, College of nursing Mahe, PGI Chandigarh, and many other institutes.
- ❖ From 1991, there on wards are numerous colleges and universities, colleges providing various courses.
- ❖ 1970 during that time getting nursing admission was difficult few Government colleges, who want to go for post Basic BSc Nursing has to wait for at least 10 years to get seat.
- ❖ After 1991 many private nursing school and colleges were started, given opportunities to join nursing due to this changes nursing profession grown that extent many postgraduate and Phd program started throughout India.

Service Opportunities

In both government and private sectors:
- ❖ Auxiliary Nurse Midwives (multipurpose health workers)
- ❖ Staff nurses
- ❖ Senior staff nurses on promotion
- ❖ Nursing officer
- ❖ Nursing superintendent Grade I, on promotion
- ❖ Nursing superintendent Grade II, on promotion
- ❖ District health nurse supervisor, on promotion
- ❖ Assistant joint director of health and family welfare services on promotion.

In Educational Institutes Job Opportunities

In both government and private sectors:
a. Clinical demonstrator
b. Clinical instructor
c. Assistant lecturer, nurse tutor
d. Senior nurse tutor, on experience
e. Lecturer
f. Senior lecturer, on experience
g. Assistant professor, on experience
h. Associate professon, on experience
i. Professor/Principal, on promotion.

FUNCTIONS OF NURSE

A function is a pattern of behavior expected from an individual in specific position/situation. Functions are the different roles a professional nurse performs in her day-to-day practice. In practice several roles often coincided. They are:

Caregiver

The caring or confronting role of the nurse has traditionally included those activities that preserve the dignity of the individual and those often referred to as the "mothering actions". In nursing, caring is the role of human relations. The nurse supports the client by attitude and actions that show concern for the client's welfare and acceptance of the client as a person and not merely a mechanical being. Caring is central to most nursing interventions and an essential of the expert nurse.

Communicator

Effective communication is an essential element of all the helping professions, including nursing communication, which shapes the relationship between nurses and clients, colleagues, and other health care providers. Communication facilitates all nursing action. Like the nurse communicates to other health care personnel. The nursing intervention is planned and implemented for each client. Planned nursing interventions are written on the clients care plan and once the interventions are implemented, the nurse documents them on the client's record.

Teacher

A teacher helps the student to learn. It is an interactive process in which specific learning objectives or desired behavioral changes are achieved. The focus of behavior change is the acquisition of additional knowledge or technical skill.

Counselor

Counseling is the process of helping a client to recognize and cope with stressful psychological or social problems, to develop improved interpersonal relationship and to promote personal growth. It involves emotional, intellectual, and psychological support. Nurse counsel's primarily healthy individuals with normal adjustment difficulties but the focus is on helping the person to develop new attitudes, feelings, and behavior rather than promoting intellectual growth. The client is encouraged to look into an alternative behavior, to recognize the choices, and to develop a sense of control. The nurse counsels clients who need to decrease activity levels, like stop smoking or to lose weight, accept changes in body image or cope with impending death.

Client Advocate

Advocacy involves concern for and defined actions on behalf of another person or organization to bring about a change. A client advocate is an advocate of client's rights. Advocacy involves promoting what is best for the client by ensuring that the client's need is met by protecting the client's rights.

Change Agent

A change agent is a person or group who initiates changes and assists others in making modification by them or in the system. Marriner Tomey 1992, describes a change agent as one who identifies the problems, assesses resources, determines appropriate helping roles, establishes and maintains helping relationship, recognizes the phases of the change process, and guides the client through these phases. The promotion of change is an essential component of nursing care, by using the nursing process the nurse helps the client to propose, implement, and maintain changes that promote the clients health.

Leader

Leadership roles are applied at different levels, individual, family, groups, communities, or the larger society. At the client level, nursing leadership is defined as a mutual process of interpersonal influence through which the nurse helps a client make decisions in establishing and achieving his goals to improve the clients well-being. Leadership valid the professional nurses' practice and enhances professional growth.

Manager

Management is often confused with leadership. Tappen 1989 defines management as "planning and giving directions, developing staff monitoring operations, giving rewards fairly, and representing both staff members and administrations as needed". Management, therefore, occurs within an organizational environment. Leadership by contrast may or may not require delegated authority within a formal organization.

The nurse manages the nursing care of individuals, groups, families, and communities. The nurse manager also delegates nursing activities to workers, other nurses, and supervisors and evaluates their performance.

Researcher

The majority of researches in nursing are prepared at the doctoral and postdoctoral level, although clinician with master degree are beginning to participate in research activities as part of the advanced practices role. ANA's standards of clinician nursing practice states that all nurses should participate in research based on their level of education, position and practice setting. Nursing students must learn to investigate the role of the nurse early in their career to bridge the research-practice gap effectively.

HISTORY OF NURSING

History of Development of Nursing Profession

Nursing profession has become an epicentric concept in the modern world, with the changing life style within the culture and thinking of the people it serves as the guiding force for service and for the peace of the society. At present, the world is experiencing major social and political change reflecting in the struggle of the people as they seek to live out their national, political, and religious aspirations. But sadly, conflict and violence are frequently the hall mark of these struggles as is evident with the worlds on going wars, uprising massacres terrorism, and extended civic unrest. The untold mission of the people who died or injured in these conflict seems to be growing as the numbers of refugees and forced migrants.

Nursing in Ancient Times

Nursing is one of the oldest arts. There always has been helplessness of one sort or another and to a greater or less degree. Wounds have demanded attention; babies and old people have needed care, and disease in some form. Due to willful or ignorant disregard of natural laws. Place of relegions workship had hospitals as part of the churches and temple, therefore many jobs for nurses. These relegional buildings would provide extensive core for the poor and needy. Nurses would be seen aideny these injured indiviuals with nurses and marks, where hospital may not take them.

Correlation of Nursing History and World History

Nurses need a foundation of general history on which to base an understanding of nursing history. One needs to have in her mind some picture of the times in which events and changes in nursing took place, to visualize, and interpret rightly those events and changes. It is for this reason that a brief chronology of general history has been placed at the beginning of this book.

Care of Sick among Primitive People

The lowest savages have a certain amount of nursing knowledge and skill. Much of this knowledge is instinct similar to that of animals. All men doubtless posses, these instincts until they lose them by indulgence in the abnormal habits that are the result of so called **"civilization"** nearly all primitive tribes practice massage in some form, with good results, sweats bath, fomentations, and other hydrotherapeutic measures are known and used. The first curative services were surgical in character, and attained a degree of perfection before cultural medicine had hardly begun.

Prehistoric Medicine

The study of prehistoric medicine relies heavily on artifacts and human remains, and on anthropology. Previously uncontested peoples and certain indigenous peoples who live in a traditional way has been the subject of anthropological studies in order to gain insight into both contemporary and ancient practices.

Different diseases and ailments were common in prehistory than are prevalent today; there is evidence that many people suffered from osteoarthritis, probably caused by the lifting of heavy objects, which would have been a daily and necessary task in their societies. The transport of, for example, latte stones, though this practice only started after 800 AD, during the Neolithic era: involving hyperextension and torque of the lower back, while dragging the stones, may have contributed to the development of microfractures in the spine and subsequent spondylolysis. Things such as cuts, bruises, and breakages of bone, without antiseptics, proper facilities, or knowledge of germs, would become very serious, if infected. There is also evidence of rickets bone deformity and bone wastage (osteomalacia), which is caused by a lack of vitamin D.

Plant materials (herbs and substances derived from natural sources) were among the treatments for diseases in prehistoric cultures. Since plant materials quickly rot under most conditions, historians are unlikely to fully understand which species were used in prehistoric medicine.

The life expectancy in prehistoric times was low, 25-40 years, with men living longer than women; archeological evidence of women and babies found together suggests that many women would have died in childbirth, perhaps accounting for the lower life expectancy in women than men. Another possible explanation for the shorter life spans of prehistoric humans may be malnutrition; men, as hunters, generally received better food than their female counterparts, who would subsequently have been less resistant to disease.

Nursing and Medicine

In this primitive and instinctive care of the sick no distinction made between nursing and medicine or surgery. Only in very recent times has there been a sharp line drawn between these two forms of service, and even today there is some confusion as to **which procedures belong to the doctor and which to the nurse.**

Among savage tribes that had medicine men there was sometimes developed a lower class, often women who applied the treatment that had been prescribed, dressed wounds, and, in general, did work which would be included under the term **"nursing".**

Medicine and Theology

Many forms of disease appear extremely mysterious. They are plainly caused by some external force of influence. In consequence, most races in their early development most races came to the conclusion that many diseases appear extremely mysterious. They caused by some external force or influence and sickness is caused by evil spirits. The medicine men then tried to make the patient body unpleasant for the spirit, in the hope that it would move out. Beating and starving making dreadful noises, sudden fright, evil smelling or tasting of drugs, etc., were used for this purpose. Remedies to be taken by mouth were often mixed with such materials cow dung and human urine. Under such circumstances, the medicine man become a species of priest, or the priest was appealed to for help in sickness, so that very soon medicine and religion became inextricably woven together, and were thought of as one science. For many centuries, the priest was the only physician.

Sickness and Sin

It is an entirely logical step from belief in evil spirits as causes of disease, to belief that it was caused by failure to do some things which the Gods wished, or by definite oral transgression. Many religions have clearly taught this. And in almost every country from the days of old Assyria until now, even among highly civilized and intelligent people, the idea is found. We still "hear" what did I do so that I should have this illness, and people still look for remedies in deeds. Medieval Christianity taught that, epidemics of communicable disease were due to the sins of the people and that work of charity or other notable deeds were indicated to stop them. Some of our most advanced thinkers of today are in accord with the first half of the idea, and believe that it is a public sin to permit such disease, as typhoid, diphtheria, malaria, etc., to exist.

The supposed causes of disease have always profoundly influenced its care and treatment. Nursing has followed more or less closely, both theology and the science of its day, and has been radically influenced by them.

The First Hospitals

Since religion and medicine were united so early, it followed naturally that the first hospitals were connected with temples or places of worship. Some of the institutions, which have been called hospitals, were merely houses for the sick, who had come to pray or offer sacrifices to God. The patient was cared for by friends who came with him.

Egypt and Babylon

The early medical history of Egypt is the oldest, dating from 2700 to 1550 BC, which was written by a surgeon called, Imhotep. He evidently learnt anatomy by dissecting human bodies. He devised splints, bandages, and adhesive tapes, and he used some form of surgical stitching. He is the first author, who speaks of the brain **and** recognized that it is the central part of the body. In both Egypt and Babylonia (present Iraq), had houses for the sick, which are poor, and were looked upon by slave boys and girls. Medicine in Egypt reached a surprisingly advanced stage of knowledge. From clinical observation, they learned to recognize some 250 difficult diseases and to treat them. They developed a number of drugs and procedures, including surgeries.

However, Egyptians lack of knowledge regarding normal and pathological physiology limited their theories. Women in Egypt had no carrier, but had some freedom. A mother had position of authority women of high rank become priests in the temple.

Burdett, in "hospitals and asylums" says that the Egyptian physicians were all specialists confirming their practice to one part of the body. In both Egypt and Babylon, it was the custom to lay the sick in the streets, and there were laws requiring that the passers by should give them what advice they could out of their own experience.

The ancient Persians had houses for the sick poor, who were waited upon by slave boys and girls.

India

In the old Hindu villages, there were hospitals for the care of sick travelers, and medical specialists were appointed to them. In Ceylon, in the fifth century before Christ, one of the kings established what a true hospital was doubtless. The King Ashok, about the year 225 BC built 18 hospitals in North India. These public hospitals were also the school of medicine. The attendants in them were men and were evidently called nurses. The nurse must be clever, devoted to the patient, and pure in body and mind must know how to compound drugs, be competent to cook food, skilled in bathing the patients, conversant with rubbing the limbs and massage, with lifting the patient or assisting him to walk about, well skilled in making and cleaning of beds ready. Patient and skillful, never unwilling to do anything that is ordered. This list of requirements must certainly have necessitated some sort of training.

The Vedas, the sacred books of India, treat of medicine of major and minor surgery, bandaging, poisons and their antidotes, and drugs. They also discuss nervous diseases insanity, children's diseases, and genitor urinary diseases. They contain much instruction in hygiene, and set forth the theory that disease is preventable. They teach that the chamber of a lying-in women should be very clean and well-ventilated and midwives shall have their nails cut short. They advise daily bathing, daily attention to the bowels, daily cleansing of the teeth with a special sort of stick, etc. They also say that physicians shall have their hair and nails cut short, wear white clothing, take daily bath, they shall not speak of what they have learned in confidence from the patient. They recommended that sweet smelling drugs be burned in the operating room to prevent devils, from getting into the wound. In all their regulations, there are unconscious hints of the germ theory of disease. The best era of Hindu medicine was 500-250 BC. Later it was taught that to touch blood or morbid matter made one unclean and the work deteriorated, until care for the sick become almost nonexistent. Inoculation against small pox was in use among the Hindus from time immemorial. Drugs to produce insensibility to pain were used, probably opium and cannabis.

Nursing in India has had many special difficulties to hamper its progress. The good technic and standards, which had existed before the Christian era in the section of the country ruled by King Ashok, were lost, and nursing was for centuries practically nonexistent. The fatalistic religions, Hinduism and Mohammedanism, which hold sway over the most of the country, discourage interference with existing conditions. Also, the caste system of the Hindus, which prevents one caste from doing work which belongs to another caste, and the presence of an enormous number of outcasts or untouchables, complicates nursing procedures, and the zenana or purdah system of the Mohammedanism, which keeps women at home or does not permit them to be seen by men, makes further difficulties.

Economic and political problems have been many, with almost universal illiteracy and appalling poverty complicating the situation. The many and fundamentally different languages interfere with mutual understanding and delay the standardization of existing work. In short, the sum total of India's problems sometimes seems greater than those of any other country.

Beginning: Nursing in India is as truly the work of Florence Nightingale as is nursing in England. Though less directly traceable to her. For 30 years or more, Miss Nightingale devoted much time to the health problems of India, and formulated plans, which were gradually carried out by the government. All later work was built more or less on her foundations.

As in many other countries, missionary doctors did the first skilled nursing they trained, dressers, mostly men to assist them.

Nursing in India

In 1871, the first school of nursing was started in Government general hospital, Madras with a 6 months diploma midwives program with four students, four female superintendents, and four trained nurses from England were posted to Madras between 1890 and 1900 many schools under either mission or government were started in various parts of India in twentieth century in 1918 training school were started for health visitors, and dais, at Delhi and Karachi. Two English nurses Griffin and Graham were appointed to give training and to supervise the nurses. 1926 Madras state formed the first registration council to provide basic standards in education and training. The first four bachelor degree program was established in 1946 at the college of nursing in Delhi and Vellore. With the assistance from the Rockefeller foundation, seven health center were set up between 1931 and 1939. In the cities of Delhi, Madras, Bangalore, Lucknow, Trivandrum, Pune, and Calcutta in 1947, Florence Nightingale efforts were instrumental in starting nursing training in India at St Stevens hospital in Delhi in 1867.

China

China had a well-developed civilization long before the civilization era, and cultivated medicine and surgery as honored callings China had a famous "Father of Medicine", is Sen. Long, who was greatly honored in the Hondganalty (200 BC–200 AD). Eminent physician, and surgeons are recorded. Chinese medical knowledge was passed on to Korea and Japan and become the foundation of their practice. Today, Europe and America occasionally announce a discovery, which was based on old Chinese practice. Unfortunately, Chinese progress was hampered by the belief of the common people. They believed that the was due to evil spirit in the patient and that it might enter into any one, who touches the sick person, thus the nursing was impossible.

The Ancient Jews

More than a million people, the principles of modern sanitation are anticipated in the Jewish law, and most surprisingly its methods are in accord with modern bacteriology, midwifery, which probably included some after care as well as assistance at childbirth, is spoken of as an established craft.

Greece

As far back as 1134 BC, there was an Epidural in Greece, a temple to Asklepios, the God of healing. It was a house for those who come to pray to the God, and was a hospital only in the sense that the sick were cared in it. The God was expected to appear in dreams and prescribe miraculous remedies. The Greeks did not feel it worthwhile to care for any illness, but those considered curable, person hopelessly ill, were often left to die in the streets. Special buildings were created in 170 AD for these patients. These are regarded as the first European hospitals.

Hippocrates

The Greek, who lived about 400 BC, is called the father of medicine. He set forth principles which have governed the practice of medicine up to the present time. He taught that disease was not due to demons or fate, but to the breaking of natural laws. He urged careful observation of the sick and taught the meaning of posture, expression breathing, etc. He also taught that fever cases should have fluid diet and to advice cold sponging. He explained the necessity for clean, smooth bed linen, and mouth washes to the sick. Most of these things, we regard as modern nursing methods.

Hippocrates approach to health care summarized in corpus Hippocratism, nearly parallel the teaching of professional nursing today. The writing of Hippocrates refer to procedures that would be undertaken in modern hospitals by nurses but do not refer to a nursing vocation as such. Hippocrates taught what we call today professional loyalty to the member of one's own craft the attitude toward one's work, which carries with it a special sense of obligation to those dependent upon one's service. The Hippocrates oath still used by medical colleges at graduation is a fine expression of the spirit. The so called Florence Nightingale pledge for nurses is modeled after it.

Rome

The Romans knew many of the principles of sanitation. Julius Caesar, in first century BC, was the first states man to recognize teaching of hygiene and he had a regular medical service in his army. Roman's medical knowledge came from Greece. Nursing was done by women and old men of Good character. In Roman ruins found in Switzerland. They were discovered many nursing utensils, enema apparatus, tubing rectal tubes, and ointments, etc.

Early Christianity and its Influence on Nursing

The coming of Christ brought into the world a new aspect of religious teaching. Kindness, to one's fellow was not a new idea, and we all know that, even in childhood a certain amount of kindness, sympathy for others is innate. **Real Christianity began to teach and has continued devotion to others, without hope of any sort of rewards, but for the sincere love of God and a desire to be like him**. This is undoubtedly the highest motive ever persecuted to mankind.

At the beginning of the first century, AD, the early Christian church and teaching of Jesus Christ expressed secure to orphans, the poor travelers and above all sick. The Christian tendency to exact women to a position enhance to that of man, and to give her a place in the world, outside her home. Real Christianity began to teach, and has continued, devotion to others, without hope of any sort of reward, but for the sincere love of God and a desire to be like him. This is—**Undoubtedly the highest motive ever presented to mankind. The entrance of pure Altruism into the world, of disinterested service to humanity, profoundly affected nursing. It is this motive which has raised nursing to a place among the profession.**

The first large Christian hospital in the strict sense of the world was probably basileus at Caesarea in Palestine, founded in the year 370. Other Christian hospitals were at Cappadocia in Asia Minor, and at Alexandra in Egypt. As Christianity spread to Rome, its good work went with it and in the early centuries there were Christian hospitals as for well as Aries in the south France.

Important Dates

5000–4000 BC	Egyptian medicine
3000 BC	Beginning of Chinese medicine
2000 BC	Babylonian medicine
1200 BC	Vedas written in India
400 BC	Hippocrates the Greek, Father of medicine
250 BC	King Asoka and the best era of medicine in India.

Modern Medicine and Hospitals

During the 18th century, magnificent hospitals were constructed throughout the modern world they were staffed by physician superiors to any in the world, because of knowledge gained and preserved from their Greek counter parts. One well-endowed hospital was in Cairo and was prized target that the Crusaders tried very hard to destroy. Physiology and hygiene were studied by Arabian scientists.

Nursing Brotherhoods

Fully one half of the nursing of medieval times was done by men, since it was thought improper for women to nurse a man, who is not a close relative, there grew up many religious orders of men that included nursing among their other duties. Some of these are the brothers of St Antony, Brothers of Holy Spirit, who lived early in the 13th century, and gave up all his wealth and social position. He is said to have been a man of boundless pity and charity.

Nursing Sisterhoods

The great numbers were founded from about 500 AD. The members were at first not bound by any vows and wore no distinctive dress. Later vows, more or less strict became customary, and the clergy assumed more authority over the members of the orders.

Influence of the Crusades on Nursing

The crusades were Christian military expeditions to recapture the holy land, were Jesus Christ had lived from inhibiting Muslims. The crusade began shortly before 1100 and lasted until almost 1300. In the year 1244, about 1900 hospitals existed throughout Western Europe. This large number was due to the spread of leprosy for a 1000 year after Christ, there were no attempts to organize nursing. But as middle age advanced, three type of organization developed. These organizations were the military orders, regular orders (religious), and secular orders.

Early American Hospitals

During the late 1700 and the first decade of 1800, definite land mark were established, namely the big general hospitals in Pennsylvania. The Philadelphia dispensary established in 1786, of the modern outpatient department and clinic for ambulatory patients. It apparently was so successful that the idea soon spread to other American cities, nursing orders in 18th and 19th century. The sisters of Holy cross and the Irish sisters of mercy, established hospitals and practiced high standard of nursing at that time.

Factors affecting the Development of Hospitals

There have been several developments that have represented major forces in the continued development of hospitals and patient care each one has played a unique role. Four of these developments are: (1) advance in medical science, (2) development of medical technology, (3) changes in medical education, and (4) emergence of professional nursing.

Advance in medical science

The first of these major developments related to advances in medical science. By the end of the colonial period, two medical schools had been established in the United States. Prior to that time physicians learned their skills through an apprenticeship with a practicing physician. As medicine became more of a science, advances occurred. One of the most significant was the discovery of anesthesia and the rapid advances in surgery that were to follow. The germ theory also did much to advance the practice of medicine because it was soon followed by the development of agents or techniques that would sterile or serve as antiseptics. The growth of hospitals in the United States was a direct result of these advances that made hospitals safer and more desirable. The discovery of sulfa antibiotics in the mid-1930s and mid-1940s, respectively, heralded even greater changes.

Development of medical technology

The development of specialized medical technology was a natural successor to the advances in medical science. The first hospital laboratory was opened in 1889, and X-ray were used in diagnosis in 1896. The electrocardiogram (ECG) was discovered in 1903 and the electroencephalogram (EEG) was discovered in 1929 (Haglund and Dowling, 1988)

Changes in medical education

Advances in medical education also had a significant impact on the development of health care. The Flexner Report was completed in 1910, and it led to changes in the structure and content of curricula in medical schools. It is also expanded the role hospitals to include education and research and resulted in internship and residences for medical students.

THE EMERGENCE OF PROFESSIONAL NURSING

The Renaissance

In the early 1300 great revival of learning and art developed in Italy and spread elsewhere throughout Europe. This period is referred to as the renaissance one of the causes for renaissance was a bubonic plague, epidemic that devastated the western world from 1347 to 1351, killing 25-50% of European population. As a result of travel and mixing of people with other lands men became more independent and new ideas brought about advance in many areas, new ideas in art, architecture, and literature were developed. The invention of printing increases of medical books. Forerunners of the great medical development of this period were (1) Leonardo Da Vinci (1452-1519), with his anatomical studies and drawing remained classic. (2) Ambroise Pore (1510-1590), military surgeons wrote a book on a natural history in general and surgery in particular. During this period, nursing reached high level of organization and efficiency in religious and military orders.

Beginning of Modern Science

William Harvey discovered circulation of the blood. Thomas Sydenham (1624-1689) was the first person to set the example of true clinical methodology. William Gilbert of Rochester introduced the word electricity. Newton invented calculus and the law of the gravity and Boyle introduced atomic theory. Thus hundreds of observations and discoveries, which often in the most unexpected way gained practical importance, the foundation for sciences were established. All these developments had an impact on nursing, perhaps not immediately but in subsequent eras, as nursing developed into a science and a protection using these theories as foundation for practice.

The Reformation

The reformation began in the early 1500s. Nursing to its lowest level in those countries, where the Roman Catholic organizations were upset by the reformation; oppression of women has a long history and indirectly thwarted any advancement of the nursing profession for centuries. Nursing existed in a low and dismal state without organization and without social standing. Nurses are considered as the most menial servants. They frequently worked 24-48 hours at a time and their pay was insufficient to support them. The future for these women looked black.

Industrial Revolution (1700-1800)

Women with social compliances and character continued to struggle against the oppression of women during this time.

Emancipation of women

The American Revolution was against British; as a result the revolution had an impact on women-women helped with boycotts, stepped into jobs, when n men were scarce, organized care for the sick and wounded soldiers. The American ethic has had its impact on nursing as well and served as the foundation for a need to be doing something. Many nurses today remember the time they spent fulfilling menial labor tasks. The model of nursing in Germany and to some extent grew as to fit into existing society and system.

Education for women

When women were recognized equal before the law in decision-making (voting), new opportunities for education opened as early in the 19th century. It was difficult for women to obtain an education except through private tutoring such education was expensive and available only to few privileged. Florence Nightingale was educated by her father and by travel and social contact at that time there were no school for women.

The dark period of nursing

In England, the reformation closed at least a hundred hospitals and put nothing in their place for sometime. As the municipal hospital hospitals grew in size, they sometimes had a matron who was no more than a house keeper and rarely knew anything of nursing an old record specifies the duties of a nurse on the wards.

During the so called "dark period of nursing" extending from about the year 1600 to the middle of the 19th century. Little that could be called nursing was done, and no women of intelligence nor refinement went into it, except where the religious orders, reopened, were cherishing their traditions. Nurses were so ill fed, over worked, and ill treated that no one would undertake the work that could get anything else to do. The average nurse was lacking both in skill and morals, some of the hospital rules set forth in 1789 suggest the state of affairs.

In England

Some of the more advanced doctors of England felt the need of help from women of a better class than most of the nurses were about 1825 Dr Robert Gooch, tried to induce either the Methodists or the Quakers to establish an order of women, selected for their good sense, industry, kindliness and piety. Let them be placed as pupil nurses in the hospitals of Edinburgh and London. Let the women thus educated be placed two together in a cottage in some country district, and villagers would soon have reason to bless the hour that they came. The germ ideas of the training school connected with a hospital, of nursing textbooks, of nurse's examinations and of district and rural nursing.

The Kaiserswerth training

Nursing was the deaconesses chief work, but they also cared for prisoners and orphans, they had a good deal of Bible study, and took their turn in kitchen, laundry, and garden, teaching, supervising play, etc.

What we owe to Kaiserswerth?

Modern training schools for nurses have inherited much from the deaconess organizations and especially from Frau Fliedner's regime the probationary system letters from clergy man and doctor as to character and health. The principles of discipline, etiquette, and ethics and insisted that all nurses be on the same social level. They required that nurses sent out to private duty be treated as members of the family, not as servants and they saw to it that they were allowed proper time for rest.

Contribution of Florence Nightingale

The dominant figure in the development of organized nursing is Florence Nightingale. At that time, she made her mark in the history. Society has changed to the point that holistic scene amenable to a new profession.

Early life and education

Her parents were well to do English people, cultured, remarkable for their sincerity, high ideals, and deep mentality. Florence, the younger of two daughters, was born May 12, 1820, in Florence, Italy, and was named for that city. Her wish to be a nurse: soon after she was twenty she asked her parents to permit her to go into a hospital and learn to be a nurse, so that she might care for the poor people of her own neighborhood. They knew something of the dreadful conditions then existing in hospitals that the majority of nurses were of a low, rough class and could not bring their minds to the thought of their daughter doing such a thing. She would not go without their consent, and the situation and the situation grieved her greatly. She believed that an earnest life must express itself in work for humanity, and that "the service of man is the service of God". She longed for the chance to be helpful in a large way. She was always deeply religious.

Young Florence never quite fit the mold of Victorian lady; she was well-educated in literature, music, drawing, and the domestic arts. A woman of her social standing was expected to marry and devote her life to her family, entertaining, and cultural pursuits. However, she felt an early calling to serve, and refused to marry. When she attempted to go to work as a nurse, her horrified family repeatedly opposed her. In those days, hospitals were often dirty and dark and nurses were untrained, sometimes drunken women. Finally, at the age of 33 years, she was able to obtain some minimal training and begin her carrier.

Training at Kaiserswerth

In 1850, when she was thirty years old she was able to stop at Kaiserswerth for a 2 weeks visit, the opportunity gave her great joy. The next year she was allowed to go there for four months training. She realized then for the first time her wish for practical instruction in nursing.

Crimean war

The Crimean war won Nightingale title of lady with the lamp. The British, French, and turkey's were fighting with Russian near the black sea and Crimean Peninsula. There were serious problems with the handling of sick and wounded soldiers, especially British leaders were needed to organize an effort to save lives of the wounded and sick. 38 nurses were recruited, condition under which these nurses worked were atrocious, even the simplest means of healthy living were absent. At first Nightingale and the nurses do not had the respect and confidence of the physicians, which required time and evidence of what the nurses could do. But Nightingale insisted that nurses not to give help unless they were asked. Finally, the nurses were asked for assistance by the physicians.

Once the Nightingale and her nurses were set to work, hospital was established. Florence divided her time between administration and personal attention to patients. She becomes famous for her night rounds. It was during her night rounds with her lantern, that she made her tour of inspection with friendly word, smile for others. She inspired a feeling of comfort by sympathizing with the patient's Nightingale's Night rounds are perhaps the most famous, which made reference to Florence Nightingale as the lady of the lamp. Her changes revolutionized British military medical care, increasing standards for sanitation and nutrition and dramatically lowering mortality rates. While visiting the front lines, she becomes ill and never really recovered.

Nightingale continued to have an influence on standards of nursing care and training. In 1859, she helped to establish the first visiting nurse association and in 1860, she established a school that become a model for modern nurses training, at Saint Thomas hospital. She published book notes on nursing to state what and what it is not. Graduates of nursing school went to various countries of the world to practice nursing. Many of them become head nurses in such countries as Germany, Norway, Sweden, Scotland, Canada, US, India, South Africa, and Australia.

The soldier's love for Nightingale

With all her fearlessness in the use of authority and all her attacks upon bad administration, she was the womanly, gentle nurse. Two famous quotations describe this aspect of her work. One of the soldiers wrote home. What a comfort it was to see her pass. She would speak to one and nod and smile too many more. She could not do it to all, you know, for we lay there by hundreds, but we could kiss her shadow as it fell and lay our heads on the pillow again content. Before she came there was such cursing and swearing, **but after that it was as holy as a church.**

As Nightingale demonstrated, statistics provided an organized way of learning and lead to improvements in medical and surgical practices. She also developed a model hospital statistical form for hospitals to collect and generate consistent data and statistics. She becomes a fellow of the Royal Statistical Society in 1858 and on honorary member of the American statistical association in 1874. Karl Pearson acknowledged Nightingale as a prophetess in the development of applied statistics. Written by Cynthia Audain, class of 1998 (Agnes Scott College).

She was considered an expert on the scientific care of the sick and was asked by the United States for her advice on caring for the wounded soldiers of the civil war, through correspondence and reports; she continued her influence throughout her last years. She was the first women to receive the British order of merit. In 1907, the international conferences of Red Cross Societies listed her as a pioneer of the Red Cross movement. She died in 1910 at the age of 90 years.

Her work for India

After her work for the army was well under way she took up the enormous subject of sanitation in India, and for the 40 years devoted much time to it. The work was planned and carried out through a Royal Commission, and her connection with it never appeared, though it was she who made the plans and saw that they were carried out.

She worked out a health program for all the millions of Indian's population, and much of it has been put into force, with far reaching results. Probably no women, and few men, have in the worlds history, planned such a masterly undertaking.

Her political influence

She was personally acquainted not only with the queen and most of the cabinet, but knew every prime minister of her time, the royalty of other nations, and such men as John Stuart Mill, Benjamin Jowett, Gladstone, Spurgeon, etc., these men came to her advice and deferred to her judgment, and she never failed to measure up to their confidence in her.

Important dates

1820	Florence Nightingale born
1851	Took training at Kaiserswerth
1854–56	In the Crimean War
1856	The Nightingale Fund
1860	Founded the Nightingale School at St Thomas
1910	Died

Nursing as a Profession

A profession is a disciplined especially one that involved systematic education with moral obligation. Ethical Standard and who hold themselves out as, accepted by the society able to meet special criteria.

Professions are occupationally related social institutions established and maintained as a means of providing essential services to the individual and the society. Each profession is concerned with an identified area of need or function (e.g., maintenance of physical and emotional health, preservation of rights and freedom, enhancing the opportunity to learn). The profession collectively, and the professional individually, possesses a body of knowledge and a repertoire of behaviors and skills (professional culture) needed in the practice of the profession; such knowledge, behavior, and skills normally are not possessed by the nonprofessional.

A profession is with moral principles that are devoted to the human and social welfare. Professional nursing is a service devoted to the promotion of human and social welfare (**Fig. 1.1**).

Orient to service for the welfare of the society, nursing is an art and science as well as humanitarian service. It is unique profession within the health care sector focused on the care of individuals, families, and communities, nurses may attain, maintain, or recover optimal health and quality of life .

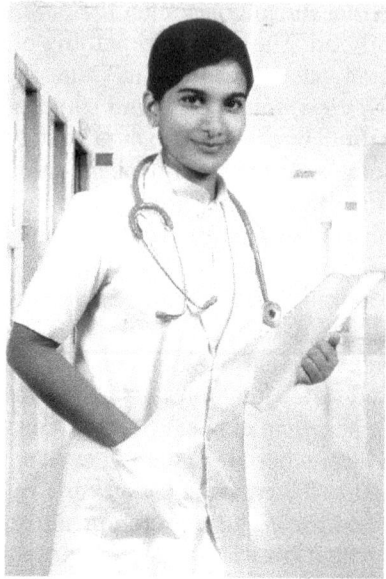

Fig. 1.1: Nursing as a profession.

Characteristics

1. **Ethical:** Means deals honestly with others, maintain confidentiality regarding professional matters. Recognizes professional's biases and bases attitude and action upon a sound rationale, believes that others recognizes the stature of a professional and doesn't misrepresent personal qualification and maintain self honestly
2. **Responsible:**
   a. Foresees possible outcomes of the professional action
   b. Make decision based on possibilities
   c. Consider the best interest of the client
   d. Support the basic tenants of the profession
3. **Theoretical:**
   a. Theoretical foundation of ideas contributes to knowledge base
   b. Shows appreciation for research and theory
   c. Evaluates own professional practice
4. **Committed:**
   a. Takes active part in professional organizational activities
   b. Identifies with professional scope based on trends
5. **Intellectual:**
   a. Keep abreast of technical advances
   b. Update about own and related professional and specialty
   c. Interact with other professionals and gain new perspectives
   d. Improve professional skills

Nursing is a **profession** within the health care sector focused on the care of individuals, families, and communities so they may attain, maintain, or recover optimal health and quality of life.

Profession is a vocation founded upon specialized educational training, the purpose of which is to supply objective counsel and service to others, for a direct and definite compensation, wholly apart from expectation of other business gain. The term is in essence a rather vaguer version of the term liberal **profession**, an Anglicization of the French term **profession** liberal.

Criteria of the profession

The criteria are—(1) education, (2) practice, and (3) research. It needs more and more criteria, for it to become a profession. They are:

1. Based on social and scientific principles, have its own body of knowledge.
2. Have a strong scientific base (academic and theoretical).

3. Have a strong service orientation in response to the social needs of human and social welfare.
4. Have a code of ethics.
5. Have a professional organization to that sets standards.
6. Conduct ongoing research to enhance the body of knowledge and to improve service to society.
7. Have autonomy (self-governance).

Values

Values are principles, and fundamental beliefs that guide or motivate attitude or actions, they help us to determine what is important to us, values are the motive behind purposeful action, they are the ends to which we act and come in many forms.

Importance of values

Our values represent our personal guiding principles or life goals, guiding our behavior in all aspects of life, including our home life, our work life, and our social life. Values guide our beliefs attitudes and behavior.

ETHICS IN NURSING, ROLES AND RESPONSIBILITIES OF A NURSE

Health is influenced by an array of demographic, socioeconomic, political, and environmental factors that are constantly changing. Most countries are currently seeking to adopt health structures and policies that will use resources more efficiently and encourage behavior that promote health. Therefore, reformed health system needs health care personnel, who can provide the essential elements on primary health care effectively, within the cost constraints. This requires the effective use of human resources, intrasectorial cooperation, and partnership between individual, and communities. Nursing practice is a valuable resource for health. It was constantly shown flexibility in its response to demographic, economic and social changes. As a result of these changes, nursing practice is now a key component of health care in every setting.

Elements of the Code of Conduct

Dignity

Dignity is a feeling of self-esteem and self-respect and is a basic value of nursing and midwifery practice. The nurse or midwife aims to promote protect and advocate the dignity of those clients who are vulnerable and incapable of protecting their own interests. The nurse or midwife respects the patient or client as an individual.

❖ Nurse must recognize and respect the role of patients and clients as partners in their care and the contribution they can make to it.
❖ This involves identifying their preference regarding care and respecting these within the limits of professional practice, existing legislation, resources, and the goals of a therapeutic relationship.

❖ Nurse must deliver nursing or midwifery care without prejudicial behavior.
❖ The professions are morally obliged to respect human existence and the individuality of all persons who are the recipients of nursing or midwifery care. Factors such as gender, age, ethnicity, personality and religious beliefs should be respected by the nurse or midwife, and care should be tailored in such a manner that personal needs as well as cultural values are maintained.
❖ Nurse must all times maintain appropriate professional boundaries in the relationship she have with patients and clients and ensure that all aspects of the relationship focus exclusively on the health care needs of the patient or client.
❖ Nurse must direct care toward the prevention and relief of suffering at all times.
❖ Care is tailored for the individual patient or client with the intention of strengthening his/her own capacity for care and recovery, thus achieving the highest degree of well-being. The professionals comfort and care for people of all ages. When life can no longer be sustained the nurse or midwife supports a dignified and peaceful death.

Code of Ethics

Nursing has developed codes of ethics that describe ideals for professionals conduct. Codes reflect ethical principles widely accepted by members of the profession, because codes are written in general universal terms, they are not designed to tell nurses what to do in specific ethical situations, rather, they give guidelines to assist nurses in their own moral reasoning. There are several codes for professional nurses.

International Council

❖ The fundamentals responsibility of the nurse is four folds, to promote health, to prevent illness, to restore health and to alleviate suffering.
❖ The need for nursing is universal inherent in nursing is respect for life, dignity, and rights of man. It is unrestricted by considerations on nationality, race, creed, color, age, sex, politics, or social status.
❖ Nurses render health services to the individual, the family and the community and coordinate their services with those of related groups.
❖ The nurse's primary responsibility is to those who require nursing care.
❖ The nurse, in providing care, promotes an environment in which the values, customs and spiritual beliefs of individual are respected.
❖ The nurse holds in confidence, personal information and uses judgments in sharing this information.

The basic terms in ethics includes:

Accountability

The state of being answerable for one's decisions and actions. It cannot be delegated.

Advocate

A person who argues or defends the cause of another. Nurses or midwifes may find they need to advocate for patient or clients.

Autonomy

Refers to independence, respecting others right to determine course of action, include in all aspect of care, in other words, nurses respect the patients "bill of rights". Clients are responsible for their own care in matter of health and illness.

Beneficence

Taking right action or providing good care to client or the act of a nurse should benefit the client do well to the patient. Act in the best interest of the patient.

Competence

Competence is related to professional roles, and the ability to perform those roles legally, safely, and with minimal supervision.

Fidelity

Refers to keep promises to reduce the discomforts, i.e., if client complain of pain abdomen, health care providers/nurse offered the pain medication, fidelity, encourages to monitor client response to pain, revision of plan of care, if necessary.

Justice

Refer to fairness. Health care providers do justice while providing care. For example, provision for resource distribution like provision for admission, discharge planning, supply of proper medication, and implants.

Legally competent person

A patient or client who is legally competent can understand and retain information and can use it to make informed choices.

Nonmalfeasance

Nonmalfeasance is the avoidance of harm nurses not only doing well to the patient, but also they should have equal commitment to do no harm to the clients.

Performance

Performance is related to the act of execution of nursing and midwifery care in the practice setting. Standards of acceptable performance are clearly defined by regulatory and professional bodies and society hold fully accountable when performance is unacceptable or questionable.

Reasonable

The test of what is reasonable is related to the standard of the ordinary skilled professional exercising and professing to have that special skill. Individual needs not possess the highest expert skill. It is sufficient to exercise the skill of an ordinary professional exercising nursing or midwifery.

Scope of Professional Practice

Scope of professional practice is related to an individual's knowledge, skill, attitudes, educational background, and abilities. Individual nurses and midwives will have their own scope of professional practice.

Obtaining consent for a child

Obtaining consent for a child will involve those with parental responsibility, but will depend on the age and understanding of the child. You must be aware of legislation relating to consent

When patients or clients have lost their capacity to consent or refuse treatment/care due to illness or incapacity:

- ❖ Should try to find out, if the patient or client had previously indicated any wishes or preference. If these wishes or preferences are not known, the criteria for treatment must be that it is in the patients or clients best interest.
- ❖ Principles of obtaining informed consent apply equally to those people who have mental illness.
- ❖ Relevant people close to the patient or client should also be involved, e.g., psychiatrist.
- ❖ Emergency where treatment is necessary to preserve life, provide care without the patients or client consent, if they are unable to give it, must follow institutional policy.
- ❖ Complementary therapy or alternative therapies must be discussed with the health care team, as part of a therapeutic process and patients or client must consent to their use.

Reflective scenarios

> A 14-year-old boy suffered from a serious neck and face deformity, which could be alleviated by surgery. He wished to have the operation so that he could have a normal life. His mother had no objections to the surgery but refused to consent for blood transfusions due to her religious beliefs. The surgeon refused to perform the operation unless he could transfuse the patient.

Reflect on the above scenario, discussing the various approaches to resolving this issue.

Confidentiality and privacy

- ❖ Confidentiality means protecting all information concerning patients/clients.
- ❖ Privacy means limiting access to a person, the person's body conversation, bodily function and objects immediately associated with the person. Unless access is necessary to give care.
- ❖ Ensure that any kind of information about a patient or client is kept confidential. This not only includes information that relates to the current health problem but also to any other information obtained about the patient/client during professional practice.
- ❖ Respect the patient's or client's wishes regarding the disclosure of information to family members and others. Only information essential for the treatment and welfare

of the patient/client can be disclosed to other members of the health care team. Disclosure of information can only be made with the patient's or client consent, or if required by law or by the order of the court.
- Report any breach in confidentiality immediately. Whenever a breach in confidentiality is suspected you must inform the person with the authority to manage the situation, so that action can be taken to prevent harm to patient or client.
- Protect the patient's or client's right to privacy. Information about patients or clients obtained during professional practice must be restricted to appropriate personnel and settings. Privacy must be ensured when getting information about a patient or client, for example, asking personal details about illness or medication on admission privacy must be protected during all care administered to the patient or client, and measures taken to ensure that unnecessary bodily exposure doesn't occur.

Reflective scenarios

> A client you are caring for has been diagnosed with a mental health problem, several friends and people who know the client in his village are generally concerned for him. They approach you as the senior nurse on duty and ask you about the client's illness and how it can be treated.
>
> A patient is admitted to a male medical ward for the treatment of right upper lobe pneumonia. Following investigations the patient is found to be HIV positive. Your colleague from the female medical ward knows the patient and asks to see his case notes.

Reflect on the above scenarios with a colleague and decide upon an appropriate way of dealing with these situations.

Working as a team

The team includes the patient or client his/her family, informal careers and health care professionals among the team. The delivery of health care is a complex process that requires a multidisciplinary approach to meet the health needs of society.
- Develop and maintain a cooperative relationship with coworkers and other disciplines involved in the delivery of health care.
- Work cooperatively within teams and to respect the skills, expertise and contributions of your colleagues. You must treat them fairly and without discrimination.
- Establish a fair unbiased and supportive working environment that is conducive to the provision of quality health care.
- Consult and collaborate with others to meet the health needs of society. To be effective, there must be mutual understanding, shared knowledge, trust, and respect for each person's contribution.
- Actively promote collaborative planning to ensure the availability and accessibility of high-quality health services to patients and clients.
- When working as part of a team, you remain accountable for your professional conduct, including any actions or omissions on your part. Nurses are accountable for any care that they delegate, or any care provides, respect the rights of the team.

Reflective scenarios

> You have been caring for a very sick child on a pediatric ward for the last week and have managed to get to know the child very well. The child, a 3-year-old boy has pneumonia and has responded very poorly to chest physiotherapy. The last time you gave chest physiotherapy he collapsed and required oxygen, so the doctors decided to abandon chest physiotherapy for the present time. The morning of the next day new doctor arrive on the ward and after viewing the chest X-ray order chest physiotherapy 4 hourly.

Reflect on the above scenario with colleagues and discuss the nursing contributions to the overall care.
- The consultant in charge of your department has decided to introduce multidisciplinary audit as part of a quality improvement program. The consultant explains that case notes will be selected. And nurses will present the patient or client's case discussions will help the whole. Team to find examples of good and bad care, and how improvements can be made to the quality of multidisciplinary care.

Reflect on the role of the nurse or midwife in such an audit, what contributions the professionals can make.

Professional knowledge and competence

Professional knowledge and competence is the knowledge, skills, and attitudes acquire though education and experience. Clinical competence is related to professional roles as defined by the scope of professional practice, standards of practice, the code of professional conduct, and guidelines that governs safe and effective practice:
- Possess the appropriate knowledge, skills, and attitudes in order to practice competently.
- Knowledge skills and attitudes needs to be relevant to the current scope and standards of practice, changing issues, concerns, and ethics.
- Have a responsibility to deliver care based on current evidence. Rather than totally base care on experience, opinion and tradition you must deliver care based on current evidence, best practice, and where applicable validated research when it is available.
- Should be committed to life-long learning, this include continuing education, self-study, net working with professional colleagues and professional reading.
- Share your knowledge—this includes providing mentorship, preceptorship, and guidance for the professional development of student nurses and midwifes and other colleagues.
- Keep knowledge and skills up to date throughout your competence and performance.
- If an aspect of practice is beyond your level of competence or outside your scope of professional practice, consultation

must be sought from a competent, or the patient or client should be referred to others for appropriate care.

Trustworthy

Trustworthy means you can be relied upon to be honest, truthful, or reliable being trustworthy means that you will uphold the reputation of the profession, and value the public confidence and trust invested in you.

* Must behave in a manner that upholds the reputation of the profession, behaviors compromising this reputation may call your registration into question at any time.
* Must acknowledge professional boundaries in the privileged relationship you obtained during the course of the patients/clients treatment.
* Must avoid any abuse of the privileged relationship with patients or client and access allowed to their person, property, residence or workplace.
* Ensure that your professional judgment is not influenced by any commercial considerations.
* Registration status must not be used in the promotion of commercial products or services.

Reflective scenarios

> You are the nurse in charge of a busy accident and emergency unit within a hospital. A representative from a large international company approaches you and offers you financial rewards in return for recommending the purchase of the company's product. You know that the product is inappropriate and would not do the job you needed it for
>
> A 68-year-old active independent, cheerful grandfather who smokes heavily is admitted to hospital for an acute exacerbation of pneumonia requiring intensive care. His diagnostic tests reveal a widespread metastasis inoperable cancer. His devoted children and wife are told the diagnosis while the patient is in intensive care. The family insists that the patient not be told the truth so that the patient's remaining time at home will be as happy as possible. When the nurse comes into the room to prepare the patient for discharged, the patient says. I know I have had lots of special tests and X-rays of my lungs. I believe something important is being kept from me. I believe I have the right to know what's wrong with me.

Reflect on the above scenarios with colleagues and discuss how the nurse should respond.

Risk reduction

* Risk implies a situation or environment that may compromise the safety of patients or clients. Risk reduction is the ability to limit or reduce those risks with the aim of protecting patients and clients.
* You must work with other team members of the team to promote health care environment that are conducive to safe, therapeutic and ethical practice.
* Where you cannot change circumstances in the care environment that could compromise standards of practice. You must report them to senior person with sufficient authority to manage the situation.
* When working as a manager, you have a duty of care toward patients and clients, colleagues, the wider community, and the organization in which you and colleagues work. When facing professional dilemmas, your first consideration in all activities must be the interests and safety of patients and clients.

Nurses and Practice

Maintaining Standards of Practice

Most nurses have learnt basic theoretical concepts and clinical skills in their nursing education. It is the responsibility of the nurses, employers, associates, and all the educators to assure the updating of these abilities by continual education and by other means. The administrative and managerial skills are frequently necessary, as these abilities must also be continuously improved.

The code recognizes that in many situations reality may impede in carrying out nursing skills at the highest level as stated in the set standards.

Examples of such situations are:
* Shortage of supplies or in an adequate supply (medicines/materials/manpower)
* Unsuitable facilities or insufficient personnel
* Language barrier or geographical isolation, etc.

Delegating and Accepting Responsibilities

The nurse uses judgment in relation to the individual's competence when accepting and delegating responsibilities. The nurse faces daily situations in which she is asked to carry out certain functions for which she feel. In adequately prepared by her colleagues, nursing administration, physicians, patients, and families. This requires a more competent person. If it is not available then it is question of convenience or the lack of knowledge of the person making the request.

The nurse may be expected to take over activities that could be done equally well by a person with less preparation, thus underutilizing the nursing competencies. In delegating activities or functions to others, the nurse must give full consideration to the dangers that are implicit in the assignments beyond the individual's competence and potentials.

Nurse and Coworkers

Cooperative Relationship

Under this heading, nurses and coworkers, the code of nurses states that the nurse sustain a cooperative relationship with coworkers in nursing and in other fields.

Implication for Nurses

1. The relationship between nurses and other workers often leaves much to be desired.
2. In nursing the traditional hierarchy often is interpreted as there are people who give the orders and there are those who carry out orders.

3. In a truly cooperative relationship especially between the staff and the administration, there should be give and take all around. This may be interpreted as harmonious relationship. But truly professional nursing calls for a true colleague relationship on information sharing and decision making among nurses, doctors, and other worker involved in certain aspects of the patient care and well-being.

Nurses and Profession

The code states that the nurse, acting under the professional organization, participates in establishing and maintaining equitable social and economic condition in nursing.
1. In the past decade international council for nurses (ICN), has promoted improved salary and better working conditions for nurses.
2. The council has helped member associations to develop programs to enhance better conditions for nurses in their countries, which are equitable to those persons who have similar qualifications and responsibilities.
3. In the international level, ICN has worked with WHO and international labor organization (ILO), to prepare a document which hopefully makes a major impact on recruiting and retraining nurses in the work force.
4. The change in the status of the nurse since the modern times are from a single women living in a nursing quarters to a married male or female nurse, required a major change in the employment conditions. Selected statements of the ICN code for nurses and their implications.

Respect for Life

The code for nurses states that the nurse should respect life. This statement was replaced by preserved life as the change was made in the light of modern technology, which enables the continuation of vital life functions by mechanical means, in situations where the irreversible damage would course immediate death without artificial intervention.

Implication for nurses

The question of respect for life is deeply routed in religion, culture, law, nursing, medicine, philosophy, and other disciplines. Each nursed holds strong faith and belief on these concepts. There are three kinds of situations, in which the nurse may face with these issues. They are heroic measures in irreversible terminal cases, preventing conception or interrupting pregnancy and decision related to respect for life, must be made by a qualified and authorized group and not by a single individual.

Conflict Related to Malformed Infant

Infants are sometimes born with defective bodies or minds. Many times these defects can be seen at birth. These infants have a very short life span and sometimes long. The quality of life depends on the nature and extent of the deformity and the infant's culture. A conflict exists between people for the appropriate care on these infants. Nurses also face such conflicts. They may follow the direction of others or follow institutional policy.

Nurses and People

The code of nurses states that the nurse provides care, promotes on environment in which the value, customs, and spiritual beliefs of an individual is respected.

Values, Customs and Beliefs
Implication for nurses

Core may meet certain individual needs, namely:
- Biological needs
- Therapeutic regime
- Provide emotional support
- Health education

Environment

Physical setting of an individual as his home, school, place of work, health center, clinic, hospital, and the psychosocial atmosphere such as interpersonal relationship, behavioral norms, socialization process, etc. They nurse cannot control or direct the total environment.

Utilizing the available resources and developing resources which are not available. The nurse is the care giver who has extensive contact with an individual and the family. She is then able to assess the values, beliefs, and the customs to incorporate her knowledge to them by directing the nursing care of other therapists.

Note: Recognition and respect to these values customs and beliefs of an individual does not mean actively accepting them, but is should not cause any conflicts with the nurse's basic beliefs or values.

Personal information held in confidence

The code of nurses states that the nurse holds in confidence personal information and judgment in sharing this information.

Implication for nurses

Patients' under stress frequently reveals thoughts and ideas, which they would not want other to know. Later they may regret or even fear of having made such confidence. Sometimes, these revelations may relate directly to the illness or affect the recovery process or they may have an indirect effect on the patient or others within the patient's family or friends, hence the nurse should use her judgment to determine when to share information.

Informing the patient

One of the rights of a man is the right to knowledge about himself in the case of a patient knowledge of a diagnosis the treatment the prognosis or other facts may help or hinder in his care. Both the physician and the nurse must be in a position to give or withhold information. The patient or his family may request such information. Sometimes those give care, relate information voluntarily.

Code of Ethics and Professional Conduct for Nurses

Statement/Guidance

1. Act always in such a manner as to promote and safeguard the interests and the well-being of the patients and the client.
2. Ensure that no action or omission on your part or with your sphere of responsibility is detrimental to the interest, condition or safety of the patients and client.
3. Acknowledge any limitation in your knowledge and competence and decline any duties or responsibilities unless you are not able to perform them in a safe and skilled manner.
4. Work in an open and cooperative manner with patients, clients, and their families, foster their independence, recognize, and respect their involvement in the planning and delivery of care.
5. Work in collaborative and cooperative manner with health care professionals and others involved in providing care, recognize and respect their particular contributions within the care team.
6. Recognize and respect the dignity of each patient and client, and respond to their need with care, irrespective of their ethics origin, religious beliefs, personal attributes, and the nature of their health problems or any other practice.
7. Report to an appropriate person, authority, at the earliest. Any conscientious objection may be relevant to your professional practice.
8. Avoid any abuse of your privileged relationship with patients and clients and of the privileged access allowed to their person, property, residency, or work place.
9. Protect all confidential information concerning patients and clients obtained in the course of professional practice, and make its disclosures only with the consent or when required by the order of a court or where you can justify disclosure in the wider public interest.
10. Report to an appropriate person or authority having regard to the physical, psychological, and social effects on clients. Any circumstances in the environment of care could jeopardize standard of practice.
11. Report to an appropriate person or authority at any circumstances in which safe and appropriate care for the patient and clients cannot be provided.
12. Report to an appropriate person or authority where it appears that the health or safety of the client is at risk, these circumstances may compromise standard of practice and care.
13. Assist professional colleagues, in the context of your own knowledge, sphere of responsibility to develop their professional competence and assist others in the care team including informal carriers, to contribute safely and to a degree appropriate to their role.
14. Refuse gifts, favors or hospitality from patients or client currently in your care which might be interpreted as seeking to exert influence to obtain preferential consideration.
15. Ensure that your registration status is not used in the promotion of commercial products or services. Declare that any financial or other interests in relevant organizations providing such goods and services will ensure that your professional judgment is not influenced by any commercial considerations.

TYPES OF HEALTHCARE AGENCIES/SERVICES

TYPES OF HEALTHCARE AGENCIES

- Hospitals
- Clinics
- Nursing homes
- Mental health and addiction treatment centers
- Birth centers
- Hospice care facilities
- Dialysis facilities
- Diagnostic center, imaging and radiology

Hospital

Like all social organizations hospitals grew out of necessity. In the past, the hospital has been a place for care of the sick. Today, the hospital has become a center of technical services for the sick and well, inpatients as well as outpatients with greater emphasis on achieving the highest standards of patient care and community health.

Definitions

The word "hospital" is derived from the Latin word hospitals, which comes from "hospes", meaning a host.
1. "The hospital is an integral part of a social and medical organization, the function of which is to provide for the population complete health care, both 'curative' and 'preventive' and whose outpatient services reach out to the family and its environment; the hospital is also a center for the training of health workers and biosocial research" (WHO Expert Committee on Organization of Medical Care).

2. The American Hospital Association (AHA) defines a hospital as: An institution with the primary function of providing diagnostic and therapeutic patient services for a variety of medical conditions, surgical and nonsurgical.
3. A hospital is a health care institution with an organized medical and professional staff, and with permanent facilities that include inpatient beds, provides medical, nursing and other health related services of patients.

Functions of the Hospital (Four Categories)

1. **Patient care: Primary function (curative function)**—Refers to any type of care given to patients, by the health team members, like Physicians, Nurses, Physical therapists, Dieticians, etc. It also includes health teaching to patients.
2. **Health personnel education: Secondary function (training function)**—Refers to the education of professional and technical personnel, who provide health services, e.g., Physicians, Nurses, Dentists, Therapists, Technicians, etc.
3. **Health promotion: Secondary function (preventive function)**—An emerging function for the hospital is that of a community health center taking an active role to improve the health of the population it serves. Hospitals as major community health centers can sponsor programs of environmental and occupational health, home care services, etc.
4. **Health related research: Secondary function (research function)**—Research that focuses on the improvement of health and/prevention of disease.

Classification of Hospital

Hospitals are classified as follows:

According to the type of service
a. **General hospitals:** They care for patients with various disease conditions of both sexes to all age groups, medical, surgical, pediatrics, obstetrics, eye and ear hospital, etc. General hospitals may contain specialized units staffed by specialized personnel, Renal Unit, Intensive Care unit, Coronary Care Unit, Plastic Surgery Unit and Burn Unit. There may be specialization at Unit level, Neurological, Urological, Orthopedic Units, etc.
b. **Special hospitals:** They limit their services to a particular condition like orthopedics, maternity, pediatrics, cardiology, renal, geriatrics, etc.

According to administration, ownership, control or financial income
a. **Governmental or public hospitals:** They are owned, administered, and controlled by government. They provide free care, to all patients. They may offer private accommodations for fee-paying patients. The Government Hospitals are guided by Ministry of Health, Director of Medical Education, and Family Welfare Services, managed by Medical Superintendent and Nursing Superintendent.
b. **Nongovernmental or private:**
- **Proprietary:** Privately owned or controlled by an individual or group of physicians or citizens or by private organization (profit-making).
- **Voluntary:** Owned and operated by nonprofit organizations, i.e., temple, mosque, or church authorities.

According to size and bed capacity

Small hospital	100 beds or less
Medium size hospital	100–300 beds
Large hospital	300–1000 beds

Organization of the Hospital

At the head of any hospital organization, there is a governing board or board of directors (policy-making body), which represents the owners. Authority for the administration of the hospital is delegated by the governing board to the director or administrator. The administrator is responsible for maintaining standards of service and patient care, established by the board. He is responsible to carry out the functions of the hospital in accordance with the philosophy and established policies set by the governing board. He delegates the responsibility for the different departments to the departmental heads, who are specialists in their field. In large hospitals, the administrator has one or more assistants to help with the administration of various departments, one of them for the business management and the other for the professional care of the patient.

MAJOR HOSPITAL HEALTH SERVICES DEPARTMENTS

A. Professional Health Service Departments

Medical Department

The medical department has within it the various clinical services. They are medicine, surgery, gynecology, obstetrics, pediatrics, ophthalmology (eye), ENT, dental, orthopedics, neurology, urology, cardiology, psychiatry, dermatology (skin), plastic surgery, nuclear medicine, etc. Medical director is a doctor, who has control over all the medical departments.

Nursing Department

The nursing department consists of nursing service and nursing education. The primary purpose of the nursing service is to provide comprehensive, safe, effective, and well-organized nursing care through the personnel of the department. The primary purpose of nursing education is to raise the standard of nursing service by providing education to nursing service personnel in the hospital.

Paramedical Departments

They include:

❖ **Laboratory:**
- **Pathology department:** The pathology department is one of the largest departments and has the responsibility for making tests and studies on blood, sputum, urine, feces, body fluids, and tissues. The following laboratories are usually found in a pathology department.
- **Bacteriology department:** This laboratory is concerned with studies about the bacteria and their toxins.
- **Biochemistry:** This is considered with the chemistry of living organisms and of vital processes.
- **Hematology laboratory:** It is responsible for making hemoglobin determinations, coagulation time studies, red and white cell counts and special blood pathology studies for anemia and leukemia, etc.
- **Parasitology laboratory:** It studies the presence of parasites, the cysts, and ova's of the parasites that are found in the feces.
- **Serology laboratory:** It does blood agglutination tests, Wassermann tests, VD.
- **Blood bank:** It has the responsibility of collecting and processing all blood used in the hospital for transfusions. It makes studies of new born infants, who may have hemolytic diseases, and does antibody studies on the prenatal patients.
- **Histopathology laboratory:** It prepares tissues for gross and microscopic studies. Small hospitals, which do not have a pathology department, send specimens to be investigated to a central pathology service or to a large hospital.

❖ **Pharmacy department:** The pharmacy department has the responsibility for selecting, compounding, storing, and dispensing all drugs and medications for inpatients and outpatients. The pharmacy should be under the supervision of registered pharmacists.

❖ **Physical medicine and rehabilitation department:** The department treats patients, who have functional disabilities resulting from disease conditions or injuries. It has several specialties such as physical therapy, occupational therapy, speech therapy and vocational training. This department is under the direction of a well qualified physician, who has special training in the field of physical medicine and rehabilitation. The staff should include therapists with qualification in the various specialties. The work of this department is one part of the total patient care plan.

❖ **Radiology department:** This department functions under the control of radiologist and qualified technical staff. It has the following diagnostic and therapeutic services for inpatients and outpatients, such as:

- Radiographic examinations and their interactions
- X-ray, radium, radioactive cobalt, and other radioactive therapies
- Radioactive isotopes tracer
- Radioactive isotopes therapy

❖ **Dietary department (catering):** In most hospitals, this department is under the direction of a trained dietician. The department is charged with:
- Ordering and preparation of food
- Tray service
- Diet teaching

The dietician is a member of the health team and works closely with nursing service personnel in meeting the patient's nutritional needs and in teaching. He/she is responsible for the ordering of supplies and the supervision of all staff engaged in the preparation and delivery of food. The kitchen should have ample light and air and should be as close as possible to the stairs, the dining rooms and the elevators. Procedures for handling dishes for communicable disease patients should be separated from general patients.

A periodic complete physical examination including X-ray of chest, analysis of stool and urine should be considered in order to detect silent carriers and take appropriate action. Daily inspection of personal appearance and hygiene also are important.

Three types of dietary services are in use:
1. Centralized services
2. Decentralized services
3. A combination of both

Outpatient Department

This is a combination of several departments. It is a miniature of the hospital except that the patients are ambulatory. Services are provided by specialists. Individuals may attend this department for the purpose of receiving treatment, or to enable a physician to assess their progress following discharge from hospital.

Accident and Emergency Department (A and E)

In most large hospitals, people who are classified as "emergency admissions" are received into this department to receive life-saving services immediately needed after thorough examination by the responsible physician, i.e., road accidents, people who become suddenly very ill, etc. Arrangements for admission to hospital are made, if necessary. Some accidents and emergency departments have their own operating rooms, where minor surgeries can be performed, a plaster room, where casts are applied, and other services, such as X-ray and pharmacy.

Operating Theater

Depending on the size of the hospital, there may be one or more number of operating rooms. In addition to the rooms, where surgeries are performed, there are sterilizing rooms, anesthesia rooms, recovery rooms, utility and storage rooms, staff amenities such as offices, toilets, etc.

In addition to these departments mentioned, large hospitals may provide other services such as intensive care, education department, blood bank, referral services to other hospitals, etc.

B. Nonprofessional Health Service Departments

Admitting Department

This department has the responsibility for admitting the patient to the hospital. It should maintain good public relations. The patient, family, and friends must be treated with utmost respect, courtesy, and tact. Appropriate answers are to be given upon enquiries about the hospital.

Personnel Department (Functions)

- Recruitment of personnel
- Interviewing
- Promotion and transfer
- Termination of employment
- In-service training
- Safety
- Health programs
- Recreation
- Remuneration and incentives

Purchasing Department

This department has the responsibility for purchasing all supplies and equipment for the hospital.

Medical Records

This is one of the important departments in the hospital. The patient's records (charts, X-rays, etc.) are valuable not only to the patient but also to the doctor and to medical and nursing education and research.

Accounts

This department has the responsibility for collecting the money, which is owed to the hospital, paying for supplies and equipment, handling all records pertaining to hospital finance, assisting with budget, etc.

Housekeeping Department (Domestic Services)

This department's main function is to keep the hospital clean. It plays an important role in hospital hygiene and infection control.

Laundry Department

The laundry takes care of the entire linen of the hospital. It has the responsibility of washing, repairing and replacing linen (if it is on contract basis). The location should be as far as possible from patient services are as to reduce noise. Linen, which requires special care should be marked, e.g., infectious or from isolation, etc. Nursing personnel should be careful and alert the laundry workers to the dangers of needles or sharp instruments sent unintentionally.

Centralization of laundry services promotes efficient and quick service.

Mechanical Department

Electricity, water supply, heat, air conditioning, etc., are looked after by the mechanical department.

Maintenance Department

The maintenance department keeps the hospital in good condition. Carpenters, painters, gardeners, etc., are included in the personnel of this department.

Central Sterile Supply Department (CSSD)

In modern hospitals, the trend is toward centralization of preparation and sterilization of supplies and equipment. The location should be as central as possible within the hospital with ample light, where space conditions permit, this department should adjoin the operating department, since it uses a large amount of surgical supplies.

Purposes of CSSD

- To prepare and furnish other departments and nursing units with sterile equipment and supplies needed in patient care.
- To ensure:
  - Standardization, and better utilization and control of supplies and equipment used for diagnosis and treatment.
  - More adequate methods of sterilization than on a nursing unit.
  - Early detection of mechanical defects in equipment through regular checks.
  - Economy of time and better care.

Modern hospitals use elevator between the CSSD and nursing units. Items not used within 7–10 days should be resterilized, as per the infection control policy.

Social Service Departments

This department assists in obtaining financial aid for patients and their families. It advises on the agencies through which help of various kinds can be arranged. It serves as a liaison between the patient and community agencies.

Nursing Service Department

The department consists of two main classifications:

1. **Professional nursing personnel:** They are the director, matrons assistants, supervisors, senior nurses, and staff nurses.

2. **Nonprofessional nursing service personnel:** They are aids, orderlies, and clerks.

Functions of the Nursing Service Department

- To plan, provide, and evaluate nursing care for patient and families.
- To define and implement the philosophy, objectives, and standards for nursing care of patients.
- To provide and implement a departmental plan of administrative authority, which delineates responsibilities and duties of each category of nursing personnel.
- To coordinate the functions of the department with the functions of all other departments.
- To estimate the requirements of the department.
- To interpret hospital and nursing service objectives to the patient and community.
- To participate in the formulation of personnel policies, to implement established policies and evaluate their effectiveness.
- To develop an effective system of nursing records and reports.
- To estimate needs for facilities, supplies and equipment.
- To participate in financial planning.
- To participate in studies and research projects for the improvement of patient care and hospital services.
- To provide and implement continuing education programs for all nursing personnel.
- To participate or facilitate all educational programs of students in the health care field.

NURSING UNIT

The nursing unit is referred to as the inpatient care unit, or the hospital unit or ward.

Definitions

- The nursing unit is the place, where patients actually live during their stay in the hospital.
- The nursing unit is a section of a general hospital that includes a nursing station, the beds it serves an associated facilities needed to carry out nursing care.

Functions of the Nursing Unit

1. Provide and maintain the highest quality patient care with the lowest possible cost.
2. Furnish the most desirable environment (safe, comfortable, and pleasant) for patients and health service personnel, i.e., medical and nursing staff as well as other hospital personnel.
3. Consider needs of patient's families and significant others.
4. Provide adequate space to facilitate the carrying out of all the activities needed, i.e., using different types of equipment with minimum waste of personnel time.
5. Promote job satisfaction of the health service personnel.

Types of Nursing Unit

1. **General units:** Where there are similar medical or surgical treatments, e.g., medical or surgical units.
2. **Special units:** Where there are similar:
   - Patient's age, e.g., pediatrics, geriatrics, etc.
   - Patient's needs, e.g., recovery room, nursery, intensive care unit, etc.
   - Medical specialty, e.g., neurology, gynecology, dermatology, ophthalmology, etc.
   - Patient behavior, e.g., psychiatry.

Recently, a system known as Progressive Patient Care has been adopted in some hospitals–Intensive Care Unit (ICU), Intermediate Care Unit, Self-care Unit, Long-term Care Unit, and Home Care Unit. This system is one of organizing the hospital units, around the medical needs of patients and grouping them according to their degree of illness and their needs of nursing care.

Though it is advantageous in terms of economy of manpower and material, it has failed to sustain practicality, due to the current trends in specialization and super specialization.

Hospice Care

Hospice is a special kind that focuses on the quality of life for people and their care givers who are experiencing an advanced life-limiting illness. Hospice care provides compassionate care for possible. The services are provided by a team of health care professionals, the nurses who maximize comfort for a person who is terminally ill by reducing pain and addressing physical, psychological, social, and spiritual needs.

Hospice is not a place, but rather a client and family centered approach to care. Nurses providing care involve all aspect of care, and coordinate and manage symptoms relief, as client death comes closer, the team provides care and support to the family.

REHABILITATION CENTER

Rehabilitation centers are functioning with patient having variety of disabilities, including brain injury, debility, amputations and orthopedic problems.

Rehabilitation Process

The rehabilitation process consists of the following staps: Identifying the disabled/injured person and their environment, setting objectives for rehabilitation efforts, planning, and implementation of suitable measures and evaluating the result.

HEALTHCARE TEAMS

Healthcare teams include:
- Group of physicians
- Nurses
- Physician support group
- Nursing assistance
- Pharmacists
- Social workers
- Radiology staff
- Administrative staff
- Transport staff
- Other nonhealth professionals
- Housekeeping staff
- Laundry staff
- Dietary section staff
- Engineering staff
- Maintenance staff
- Health assistant
- Medical assistance (medical orderly), sanitary workers

MODERN APPROACHES TO NURSING CARE

Modern approaches endorse the holistic approaches for all nursing practices. In holistic nursing, nurses foster relationships with their patients to promote healing and wellness. Holistic nursing are based on the principle that a patient's biological, social, psychological, and spiritual aspects are interconnected.

Holistic Nursing

Holistic in nursing is a philosophy that guides the care that patient receives, which emerged from the concepts of humanism and holism. It refer to the provision of care to patients that are based on a mutual understanding of their physical, psychological, emotional, and spiritual dimensions.

HEALTH AND DISEASE

Concept

Traditionally health means absence of disease, this concept ignores the state of health, health must be viewed in broader prospective based on individual physical, psychological, and emotional states. Understanding the relationship between the concept of health, **wellness, and illness**, one should understand individual health depends on many factors and maintaining optimal level of health know the meaning of health.

Illness

Illness is a state in which, a person physical, emotional, intellectual, social, developmental, or spiritual functioning are diminishes or impaired. Tuberculosis is a disease process, but who is responding to treatment may continue to function as usual, where another client with intestinal problem and who is preparing for surgery may be affected in dimension other than physically. Illness, therefore, is not synonymous with disease. There are two kinds of illness—acute and chronic. Acute illness is usually as a short duration and is severe. The symptoms appear abruptly or intense and often subsides after a relatively short period. The chronic illness persists usually longer than 6 months and can also affect functioning in any dimension. A person with a chronic illness is similar to a person with disability.

Illness Behavior

People, who are sick, generally act in a way that health care provider calls illness behavior. It involves how people monitor their bodies, define and interpret their symptoms, take remedial actions, and use the health care system.

There is a large difference in a way people react to an illness, depends on people pursue themselves to be ill. These sickness behaviors influenced by types of symptoms, cultural background, socioeconomic status, and availability of health care systems.

Examples of illness behavior are fatigue, sleep disturbance, anorexia.

Wellness

A dynamic state of health in which, an individual progresses toward a higher level of functioning, achieving an optimum balance between internal and external environment. Wellness education, teaches people how to care for themselves in a healthy way and include topics such as physical awareness, stress management, and self-responsibility. Wellness strategies are designed to help person achieve new understanding and control of their lives.

Wellness Behavior

Wellness behavior is an important form of health care, because they assist client in maintaining and improving health. Wellness can be influenced by individual practices such as eating habits, exercises, avoiding stresses, improving environment, avoiding pollutants, and unsafe practices.

DEFINITION OF HEALTH

Health is a state of complete physical, mental, and social well-being, not merely the absence of disease or infirmity (WHO, 1947).

Individual views of health depends on different group or society where they are residing, not to assume people free from disease are not healthy may be they are suffering systemic disease, which is a symptomatic (person not experiencing signs and symptoms), if health screening take place we can identify the specific health condition.

DETERMINANTS OF HEALTH

Determinants means, a thing that decides whether or how it happens. Health is influenced by many factors, the factors which contribute to lay both internally and externally, where the individual lives. Health and illness depends on various factors.

The following factors determine individual health and illness status.

Heredity (Biological)

Genetic: Pertaining to reproduction, birth, or origin. The genetic material transferred from one generation to next generation or from parent to children, the genetic make up cannot be altered after conception. Quite a number of diseases are known to be genetic origin, e.g., diabetes mellitus, hypertension, cancer, etc. Hence, determinants of health or the state of health depends partly on the genetic constitution of man. In case of mental retardation scientists advice the genetic counseling to avoid future mental retardation.

Sociocultural Conditions (Lifestyle)

Sociocultural conditions reflecting a whole range of social values, attitudes, and activities. It includes cultural, behavioral, and lifelong personal habit otherwise is called lifestyle.

Lifestyle; is the way, in which an individual or a group lives. Lifestyle induced health problems, disease with natural histories that include conscious exposure to certain health, compromising or risk factors. An example is heart disease associated with cigarette smoking, poor dietary habits, lack of exercises, and also involving in risk-taking activities, which induces stress. Lifestyles are learnt through social interactions with parents, peer groups, friends and siblings and through school and mass medias.

Health and illness are affected by choices made by individuals. An individual takes responsibility for health and wellness by making appropriate lifestyle choices. Lifestyle choices are important in that they affect a person quality of life. Positive lifestyle choices and avoidance of negative lifestyle choices may also play a role in the prevention of illness. The categories, which are identical as determinants of health status are, poor nutrition, alcohol, and drug abuse, use of tobacco, lack of exercise, insufficient rest and sleep, poor personal hygiene, unsafe sexual activities and multiple sex partners.

Environment (Internal and External)

Environment is the place where we live and the condition of that area include air, water, and soil determines how we live, what we eat, and the condition to which (organism) we exposed.

Environment is classified as "external" and "internal". Internal environment of man pertains to each and every component part, every tissue, organ, and organ system. External environment consists of those things to which man is exposed. The physical environment in which a person works or lives can increase the likelihood that, certain illness will more likely to develop when industrial workers are exposed to certain chemicals or when people live near to toxic waste disposal sites.

It is a known fact that the environment has a direct impact on the physical, mental, and social well-being. The environmental factors range from housing, water supply, psychological stress, family system, and social welfare services in the community.

Socioeconomic Conditions

Social and psychological factors can increase the risk for illness. A person generally seeks approval and support from peers, neighbors, and coworkers. Social variables determine how the health care system provides medical care and how clients can obtain care, the treatment method, the economic condition of the client. The economic status determines the purchasing power, standard of living, quality of life, family size, pattern of disease, and deviant behavior in the community. It is also important in seeking health care facilities. Like social variables, economic variable may affect a client level of health by increasing the risk for disease and improve health status also affected by economic status.

Economic status of the Government system often is the main obstacles to the implementation of health technologies and concerning resources allocation, manpower, policy technologies and degree to which health services are more available and accessible to the society. Social, economical and political actions are required to eliminate health hazards in people's living environment.

Health Services Available

Health service is a service available to community for the treatment of diseases, prevention of illnesses, and promotion of health. The purpose of health service is to provide health care services to community, improve the health status of the population, e.g., immunization to children can influence the incidence/prevalence of particular disease, the care of pregnant women and children would contribute to the reduction of child morbidity and mortality to be affective. The health service must reach the social periphery and it should include whether it is available, timely and convenient affordable, affects healthcare utilization.

Patient/Client as an Individual Member of the Family, Society

Family can be determined biologically, legally, or as a social network with personally constructed ties and ideology. The nurse personal belief, do not have to coincide with those of the client, to provide individualized care. The nurse understands that family take many forms and have diverse culture and ethniques orientations. In addition no two families are alike; each has its own strengths and weakness, resources and challenges. In other words, nurse can think of the family as a set of relationships that client identifies as a family or as a network of individuals who influence each others lives.

Family is an open social system that exits in and interacts with the larger systems of the community (e.g., political, religious, schools, and health care systems) as with all systems. The family system has both implicit and explicit goals, which vary according to the stage in the family life cycle, family values, and individual concern of the family members. The family health services include improved family health or well-being. Family management of illness condition and achievement of health outcomes related to the family areas of concern.

DIMENSIONS OF HEALTH

Health is an ongoing process of being conscious and making the right choices for a balanced healthy life. Health is more than being free from illness.

There are seven dimensions of health they are:
1. Physical
2. Social
3. Emotional
4. Spiritual
5. Environmental
6. Occupational
7. Intellectual

Physical Health

Refers to the healthy life style, overall well-being, which includes regular exercise, healthy diet, rest, and sleep all these aspects protect individual from illness and enhance healthy life only healthy body can bring an active mind.

Social Health

Social needs are equally important as biological needs, being mixed with family and social networks we feel we belong to them; this makes individual socially protected changes the way we react to failure, disappointment, and other negative circumstances. Social support includes family, friends, peers, working place, it is important to keep social support group in balance.

Emotional Wellness

When individual emotionally balanced individual feel equipped to cope with any emergency or any unpredictable life events.

Spiritual Health

Spiritual wellness involves owning a set of principles, beliefs, or values that gives directions to ones life. It includes a high level of trust, hope, and assurance. To obtain spiritual wellness needs rigorous practice learn how to be more compassionate, thankful, forgiving, and less judgmental. It also helps to cope up with tough time.

Environmental Health

Environment refers to surrounding the individual is important to health. Environmental wellness is to understand the fact that every action of human beings impacts the quality of nature and its surrounding. Environment includes water contamination, air pollution, chemicals, and noise.

Occupational Health

Occupational health refers to branch of medicine dealing with the prevention and treatment of job-related injuries and illness. Occupational health is an area of work in public health to promote and maintain highest degree of physical, mental, and social well-being of workers in all occupations. The main objectives of occupational health are the maintenance and promotion of workers health and working capacity.

Intellectual Health

Intellectual health refers to being open to new ideas and experiences, and the desire to increase understanding, improve skills, and continually challenge you.

Example of Intellectual Health
- Development of good study skill
- Ability to challenge
- Becoming a critical thinker
- Exposing to new ideas

Intellectual wellness recognizes creative abilities and encourages us to find ways to expand our knowledge and skills, intellectual wellness can be developed through personal and professional development, cultural involvement, and community involvement.

MASLOW'S HIERARCHY OF NEEDS

Basic Human Needs

A basic human need is want of something or requirement for biological, psychological social, or spiritual functioning experienced by a person without which a person cannot survive.

Hierarchy

Hierarchy means that in any list of items some items are classified as more important than others.

Abraham Maslow identified in 1968, five basic levels of basic human needs that are arranged in the order of priority for satisfaction. They are:
1. **Physiological needs**
2. **Safety and security needs**

3. **Love and belonging needs**
4. **Self-esteem needs**
5. **Self-actualization needs**

According to Maslow's theory, the lower level needs must be satisfied before the individual attempts to satisfy needs of a higher level. He found that all these needs are interrelated and some needs cannot be met unless related needs are met. For example, the need for hydration (the normal water volume in the body) can be seriously changed, if the need for elimination of urine is not met. A need can make itself felt either by internal or external stimuli, e.g., the need for food. He also found individuals who satisfy their basic needs are healthier, happier, and more effective than those whose needs are unsatisfied.

Basic Human Needs and Related Nursing Actions

Physiological Needs

They are the lower level needs. They have the highest priority overall the other needs because they are essential to life. They include the need for air, food, water, temperature maintenance, rest or sleep, elimination, sexuality, and avoidance of pain. Some physiological needs are more important to survival than others, e.g., the need for oxygen takes priority over the need for food or water. Also the body can survive longer without food than without water. A primary nursing function is to meet these needs as they are vital to the survival of patients.

Safety and Security Needs

These needs come next in priority. They can be attained through adequate shelter and protection from harmful factors in the environment. Safety means physical as well as psychological safety. Individuals usually feel most secure in familiar environment (e.g., home), with familiar routines and with people they can trust and the things they can know. An important function of the nurse is the promotion of patients' physical safety and emotional security in a health care setting, e.g., bed railings for an unconscious patient.

Love and Belonging Needs

Once individuals have satisfied with the basic physiological safety and security needs, they seek their need for love and belonging (higher level needs). These needs include understanding, group acceptance, affection, mutual trust, and the feeling of belonging to others. Every individual either sick or well desires the companionship and recognition of others, e.g., his family or friends. The nurse should always consider love and belonging needs of the patients by the way of care and by establishing a nurse-client relationship based on mutual understanding and trust.

Self-esteem Needs

It is needed to feel good about one to feel pride, to feel a sense of accomplishment in what one does, and to believe that others also hold one in high regard. Self-esteem gives the individual confidence, independence, worth, strength, adequacy, and usefulness and importance. Lack of self-esteem gives a feeling of inferiority, inadequacy, weakness, and helplessness. The feeling of self dislikable adds to frustration and a sense of failure. Nurses can meet patient's self-esteem needs by accepting their values and beliefs, encouraging them to set attainable goals and facilitating support by family or friends.

Self-actualization Needs

Self-actualization is the highest level of human needs. When the need for self-esteem is satisfied the individual strives for self-actualization, i.e., the need to reach one's potential through full development of one's unique capabilities. Cognition (the need to know and understand) is a strong desire of a human being. The intelligent individual seeks information, analysis it, and searches for its meaning. Esthetic needs vary by its importance from individual to individual. A patient with highly developed esthetic sensibilities will be distressed by unpleasant sights, sounds and odors. The nurse must focus on the strengths and capabilities rather than on problems to meet patient's self-actualization needs. She must aim at coring the total individual need (holistic core), and must provide a sense of hope to maximize his potentials.

HEALTH ILLNESS CONTINUUM

Illness-wellness Continuum (Table 1.1)

Health illness continuum is showing one side wellness another side illness or early death. It gives warning to take care of health, if not taking care any time untimely death will occurs. Health fluctuate throughout individual life, if person not taken precaution he may suffer illness, if he take precaution he will enjoy wellness, if not taken care of health because no symptoms that is not the indication for good health.

FACTORS INFLUENCING HEALTH

Factors influencing health are:

Socioeconomic factors: It includes education, family income, occupation, and support from social network, neighbor, peers, and coworker. Healthcare utilization includes poverty and its correlates, geographic area of residence, race and ethnicity, sex, age, language spoken and disability status.

Table 1.1: Illness-wellness continuum.

Illness	Neutral or maintaining health	Wellness
Disease developing Poor health	No symptoms	Awareness, education
Premature death	Not taken seriously	Optimal health

Life style: Eating habit participating in exercise program or sedentary life (which is a risk factor for disease), poor living environment like stressors, alcoholism, and smoking, consuming fatty food substances, environmental exposure to air pollutant, overweight, obesity, tobacco chewing and substance abuse.

Culture: Cultural practice beliefs influence the personal health practices and remedies. Cultural understanding of illness may affect the way of individual health report. When assessing health care providers should consider beliefs, value, and traditional health care practices.

Family: Family support system is important for maintaining health and care during illness. Family health care practices will be followed by next generation.

Emotional factors: Individual health depends on health belief and practices in which person handles stress through each stage of life.

Developmental factors: Development influences the health practices. Belief about health and illness influence during development experiences depends on individual developmental exposure based on lack of information or miss information.

Spiritual: Healthy practices depend on ones one belief that the spirituality establishes with family and friends and ability to find hope and meaning in life. People live joins with religious practices.

Diet and nutrition: Health can be maintained, if individual adhere good diet and nutrition. A good diet reduces the risk of developing the disease. One of the problem in taking excessive fat intake has been linked to raised cholesterol level in the blood leading to increased risk of cardiovascular disease the diet should be balanced with less saturated fats and oil should contain lots of fruit and vegetables, salt, and sugar should be avoided.

CAUSES AND RISK FACTORS FOR DEVELOPING ILLNESS

Risk Factors for Developing Illness

- ❖ **Genetic factors:** Genetic predisposition to specific illness example a family history of cancer or hypertension is at risk for developing the disease later in life.
- ❖ **Age:** Younger children and elderly people more prone to developing illness.
- ❖ **Environment:** When individual exposed to environment like air pollution, water pollution, vegetable pollution, excessive temperature like hot and cold or occupational exposure to pollutant, chemical, stress in the life, physiological stress like pregnant, person will develop illness.
- ❖ **Lifestyle:** Major risk factors for developing illness is lifestyle of person, which include sedentary lifestyle, alcoholism, smoking, high fat consumption, specially young generation adopting western food style, more vulnerable to develop illness. Additional any individual present with familial risk factors and unhealthy eating they will prone to develop illness.
- ❖ **Other factors:** Emotional stress may include working environment, marital disharmony, and financial difficulties, associated with illness.

Illness

Illness in which person's physical, psychological, emotional function is affected.

Types

Acute illness and chronic illness

Acute illness: Immediate onset and remain short duration, sometime life threatening.

Chronic illness: Appear after long duration of disease in the system. Person may suffer all dimensions with functional disabilities.

Illness Behavior and Emotional Changes

Reaction to illness depends on the nature of illness, the client attitude toward it, and the reaction of others to it. Depending on severity and duration of illness, the family and client will react, e.g., if a client is a bread earner of the family, the emotional or behavioral changes will be severe.

Adjustment to Change of Body Images

Some illnesses results in changes in physical appearance. Client and family react differently to these changes. The reaction depending on type of changes, e.g., amputation of leg or hand, disfigure caused by burns, injuries, etc. Generally clients adjust in the following phase, shock, withdrawal, acknowledgment, acceptance, and rehabilitation. As the client and family recognize the reality of the change, they become anxious and may withdraw, refuse to disease. When they acknowledge the changes, they more through period of grieving, and the client will try to adjust and adapt to the change in body image.

Change in Self-concept

The composite of ideas, feelings, and attitude that a person has about his own identity as client whose self-concept changes because of illness may no longer meet family expectations, leading to tension and conflict. As a result family members may change their interaction with client in the house of providing care.

Change in Family Roles

Family role of a person depends on position in the family like husband, wife, children, parent, etc. When illness occurs family members try to adapt to major changes, to save time and role reversal is common at that time, e.g., when husband admitted wife role will be changing to make decision in the family. Such a reversal of the usual situation can lead to stress and conflict among the family members temporarily. An individual and family generally adjust more easily to short-term changes. Long-term changes may require an adjustment process. The client and family often require guidance and counseling. Illness behavior influenced by merely variables and must be considered by the healthcare providers, specifically nurse while planning care.

Effect of Illness

The client and family must deal with changes resulting from illness and treatment, each client responses differently to illness. The family and client commonly experiences:
- Behavior and emotional changes
- Adjustment to change of body images
- Change in self-concept
- Change in family roles

Impact of Illness on Individual

Chronic illness carries the potential to impact on the life of the family compared to parents of healthy children, or any family members. If any member report sick they will have lower self-esteem, it will affect the emotional stability and their family daily functioning.

Some studies suggest that having a child with chronic illness has a negative impact on the relationship, including lack of time with the spouse, communication problems, higher divorce rates, relationship conflict, and decreased relationship satisfaction.

EFFECT OF HOSPITALIZATION

The hospital milieu is a strange environment for most of the patients. It is an anxiety producing, environment due to health problems. Therefore, the patient fears and has anxiety as he enters the hospital, which must be dealt with an empathetic nursing, intervention to help the patient feel comfortable. An alert nurse should be aware of the factors in the hospital environment.

Common Anxiety Factors

Regimentation

The patient in the hospital is told when to bathe, sleep, what to eat, and drink, as per the decision made for the patient. The patient feels that hospital rules are more important than he is. The nurse should allow the patient to make decisions regarding his care to the extent that he can, unless contraindicated, e.g., patient can bathe at night instead of morning. In other words, the nurse should allow the patient to perform his Activities of Daily Living (ADL), at his accustomed time.

Dehumanization

- The patient can be referred to be diagnosis, e.g., coronary or by room or by bed number
- The patient is not involved in decisions about his care.
- Health care personnel discuss about the patient in his presence without talking to him. Hence, the nurse and the health workers should note the following:
  - Take time to consider each patient as an individual person with his own needs
  - Consider the patient as whole, who reacts always physiologically and psychologically

Separation from Significant Others

Hospitalization can be a lonely experience for the patient. Separation from family and friends contribute to the patient's anxiety. A careful review of hospital rules regarding visiting hours is essential.

Lack of Privacy

- Patient's conversation can be overheard
- Functions carried out in private, e.g., elimination, may require assistance from others
- People come and go from the patient's room at any time
- The nurse should make provisions for privacy.

Lack of Understanding of the Hospital Language

The health team members often speak in the language that the patient cannot understand. The patient feels that he is entering a foreign country. Hence, the nurse should communicate effectively with the patient in the language he understands.

Strange Sights and Sounds

The presence of different equipment, in the hospital and in the patient's room, e.g., oxygen cylinder, oxygen humidifier, cardiac monitor, and the unusual sound of equipment and procedure may give threat to patient. The nurse should explain to the patient about these things and assist patient to become comfortable in his strange environment.

UNIT 2

Nursing Care of the Patient

LEARNING OBJECTIVES

After completing this unit, learner will be able to:
- Explain patient's adjustment to the hospital:
  - Explain understanding the patient as a person, the patient as a person's socioeconomic, cultural background, health status, etc.
  - Effect of hospitalization on patient and family.
  - Admission, transfer, and discharge procedure.
- Discuss basic nursing skills:
  - Communication
  - Nursing interview
  - Recording and reporting
- Describe nursing process:
  - Meaning and importance
  - Assessment, nursing diagnosis, planning, implementation, and evaluation
  - Nursing care plan

INTRODUCTION

It is imperative that all people attend to the maintenance of a safe environment in which to carry out their activities of daily living. People throughout the world are exposed to a variety of environmental hazards, which endanger their safety, health, happiness and needed survival.

Safety Knowledge

Information is crucial for safety. Patients in hospital and other unfamiliar environments frequently need specific information. Lack of knowledge about physical (use of equipment), chemical (drugs/disinfectants), and biological (infections) safety, is potential hazard.

Environmental Safety

Environment contributes to the patient's sense of well-being. It is important for the nurse to ensure that the bedside environment is clean, safe, and pleasant. A nursing responsibility is ensuring that necessary equipment and items are in their proper place and function properly. On admission, the patient and the visitors will be oriented to the hospital environment, the equipment including the beds, call lights, and the layout of the room and unit. Arrange the equipment in the patient's room, so that he or she is able to reach the needed articles in his bed-side locker. The nurse is responsible for allocating the type of bed/crib needed in accordance to patient's age needs, mental status, and capabilities.

Safety Guidelines in Nursing Unit

Safety and security are major concerns in nursing care. The responsibility of nurse is to provide safe, secure environment, and to identify the harmful environment. Promoting safety and preventing injury are primary concerns in nursing. Many patients experience falls especially when they need to go to the toilet. Any limitation in mobility is dangerous, like when an elderly patient with unsteady gait is prone to falling and the hospital setting may increase the risk. The patient with paralysis or spinal cord injury needs support such as walkers, wheel chairs, and they need careful guidance. Nurses must assess the risk for injury in order to support and boost self-esteem of the patients.

Safe bedside unit includes the following:
- Patient calling lights should be functioning and always within reach
- Bed positioned properly
- Side rails and restrains safely used

- Provide uncluttered walk space
- Attention to ventilation, odors, room temperature, lighting, and noise
- Odors may be decreased by promptly emptying bedpans, urinals, and emesis basins, not to dispose off soiled dressing in client's room or near the bed.

Therapeutic Environment

Assessing Patients at Risk for Physical Injuries

The ability of people to protect themselves from injury is effected by a number of factors. Nurses need to assess each of these factors when they plan care to provide safety.

Most Common Factors Age

Learning about the environment is very essential from the childhood. Through knowledge and accurate assessment of the environment, people learn to protect themselves from many injuries. Usually, elderly people have special problems in protecting themselves from injuries. Often the balance of elderly people is impaired by their flexed posture. Slowness of movement and diminished sensual acuity also contribute to the likelihood of injury.

Lifestyle

Lifestyle factors that place people at risk are unsafe work environment, where workers are in danger from machinery and chemicals, residence in neighborhoods with high crime rates, access to illicit drugs, etc. Risk-taking behavior is a factor in accident.

Sensory/Perceptual Alterations

Accurate sensory perception of environmental stimuli is vital to safety. People with impaired touch perception, hearing, taste, smell, and vision are highly susceptible to injury. Paralysis and other neurologic impairments diminish perceptions. Some neurologic diseases cause changes in kinesthetic (movement) sense and tactile (touch) perceptions. For example, disease of the inner ear can cause loss of kinesthetic sense and tactile perceptions. Spinal cord injuries can cause paralysis and loss of tactile perceptions.

Level of Awareness

Awareness is the ability to perceive environmental stimuli and body reactions and to respond appropriately through words and action. The normally alert person assimilates many kinds of information at one time, perceives reality accurately, and acts on those perceptions. Occasionally, people exhibit abnormalities of thoughts; they become absent minded or lose their sense of direction. Patients with impaired awareness include persons lacking in sleep, unconscious or semiconscious persons, disoriented persons, and persons whose judgments have been altered by medications, such as narcotics and sedatives.

Mobility Status

Persons who have impaired mobility are obviously prone to injury. Patients weakened by illness or surgery are not always fully aware of their conditions. It is not uncommon for patients to believe them able to walk and fall while trying.

Emotional State

Extreme emotional state can alter the ability to perceive environmental hazards. The acutely anxious or angry person has reduced perceptual awareness. Depressed persons may think and react to environmental stimuli more slowly than usual.

Ability to Communicate

People with a diminished ability to communicate are also at risk for injury. Aphasic (not able to speak) patients, people with language barriers, and those unable to read are among them. For example, the person unable to interpret the sign "No smoking—Oxygen in use", may cause a fire.

Previous Accidents

It has been recognized for sometimes that some people are accident prone.

Lighting

Many patient's find it difficult to sleep in the hospital as they are frequently disturbed for assessment or for treatment purpose, the nurse should be careful to reduce harsh lighting and noises, whenever possible.

Beds

Patients spend most of their time on bed. The bed is an important part of the client's environment. Nursing responsibility include ensuring a safe and comfortable bed, if the hospital has adjustable bed to raise or lower the head or foot, it is important that the nurse to know how to operate the bed and explain this to the patients.

Whenever the patient's condition indicates raise lower side rails, these should be used to prevent falls and the wheels on the beds should be locked to prevent the bed from slipping away.

Ensuring patient's comfort is always a priority in nursing and to create a comfortable bed environment, the nurse should provide the following:
- Line is clean and wrinkle free
- See that the patients feel comfortable
- Pressure point on patient is protected from rough sheet.

Sleep

Providing comfortable beds promotes rest and sleep. The bottom lines should be tight and clean, while the upper lines should allow freedom of movement and not exert pressure.

A quiet and darkened room with privacy is essential for relaxing. In a strange environment with unfamiliar noises, such as people walking, entering or leaving the room, and closing the windows or doors are disturbing. Effort should be made to reduce disturbances; the nurses should be aware of the patient's rituals and make every effort to meet them. One of the main problems for sleep is pain. Depending on the cause, severity, and the discomfort, appropriate measures have to be taken. Comfort and care should be considered when patient is sleeping. When care cannot be taken, nurses should explain that checking vital signs or specific nursing measures are more important than sleep.

Noises

- Unfamiliar noises should be explained to the patient on an ongoing basis.
- Nurse will help to keep noises to a minimum range by wearing shoes, which do not cause excessive noise while walking, closing doors quietly, handling the equipment smoothly, avoiding dropping of any objects, and talking and laughing loudly.

Exposure to microorganisms

- Nurses will liase with housekeeping to keep the patient's room, bathroom, and nursing units clean and tidy.
- Washing and drying of hands should be practiced before and after contact with each patient.
- Isolation procedure should be utilized and explained to the patients and visitors. For the patients suffering from communicable diseases or for protective isolation. All policies and procedures on "isolation" should be followed.
- Visitors of isolated patients will be taught hand washing, use of mask, gowns, and gloves, and other precautions as necessary.
- Disposable dishes will be used for isolated patients.
- All patients discharged with continued isolation will be taught the techniques that the patient and the family need to follow at home.

Electrical Safety

- As new machines and equipment are introduced into the hospital, nurses will have to learn the potential dangers before using.
- Inspections on all the equipment, plugs, and outlet should be done daily and suspected defects should be reported to the maintenance immediately and repaired. A sign will be placed on the defect items until repaired.
- Water and electricity should not come in contact. Prevent dampness near switches, wiring, and appliances items until repaired.
- Protect electrical cord from heat or oil, to prevent the damage in the electrical insulation.
- Any electrical cord should always be placed high enough, so as to prevent the tripping hazards.
- Nurses should make rounds with maintenance personnels to inspect cords, plugs, switches, socks, etc., and outlets for damage. Problems should be alleviated immediately by maintenance.

- Defibrillation paddle should be checked in each shift when the crash carts are checked.
- Some patients are especially sensitive to electrical hazards. Nursing staff should be aware of the existence of patients with a particular sensitivity, which may result from aware of the existence of patients with a particular sensitivity, which may result from:
  - Debilitating medical condition
  - Major loss of skin resistance due to wet dressings

Oxygen Safety

Prevention of electrical hazards

When oxygen is administered, the following precautions shall be followed:

- Smoking is strictly prohibited in health institution.
- "No smoking-Oxygen in use", signs shall be placed on the door of the patient's room.
- Flammable or combustible or vapors such as alcohol, oil, grease, or other flammable materials should not be used while oxygen is being administered.
- Nylon, silk, rayon, and woolen clothing should not be used by patients, when oxygen is being administered.
- Ether or any other explosive anesthetics should not be used.
- Oxygen administered should be humidified.
- Nurse should understand and be constantly educated on the use of oxygen cylinders, regulators, humidifiers, catheters, inhalers, facemasks, tents, and ventilators.
- Any new respiratory equipment should be explained to the nursing staff. In-services on new equipment will include the use and the safety precautions as needed.
- Oxygen cylinders should be stored in a cool temperature away from the inflammable materials and where they are not likely to be knocked over.
- Any problems or questions about respiratory equipment should be immediately reported for in section and repairs.

Incidents involving patients, visitors and employees

- All nurses should be aware of correct procedure to follow, if a patient is injured in the hospital. The patient's attending physician will be called immediately to examine the patient. The incident will be relayed to the nursing officer/supervisor and an incident report form will be filled out immediately and submitted to the appropriate authority.
- All nurses should be aware of the correct procedure to follow, if a visitor is injured in the hospital. The nurse will immediately take him/her to the accident and emergency department and an incident report form will be filled out immediately after examination and submitted to the appropriate authority.
- All nurses should be aware of the correct procedure to follow, if he/she is injured while on duty, he/she will be examined by the appropriate person, and an incident

report will be produced to the higher authority for needful action.

Safety in moving patients and equipment

When moving heavy equipment always has sufficient help to:
- Prevent injury to persons and equipment.
- Push but do not pull heavy equipment to prevent injury to feet, legs, and back.
- Open and secure swinging doors before proceeding.
- Keep hands and fingers away from the edge of equipment to prevent injury.
- When lifting patients and equipment, seek help, when needed.

Observe the following precautions:
- Keeps pine vertical and straight, use leg muscles not back muscles.
- Stand close to the person/object being lifted with feet apart, for balance bend at knees to use leg muscles to lift.
- Use a safe, firm pressure when lifting, do not jerk.
- When lifting as a team, maintain constant level of the object by doing it gradually and gently.

Safety in Transporting Patients

When transporting with stretchers, beds carts, and other wheeled equipment, safety precautions must be followed as listed below:
- When assisting patients on to stretchers, beds, or wheel chairs be sure that the equipment is properly secured and brakes are set on the wheels.
- Any patient being transferred through stretcher must have side rails in position and safety straps fastened.
- First transport patient on a stretcher or bed feet.
- Push the vehicle from the end to avoid hand injury.
- Move slowly and always have clearance.
- When patients are being transported from one room to another by stretcher, they should be secured to are straining belt and to keep their feet, arms and hands the covering blanket and on the stretcher. At doorways, stretchers and carts be pulled through rather than pushed in blindly.

Safety from Insects

Flies, mosquitoes, and cockroaches should be kept away by spraying. Make use of the number of insecticides available or supplied from the institute.

Preventing Patient Fall in the Hospital

Falls may be caused while shifting patients. It can be prevented by keeping floor dry to prevent slipping, securely holding stretchers and wheel chairs while transporting the patient.

Tips to Prevent Fall in the Hospital
- Orient the patient on admission to their surrounding and explain the call system.
- Encourage the patient to use call bell and ensure call bell is within reach.
- Place bed side tables and over bed tables near the bed or chairs, so that patient do not over reach and lose their balance.
- Assess the patient's ability to ambulate and provide assistance as required.
- Instruct the patient to be careful while using toilet.
- Encourage the patient to wear nonskidding footwear.
- Keep the environment tidy.
- Maintain clutter-free area.
- Ensure adequate lighting.
- Attach side rails to the beds of confused, sedated, restless, and unconscious clients.

Safety for Preventing Cross-infection in the Hospital
- Wash hands before and after each procedure.
- Ventilate the patient's room.
- Use damp dusting to prevent the raise of dust in the environment.
- Provide disinfectants for cleaning the floor.
- Keep the environment clean, e.g., bed locker, bed linen, over bed table, floor, etc.
- Cover the mattress and pillow with plastic cover, so that it is easy to disinfect after a patient is discharged.
- Wear disposable gloves while handling body fluids and secretions, e.g., urine, stool, vomit, pus, etc.
- Complete all the cleaning activities, e.g., bed making, dusting, etc., at least 1 hour prior to the commencement of aseptic procedures, e.g., wound dressing, IV, infusions, injections, etc.
- Wash hands before handling foods.
- Serve the food hot in a covered container.
- Protect the kitchen and pantry from files, insects, and cockroaches.
- Clean and disinfect bed pans, urinals, and sputum cups.
- Dispose all waste materials properly following hospital with infectious diseases.
- Immunize all nurses, who are taking care of patients with infectious diseases.
- Cover all used sharp instruments and discard in an appropriate container.
- Regular health check-ups for all health personnel.
- Keep the toilets clean.
- Instructs people to cover the nose and mouth while sneezing and coughing, to prevent droplet infections.

Patients and Visitors Information

- The nurse should give anticipating guidance and counseling to patients about the type of accidents likely to happen to their children at different ages.
- Children should be safeguarded from fire, gas stoves, oven, and hot water to prevent burns.
- Plastic bags and small objects that could air passage should be kept away from children.

- ❖ Poisonous substance, household cleaning agents and medications should be kept out of reach of the children. If a child has swallowed any poisonous substance or medication he/she should be taken to the hospital with the ingested substance or medication immediately.
- ❖ Children should not be left alone at home.
- ❖ Children should be supervised when riding tricycle.
- ❖ Adults should be counseled to teach the children safety measures.
- ❖ The nurse should begin to assess the patient's home environment on admission and conduct patient teaching throughout the patients stay.
- ❖ Prevent fire by proper use of gas stoves, kerosene lamps and electrical appliances.
- ❖ Prevent fire by proper disposal of cigarette buffs.
- ❖ Prevent accidents while traveling by not overloading the car and by following traffic rules.
- ❖ All chemicals should be kept in a safe place, which will probably be in a glass container.
- ❖ Sharp equipment (pins, needles, razor blades, sharp knives, electric and sharp gardening tools).
- ❖ Safety should be considered while arranging lighting in houses and access areas, particularly where there are steps or stairs and when there are children or elderly people.
- ❖ Provision of stair guard and secure locks on doors and windows.
- ❖ Use of nonslip mats in the bathroom.

Safety Precautions in the Hospital

- ❖ Read the bulletin board in order to keep up with change and improvement in the hospital policies and procedures.
- ❖ It is the responsibility of each employee to report unsafe condition to his supervisor.
- ❖ All safety measures for disoriented or emotionally disturbed patients should be utilized. Safety measures; both for patients and employees shall be put forth into practice while caring for these patients.
- ❖ Hospital personnel, visitors, and patients should be warned when doors are wet and movable object has been kept in the passage.
- ❖ **Always read warning signs such as "radiation precaution, isolation, etc.**

Patient's Adjustment to the Hospital

- ❖ Understanding the patient as a person the patient as a person socioeconomic, and cultural background, health status, etc.
- ❖ Admission, transfer, and discharge procedure.

Effects of Illness and Hospitalization on Patient and his Family

Effects of illness

The client and family must deal with changes resulting from illness and treatment, each client responses differently to illness. The family and client commonly experiences:

Behavior and emotional changes: Reaction to illness depends on the nature of illness, client attitude toward it, and reaction of others to it. Depending on severity and duration of illness, the family and client will react, e.g., if a client is a bread earner of the family, the emotional or behavioral changes will be severe.

Adjustment to change of body images: Some illnesses results in changes in physical appearance. Client and family react differently to these changes. The reaction depending on type of changes, e.g., amputation of leg or hand, disfigure caused by burns, injuries, etc. Generally, clients adjust in the following phase—shock, withdrawal, acknowledgment, acceptance, and rehabilitation. As the client and family recognize the reality of the change, they become anxious and may withdraw, refuse to disease. When they acknowledge the changes, they move through a period of grieving, and the client will try to adjust and adapt to the change in body image.

Change in self-concept: The composite of ideas, feelings, and attitude that a person has about his own identity as client whose self-concept changes because of illness may no longer meet family expectations, leading to tension and conflict. As a result family members may change their interaction with the client in the course of providing care.

Changes in family roles: Family role of a person depends on position in the family like husband, wife, children, parent, etc. When illness occurs, family members try to adapt to major changes, save time, and role reversal is common at that time, e.g., when husband admitted wife role will be changing to make decision in the family. Such a reversal of the usual situation can lead to stress and conflict among the family members temporarily. An individual and family generally adjust more easily to short-term changes. Long-term changes may require an adjustment process. The client and family often require guidance and counseling. Illness behavior influenced by merely variables and must be considered by the health care providers, specifically nurses while planning care.

EMOTIONAL NEEDS OF PATIENTS

Every individual is the sum of the physical manifestation (body), mental process (mind), feelings (emotions), and relationship to God (spiritual). Effective patient care requires attention to all these aspects (total patient care) and it depends on:

- ❖ The nurse's skills in the performance of procedures.
- ❖ The nurse's ability to establish a therapeutic relationship with patients by recognizing the emotional needs of the patient provides the foundation for a therapeutic relationship.

Definition of Emotion

An emotion is a strong feeling such as love, hate, or fear. Therefore, a helping relationship may be strengthened when emotional responses are handled appropriately.

Types of Emotion

- **Positive emotion:** Includes happiness, pleasure, joy, etc.
- **Negative emotions:** Includes fear, anger, grief, anxiety, etc.

Ways of Expressing Emotion

- Facial expression
- Movement
- Posture and body orientation
- What people say and how they say it?
- What people do not say?
- The use of silence.

Note: Emotion can be expressed in constructive ways.

Physiological Effects of Emotions

Some of the following physical effects that occur are:
- Increase in heart rate
- Increase in respiratory rate
- Increase or decrease in BP
- Cold
- Sweat in hands
- Blushing or paleness of skin
- Dry mouth
- Trembling
- Nausea
- Urination or diarrhea

Note: The severity of these physiological effects depends on the intensity of emotion.

Factors that Influence the Emotional Response Patterns

- Past experiences
- Beliefs
- Attitudes
- Self concept
- Self-esteem
- Various personality traits.

COMMON EMOTIONAL RESPONSES TO ILLNESS AND NURSING IMPLICATIONS

See **Table 2.1**.

Table 2.1: Common emotional responses to illness and nursing implications.

Emotional responses	Definition	Nursing implications
Anxiety	An emotional state characterized by feelings of uneasiness about the unknown, generalized fear of the unknown (some factors arouse fears as well as anxiety)	Allow the patient to explore anxiety and worry. He can often describe a reason for worry. But usually cannot explain why he is anxious
Worry	A mild form of anxiety characterized by the preoccupation of a problem. The patient is able to communicate the cause of the concern	Listen while the patient describes his feeling of anxiety and worry. Avoid talking to the patient out of anxiety and worry with a avoid comment such as "Don't worry, everything will be all right".
Fear	An emotional state characterized by expected harm or unpleasantness. Fear of the unknown, the hospital environment causes fear (first admission) sounds, equipment, separation from family and friends, and unfamiliar environment causes fear	• Allow the patient to describe his feelings. Some express them freely while others do not • Try to identify what is frightening the patient and offer appropriate explanations • Demonstrate that you are interested in the patient and wish to help him
Anger	An emotional state characterized by the feeling of frustration and struggling with a threatening or unpleasant situation. Why am I sick? Common reaction. Lack of patient cooperation, patient resents hospital routine, e.g., vital signs early morning or during night	• Allow the patient time to express his anger in a nonjudgmental atmosphere • Show acceptance of the patient's behavior even if the anger is directed at you • Try to determine the cause of the anger and then deal with it as realistically as possible • Be aware that it is almost impossible to reason with an angry person, if possible, wait until the anger has subsided before intervening • Expect that anger may be masked with other responses to frustration, such as hostility
Denial	Refusal or restriction for something requested. Claim or need, often resulting in physical or emotional deficiency	• Recognize that a patient using denial protects himself from something he does not wish to face • Deal with denial carefully and in cooperation with other health personnel • Confirm that denial is present and then give the patient accurate information, to the extent that the patient can accept it • Be prepared to offer emotional support as the patient comes to recognize his denial • Expect that reversing denial to a state of acceptance of reality take time and cannot be forced.

Contd...

Contd...

Emotional responses	Definition	Nursing implications
Feeling of over dependency	An emotional state characterized by feelings normal	• Be prepared to note that feeling of helplessness increase during illness, but if exaggerated it will stand in the way of recovery and well-being • Try to determine the reason for over dependency. Is the patient fearful of overdoing? Does the patient seek attention? Do the feelings conceal anger? • Encourage activities that are suitable for the patient and personal care • Offer praise in a sincere and appropriate manner as the patient makes progress toward independence

ADMISSION, TRANSFER, AND DISCHARGE PROCEDURES

HOSPITAL ADMISSION AND DISCHARGE

Admission of a Patient

Definition

Admission of a patient is a hospital policy, which requires nursing steps to be accomplished.

Types of Admission

- Routine admission
- Emergency admission
- Transfer
- Last office

Purposes

- To establish guideline regarding admission of patients
- To make the patient feel welcome, comfortable and at ease
- To acquire vital information regarding the patient
- To assess the patient from which a nursing care plan can be initiated and implemented
- To care for the patients valuables and personal belongings
- To meet patient's individual needs

Admission to the Hospital Unit and Preparation of Unit

Each institution follows a different set of policies and procedures for admitting clients. A client's condition determines the extent of the admitting procedures. Admission officer and technicians are involved with the preliminary procedures for admitting the client into a ward.

Clients usually experience considerable anxiety about the admission process, so that all personnel's should treat them courteously and professionally. This is where customer service begins. If any one person shows an uncaring attitude, clients may assume that all the personnel are unprofessional. By making the client and their families feel welcomed, nurses, and the other staff members begin to establish a therapeutic relationship with the client.

First Step in Admitting Clients

This is to acquire identifying information including full legal name, age, date of birth, addresses, next of kin, admitting physician, religion, and occupation, each clients receives a permanent identification number for hospital records, if institution has the policy.

The hospital is responsible for ensuring the client's legal rights at admission, each hospital has policies and procedures of which the clients should be informed usually the client or family receives a brochure explaining available services. Visiting hours, meal schedules, smoking policies, rules that affect the persons conduct as a patient.

In some cases clients, may undergo laboratory X-ray testing in the OPD such test can be performed safely before admission, after all necessary information has been collected and the client is thoroughly informed, the next step is transportation of the client to the nursing unit.

To begin ensuring continuity of care, the admission office notifies the nursing unit of client's admission current status and room assignment, this allows nursing staff to prepare a room and obtain necessary equipment for the arrival.

Admission of the Client to a Nursing Unit

Member of admission office transport service or emergency department transports the client to the nursing unit. The client condition determines whether ambulating or the use of a wheel chair or structure is most appropriate. Upon arrival at the unit the client and family are introduced to the nurse responsible for the client care. The initial movement spent with a client begins the orientation phase of the client-nurse relationship.

Admission process includes:

- Introduction
- Orientation
- Procedures
- Collection of a nursing history
- Physical assessment
- Collection of specimen
- Clarification of client questions and their expectation

If the client is experiencing physical or psychological symptoms the nurse determines whether any portion of the admission process can be completed later.

ROOM PREPARATION

- Wash hands
- Prepare assigned room with necessary equipment and personal care items
- Bath towel and wash cloth
- Toiletry items
- Tissue paper
- Water and drinking glasses
- Kidney basin
- Thermometer
- Sphygmomanometer
- Bedpan with urinals
- Prepare bed
- Arrange room furniture
- Assemble special equipment such as suction equipment, oxygen supplies and IV poles, etc.
- Appropriate hospital dress, foot wear, and towel

Admission Procedures

Procedure: Admission of the client to a nursing unit (Table 2.2).

Table 2.2: Admission procedure of client to a nursing unit.

Sl. No.	Nursing action	Rationale
1.	The admitting office or relevant authority will notify the nursing unit regarding the admission	Prompt response to the patient arrival on the unit is important
2.	Greet and accurately identify the patient	To instill confidence and to avoid unnecessary confusions
3.	Escort the patient as appropriate to his/her assigned bed. Introduce her/him to roommates and new environment including use of lockers, bed and how it works, television, telephone, and call light/bell, emergency signals, and bathroom. Explain policies related to no smoking. Visiting hour's attendants, and meals. Assess client general appearance, noting signs and symptoms of physical distress. Assesses client and family psychological status. Orient client to nursing division.	To enhance a feeling of belongingness. Helps to adhere to the policies and to avoid confusion to the new situations
4.	Assist patient to undress. Observe for any unusual characteristics or disabilities, e.g., bruises, cuts, color level of awareness general survey, and assessment	Helps the nurse for proper observation (from head to toe)
5.	Hang clothing neatly in close/cabinet provided for the patient (bedside locker). Encourage the patient to send home all belongings not needed with a relative.	For the safety of patient belongings
6.	Check personal property and maintain appropriate record. Keep appropriate records of the jewelry and valuables possessed by the patient	Proper record keeping legally saves nurse and the institute
7.	Check disposition of medication the patient may have brought to the hospital. Record the medications, place in a bag, and label marked as patient's own medications	Medication will be returned to the patient upon discharge. Encourage the relatives to take medications home.
8.	Complete admission procedures (bed number, Identification band/IP no.), etc.	
9.	Complete the nursing assessment form and admission record. Review the health status, screen elimination, nutrition, metabolic activity, and exercise	Detailed review helps in proper diagnosis
10.	Check records and arrange for special investigation and procedures that the patient has undergone before or on admission. Instruct client on proper techniques to collect specimen and attach requisition	Proper techniques avoid falls report
11.	Check baseline vital signs and record it in appropriate records	Proper recording guides the healthcare personnel in planning the care
12.	Check physician's order, progress notes and other documents for treatment; measures should be verified immediately	To obtain specific instructions and information
13.	Inform the attending physician of the arrival of patient	Notification helps the physician to attend the patient as per the need
14.	Inform catering department of the arrival of patient	Patient will be provided food as per schedule
15.	Activate appropriate nursing care plan. Demonstrate equipment use. Show client how to use nurse call light	Appropriate plan helps to give care as per the need. Aid in giving attention on time

Contd...

Contd...

Sl. No.	Nursing action	Rationale
16.	Inform the client about procedures or treatment scheduled for next shift or day	Client has the right to be informed of any scheduled procedure
17.	Document the procedures in the appropriate charts. Report to concerned about patient condition treatment and to be carried out or any pending procedures surgery, etc.	Helps to guide the next shift person about the completed treatment. To avoid confusions, and to give treatment as per order

ADMISSION OF PATIENT TO AN EMERGENCY DEPARTMENT

The first hour after an injury is a "Vital Hour" or "Golden Hour". Immediate, prompt, and forceful resuscitation and treatment will save the patients' life. Nurses play an important role in patient care during the "Golden Hour".

Purposes

- To meet the emergency need of the patient
- To save the life of the patient
- To help to secure a prompt and correct diagnosis.

Preparation of the Accident and Emergency Department

- Keep the emergency trolley ready
- Keep the resuscitation equipment ready
- Keep the equipment and supplies in its proper place for easily visible and accessible
- Check the emergency drugs for its immediate use.

Equipment and Supplies Required for Meeting the Emergencies

- Ventilator
- Laryngoscope handle with various sized blades and bulbs
- Various sized endotracheal tubes with stylets
- Oral and nasal airways
- Drugs for induction
  - Succinylcholine
  - Savlon
  - Pentothal for sedation
  - Morphine
  - Pethidine
- For cardiac arrest
  - Sodium bicarbonate
  - Adrenaline
  - Atropine
  - Lidocaine (Xylocaine)
  - Calcium
  - Dextrose 50%
- Heparinized syringe for ABG
- Respiratory equipment (Ambu bag) with tubing connected to oxygen source, various sized masks, and corrugated tubing
- Tracheotomy tubes and sterile suction catheters
- BP instrument
- Torch and spot light
- Stethoscope
- Thermometer
- Auto scope
- Knee hammer
- Pin
- Splint
- Dressing set
- Suturing set
- Suction apparatus
- Monitor with defibrillator
- Syringes all size
- Gloves
- Chest tube with closed drainage systems
- Blood tubing
- Plasma I/V fluids
- Other essential supplies

Equipment Kept in the Ambulance Bag

- Endotracheal tubes with stylet and syringe to inflate the balloon (sizes 7, 8, and 9)
- Laryngoscope with a curved and straight blade
- One bottle (500 mL) of human plasma protein fraction
- Various sizes of oral and nasal airways
- Spinal needle 18 gauze and 10 mL syringes
- Esophageal obturator airway and penlight
- 12 mL syringes –2
- Penlight
- Roll of ½ inch adhesive tape
- Oxygen tank wrench
- A locked box of emergency resuscitation drugs is kept in the ambulance at all times and key will be kept with responsible person.

Priorities of the A and E Unit

- Airway
- Breathing (control of cervical spine fracture)
- Circulation (cardiac dysrhythmias)
- Do not hyper extend the neck in suspected cervical injury, give cervical immobilization using cervical collar or sandbags
- Perform nasal intubations
- Monitors with multiple parameter [heart rate arterial line pressure, central venous pressure (CVP), intracranial pressure (ICP)]
- Control of hemorrhage
- Treatment of shock
- Splinting of fracture
- Evaluation of further injuries
- Continuous monitoring (all parameter).

Roles and Responsibilities of the Nurse

- Maintain patient comfort
- Initial and continuous assessment of physiological parameter
- Assist in resuscitative procedures
- Monitor fluid and electrolytes balance
- Follow aseptic technique
- Administer medications according to doctor orders
- Meet the physical, psychological, social, and spiritual needs of the patients and relatives
- Give overview of patient to the receiving unit and transferring patients.

Initial Assessment of A and E Patient by the Nurse

- Observe the clothing for signs of damage, which indicate the sites of the injury
- Observe the position of patient
- Find out from the ambulance staff about.
  - The type of accident.
  - What injuries or condition has the patient been found and whether the relatives know about the patient whereabouts.
- Reassure the patient and explain what is being done
- Ask the patient what has happened and about the pain
- Observe the entire body, from head to foot
- Place an identity bracelet on the patient.

Lifting the Patient

- Lift the patient and place him on the accident trolley
- Support the head and neck or use cervical collar in case of neck injury
- Keep the patient in the accident trolley for X-ray or plaster room tilt the patient is transferred to the bed.

Removal of Clothing

- Provide privacy and be gentle
- Use scissors and cut the clothing, if urgency is required
- Use a scalpel and cut through the sleeves
- Unbutton and remove all the upper cloths first
- Take the uninjured limb and outmode the clothing first
- Remove the clothing completely for thorough examination.

Patients Property and Valuables

- Prepare a list of valuables, handover to relatives, and get witness signed
- If no relatives nearby follow agency policy for the safety of the belongings.

Doctor's Examination

- Help the doctor in examining the patient thoroughly from head to foot
- Carryout treatment before a diagnosis made assign case of emergency
- Observe the patient with the doctor "two pairs of critical eyes are better than one pair".

Head

- Inspect and feel for lump, lacerations, and injuries
- Inspect the nose, ears, and mouth for bleeding
- Observe the facial asymmetry caused by facial paralysis or swelling due to fracture
- Test pupillary size and reaction to light, in case of head injury.

Limbs

- Compare both sides
- Observe the length, position, swelling, and injury
- Test the range of joint movements.

Chest

- Observe for paradoxical respiration
- Observe for any injury steering-wheel marks and fracture
- Look for emphysema (air leaking from the lungs into the tissues of the chest wall).

Abdomen

- Inspect the abdomen for any bruises and steering-wheel mark
- Take abdominal girth.

Baseline Vital Signs

- Temperature, pulse, and respiratory rate (TPR), BP
- Level of consciousness
- Pupillary size and reaction.

Meeting Patient's Social and Spiritual Needs

- Contact the patients next/immediate kin or friend
- Get the help of police or friends to inform the relatives
- Prepare the patient's and relatives' waiting room adequately and inform about the patient's progress.

Documents

- Prepare documents quickly and accurately
- Avoid mistakes by properly identifying the patient.

Final Checklist before Transferring the Patient to Ward

- Drug allergies noted
- Tetanus toxoid given
- Wound dressing done
- All treatments carried out
- Ward staff informed
- Final document ready
- All investigations done and reports ready or waiting
- X-ray and ECG ready
- Relatives informed
- All property safe.

INTERNAL TRANSFER OF PATIENTS

Purpose

To transfer the patent into a unit that provides special care or care suited to his needs (e.g., from general ward to ICU).

Procedures

Determine for transfer in collaboration with patient, physician (e.g., change in patient's condition, resources available at agency, and patient/family, preference regarding patient location).

Assess Patient's Current Physical Condition, Gather Patient's Personal Belongings

- Assess the method for transport, inform receiving nurse.
- Maintain patient physical well-being during transport to new nursing unit.
- Provide verbal report about patient's condition to receiving unit nurse.
- Be sure all documents including care plan is completed.
- Assist patient in transferring to wheel chair or structure.
- Announce patient's arrival to the new unit.
- Transport patient to new room and assist in transfer to bed.
- Handover to receiving nurse.

DISCHARGE FROM THE HOSPITAL

Definition

Discharge planning is the plan evolved before a patient is transferred from one environment to another. This process involves the patient, family, friends, and the hospital and community healthcare teams. Discharge planning is an integral part of the continuity of nursing care for patients through their hospital stay.

Purposes

- To ensure continuity of care by providing instructions, information, and guidelines.
- To promote continuity of coordination within the health care environment on discharge from hospital.
- To prepare the patient physically and psychologically for transfer to the changed environment.
- Prepare the family emotionally and psychologically for a changing environment.

Discharge against Medical Advice (DAMA) or Left against Medical Advice (LAMA)

Occasionally, a client chooses to leave a hospital against medical advice, in this situation, there is a risk that the client will suffer complication after leaving the hospital. The client must sign a form that releases the physicians and hospital from any legal liabilities for client health explains the risk of DAMA.

Discharge Procedure (Table 2.3)

Table 2.3: Discharge procedure.

Sl. No.	Nursing action	Rationale
1.	Assess the patient for home care needs and formulate a plan of care to meet the individual's physiological and social needs. This must begin on admission and is an ongoing process	To enable planning to start well in advance of discharge to home
2.	Document all relevant information (social, communication, home address, telephone number, etc.)	To facilitate planning, coordination, and communication
	Ensure that the next of kin or sponsor is the person who is willing to accept the responsibility of care	Personal information may not have been entered or updated in nursing and medical records
3.	Establish whether hospital/health center will be involved following the patients discharge document names and telephone number	To enable contact for exchange of information to assist in assessing potential needs on discharge
4.	Review patient's activity of daily livings	To establish the actual and potential activities that the patient can perform
5.	Plan discharge with patients care givers and other members of healthcare team	To collect information and coordinate planning
6.	Ensure that any essential aids or equipment have been obtained adaptations made, and orientation given to patient and care givers before discharge	Some equipment may not be available or may take a long time to be obtained. The patient may be at risk at home and suffer unnecessary discomfort and stress
7.	Teach patient/family the necessary skills required for rehabilitation, allowing sufficient time to practice before discharge	To enable the patient to be as independent as possible and promote an understanding of self-care techniques
8.	Reinforce any special instruction with written information, e.g., health education sheet and precautions	To enhance the patients understanding and knowledge of disease process, prescribed treatment, and precautions
9.	Review the physician progress notes, physician order notes, nursing progress notes, and nursing care plan	To obtain specific instructions/information regarding discharge planning

Contd...

Contd...

Sl. No.	Nursing action	Rationale
10.	Consult and finalize the arrangement for discharge, e.g., physiotherapist, social worker, dietary therapist, public relation officer, etc.	To enhance holistic approach
11.	On the day of discharge check physician's discharge orders for prescription/change in treatments. Determine whether client or family has arranged for transport, provide client with medication prescription. Document discharge on discharge summary form	Help in proper follow-up and continuity of care

Medicolegal Issues in Admitting Patient

Cases that are to be treated as medicolegal are:
1. All cases of injuries and burns
2. The circumstances of which suggest commission of offense by somebody (irrespective of suspicion of foul play)
3. All vehicular, factory, or other unnatural accident cases specially when there is a likelihood of patient's death.

Care of the Unit after Discharge

Care of patient unit is defined as keeping the patients unit clean, neat, and tidy. It also helps to provide maximum comfort to the patient. Patient unit is the area furnished and equipped according to the need to give adequate care to the patient.

Disinfecting the whole external environment of the patient and rendering it free from pathogenic organisms.

BASIC NURSING SKILLS

COMMUNICATION

Communication is the basic element of human interactions. It is one of the most vital components of all nursing practice. A great deal of nursing practice involves interpersonal communication skills and the establishment of relationships essential for successful functioning. For example, communication between the nurse and other members of the health team, personnel in other healthcare agencies or the public. Communication is also a component of therapy, nurses who communicate effectively are able to initiate change that promotes health, establish a trusting relationship with patients and with others, and prevent legal problems associated with nursing practice (**Fig. 2.1**).

Definitions

* Communication is the process of exchanging information, thoughts, ideas, and feelings from one individual to another.

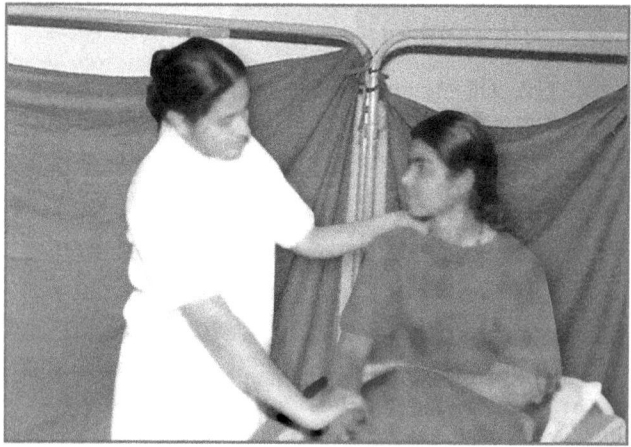

Fig. 2.1: Nurse uses touch to communicate with patient.

* Communication is the process by which a message is passed from the sender to the receiver with the objective that the message sent is received and understood as intended.

Levels of Communication

Communication takes place in:
* Intrapersonal communication
* Interpersonal communication
* Public communication
* Mass communication
* Small group communication

Kinds of Communication

Nursing practice involves three kinds of communication:
1. **Social communication:** It is the unplanned communication that gives satisfaction to patients. It is often carried out while performing nursing procedures like bath.
2. **Structured communication:** It is the planned communication, e.g., teaching a diabetic patient self-administration of insulin injection.
3. **Therapeutic communication:** It is the planned or unplanned communication that is used by nurses in many situations to relieve anxiety and fear in the patients, e.g., preoperative teaching.

Communication Process

Communication is a two-way process involving the sending and receiving of a message. Since the purpose of communication is to elicit a response, the process is ongoing. The receiver of the message becomes the sender of the response and the original sender becomes the receiver.

Basic Elements of Communication Process

There are seven major elements of communication process. The basic elements are:
1. Sender
2. Message
3. Encoding
4. Communication channel
5. Receiver
6. Decoding
7. Feedback

Sender: The sender is on the individual or group who wishes to convey the message to another. He is the initiator of the communication process and is sometimes called the "source encoder". The individual or group sending the message must have a reason for communicating and must put it in a form that can be transmitted. Encoding means translating the thoughts into specific signs and symbols. Effective encoding depends on a clear message delivered at the right place, at the right time, and phrased in such a way as to attract the receiver's attention, e.g., clear, complete, concise, concrete, and correct (5 C's of communication).

Message: It is the information that is selected and conveyed by the sender. It requires the sender's decisions about what will be said, how, when, and where it will be said and the selection of words in a language that can be understood by the receiver, e.g., in a hospital setting, the physician communicates new orders to the nurse supervisor (receiver) about patients for the purpose of implementing them. Without any purpose or goal there is no need for the physician (sender) to begin the communication process.

Channel: It is the means by which the message is transmitted. For example, through the visual, auditory, and tactile senses. It is important that the channel be appropriate for the message to make the intent of the message clear. Talking face-to-face with a person may be more effective in some instances than telephoning or writing the message. Recording message on tapes or communicating by radio or television may be appropriate for larger audiences.

Receiver: The receiver is the individual to whom the message is transmitted. This individual is sometimes called the decoder. He interprets and decodes the sender's message into information that has meaning. Understanding is the key to the decoding process. The intended meaning will be communicated when the sender and the receiver have common knowledge and experience. For example, when people with different experiences communicate as in patient teaching the sender (nurse) must speak the language of the receiver (patient).

Decoding and feedback: It is the message that the receiver returns to the sender. It is also called feedback. The receiver's verbal and nonverbal response to the sender reveals the receiver's understanding of the message. It helps the sender to recognize whether the meaning of his message has been received as intended. Communication is not successful until the message received has been understood and acted upon it appropriately.

Modes or Forms of Communication

Communication is generally carried out in two different modes or forms.

Verbal Communication

The spoken and/or the written words are the most frequent modes for conveying information of one's ideas, thoughts, and feelings to others. The words used vary among individuals according to culture, socioeconomic background, age, and education. Examples of written words are—notes, letters, records, forms, newspapers, books, and magazines. Examples of spoken words are—face-to-face meeting, recording messages on tapes, telephoning, radio, and television.

Nonverbal Communication

It is the exchange of a message without the use of words. About 80-90% communication is nonverbal. It tells others more about what a person is feeling than what is actually said because it is controlled less consciously than verbal behavior. Nonverbal communication either reinforces or contradicts what is said verbally, e.g., a nurse may say to a patient "I am happy to sit and talk to you for a while". Yet, if she looks on at her wrist watch nervously every few seconds, her action contradicts the verbal message. Nonverbal communication is sometimes called body language.

Means of nonverbal communication

a. **Physical appearance including adornment:** Personal appearance, body shapes, size, hair styles, clothing, and adornments are sometimes rich sources of information about a person. Clothing may convey social and financial status, culture, religion, and self-concept. Adornments such as jewelry, perfume, or cosmetics may reveal additional information. How a person dresses is often an indicator of how the person feels. The nurse needs to be alert to sudden changes in a patient's dress; that may be a signal of loss of self-esteem or feeling better.
b. **Posture and gait:** The way people walk and carry themselves are often reliable indicators of self-concept; mood and health, e.g., erect posture and on active, purposeful walk suggest a feeling of well-being, while tense posture suggests anxiety or anger.
c. **Facial expressions:** The face is the most expressive part of the body. Feelings of joy, sadness, fear, surprise, anger, and disgust can be conveyed by facial expressions. Many facial expressions convey a universal meaning, e.g., a smile conveys happiness.
d. **Eye contact:** The eyes may provide the most revealing and accurate of all communication signals, because they are a focal point on the body. Mutual eye contact acknowledges

recognition of the other person and a willingness to maintain communication. Total lack of eye contact may signal low self-esteem, while too much eye contact (staring) is inappropriate, e.g., a patient who feels weak or defenseless often avoids eye contact.

e. **Body movements and gestures:** Body movements may sometimes take the place of speech, e.g., a shrug of the shoulders to say, "I don't know". Some of the basic communication gestures are the same throughout the world and convey the same message, e.g., nodding the head is almost universally used to indicate yes, and the hand shake is a victory sign.

f. **Touch:** Touch is the most personal form of communication because it brings people into a close relationship, e.g., hand patting.

In nursing, touch may be the most important of all nonverbal behaviors. It is one of the most powerful means of expression; it may be performed with or without words. It is used to comfort, to evaluate some physical symptoms, e.g., determining the rate, the rhythm, and the volume of pulse. (Touch must be used at the right time and in the right way, otherwise, pause. Touch must be used at the right time and in the right way, otherwise misinterpretation of the message will occur).

g. **Tone of voice:** It can cause people to listen to speech or to be inattentive and unresponsive. An individual's personal warmth, honesty, and competence is often displayed by the tone he uses with others.

h. **Symbols:** A symbol is a sign that represents an idea, e.g., O+ means female, and O means male.

i. **Signals:** A signal is a sign to give instructions or warning, e.g., the patient puts on the signal light when he wishes to call a nurse, traffic signals, etc.

Communication Model

Elements of communication are explained in the beginning of this chapter. It is easy to tell people that they should be good communicators; it is much more difficult to tell them how to be good communicators with the elements of the communication process are sender, receiver, message, encoding, transmitting, decoding, action, and feedback.

Sender and Receiver

The sender is the source of information and the initiator of the communication process. The sender tries to choose the type of message and channel (such as computer, telephone, written memo) that will be most effective to meet the needs of the receiver. The receiver is the person who receives the sender's message and translates it into a form that has meaning.

Message

Senders must have something to say before they send a message. The first step for the sender is to choose fact, concept, idea, or feelings to communicate. This is the basis of a message.

In an organization the nurse manager is a person with needs, feelings, information, and a purpose for communicating them. A nurse manager wishes to communicate information about patients/clients or organization matters for the purpose of informing or motivating other members of the nursing team. Without any reason or goal the sender has no need to begin the communication process.

Encoding

The second step encoding means translating the message into words, gestures, facial expression, and other symbols that will communicate the intended meanings to the receiver as words have many meanings.

Encoding the message requires decisions not only about what will be said, but how, when, and where it will be said. Encoding may also involve decisions about expressing or concealing emotion. Effective communication depends on the appropriate degree of intensity for the message. For example, the nurse manager may decide not to show fear or frustration and to communicate in a matter of fact, in an unemotional manner while working in an emergency or a situation of crisis. The manager may ultimately decide to talk to the patients and the nursing personnel later, tailoring the message to the circumstances of each and communicating with them informally when the appropriate occasion arises.

Transmitting

It is the channel used to communicate a message, i.e., what form it will take. A manager would certainly use different language in a phone call than in a format report. The number of receivers to be addressed is also important. Usually, the greater the number of receivers, the more formal the language should be, the message may be in any form that can be experienced and understood by one or more of the receiver's senses—speech may be heard, written words may be read, and gestures or facial expressions may be seen or felt. A touch of the hand may communicate message ranging from love and comfort to anger and hate. A wave of the hand can communicate widely diverse messages, depending on the position ("come here!" or "get lost!"). Nonverbal messages are often more honest or meaningful than verbal or written exchanges. For instance, the patient who smiles and laughs while saying "I have an unbearable headache" and the staff member who frowns and is uncooperative while saying "Everything is fine" are transmitting nonverbal messages that are different from the spoken word.

Decoding

In the decoding step of the communication process the initiative transfers from the sender to the receiver who perceives and interprets or decodes the sender's message into information that has meaning. Ideally, the information communicated consists of what the sender believes the receiver should know and what the receiver wants to know. Understanding is the key to the decoding process. Words and symbols have multiple meanings and there is no assurance that the intended meanings of the sender have been encoded to mean the something to the receiver who decodes or interprets them.

The decoding process is affected by the receiver's experiences, personal interpretations of the symbol used expectations, and mutuality of meaning with the sender. Normally, receiver makes a genuine attempt to understand the intended message. Even with the best of intentions; however, a receiver may not understand the intended message because perceptions of the two people are different. (The more experiences the sender and receiver have in common, the more likely is that the sender's intended meaning will be communicated. So, for people with different experiences like the sender and receiver have in common, the more likely, it is that the sender's intended meaning will be communicated). In order for people with different experiences to communicate they must have shared language. Nurse managers who aspire to communicate with members of the nursing staff with varied fields of preparation and experience must learn how they think, feel, and respond in a variety of nursing situations. By applying such knowledge, nurse managers are able to predict with acceptable accuracy how a given message will be decided.

Action

Action, the next step in the communication process, is the behavior undertaken by the receiver as a result of the message sent, received, and perceived (Action is the process of doing or performing something; rather it is behaving or functioning in a certain way). The sender of the message has no guarantee that what has been heard and decoded will be put into the action intended. The receiver may listen but may or may not choose to act on the message. Many nurse managers overlook this important fact when giving instructions or explanations. They assume that merely giving a staff member a message ensures that the intended action will take place. Communication is not successful until the message received has been understood and acted upon appropriately.

Feedback

The communication process is not complete until the last step feedback occurs. Feedback is an integral part of the communication process whereby senders and receivers exchange information and clarify the meanings of the message sent. Two-way rather than one-way communication allows both sender and receiver to search for verbal and nonverbal ones. Effective two-way communication occurs when the receiver acknowledges a message and sends a meaningful feedback to the sender.

Therapeutic Communication Technique

Analysis of your communication pattern will help you to improve your methods. Realize that you cannot become skilled in therapeutic communication without supervised and thoughtful practice. However, when you are talking to another person does not get so busy thinking about a list of methods so much, so that you forget to focus the person. Your keen interest on the other person and your use of personal style are essential if you want to be truly effective.

To be effective while communicating with the patient or family, use simple, clear wards geared to the person's intelligence and experience. Develop a well-modulated tone of voice, especially with the sick person since auditory sensitivity is increased during illness. Principles, attitudes, and methods are essential.

Effective Methods

The quality of any technique adopted depends on the degree of mutual trust in the relationship. Techniques can be highly successful or they can be misfired or be abused depending on how they are used and the other person's interpretation. Techniques are stepping stones for better understanding that nurtures the trust, relationship, and expression of feelings. There must be a feeling of care, safety, and security in your company and a feeling that you want to help the person help him/herself. The more important or highly personal a feeling or idea is, the more difficult it is to say. This situation causes hesitancy in revealing thoughts, feelings, or intimate needs. By using therapeutic principles such as those previously listed, you will help the person and the family identify you as someone to whom ideas and feelings can be safely or productively revealed.

Barriers to Effective Communication

Communication in an organization is a difficult process because of the many departments and interpersonal aspects that must be considered. Comprehending barriers while communicating on healthcare facilities and taking steps to minimize them improves a nurse manager's ability to communicate effectively. There are three types of barriers, which are prevalent in nursing services.
1. Physical
2. Sociopsychological
3. Interpretation of meanings or semantics.

Physical barriers: Physical barriers are environmental factors that prevent or reduce opportunities for the communications process to occur. Some examples include physical space or distance, temperature, and ventilation, structural, or equipment problems and distracting noise.

Sociopsychological barriers: Sociopsychological barriers are blocks or inhibitors in communication that arise from the judgment, emotions, and social values of people. Just as physical interference may create barriers between people psychological and social distance can prevent communication or cause a misinterpretation. Message may not be given or received accurately while the communicators are experiencing stress. Life's experiences and emotions act as filters in nearly all communication, individuals see and hear what they are emotionally tuned to see and hear. Thus, communication cannot be separated from personality and social implications.

  i. **Take time to listen:** Many people experience difficulty in expressing what they want to say, making careful listening is essential for the receiver. If possible, set a side what you are doing and establish eye contact with the communicator. Provide cues that you understand the message by nodding or by asking questions as needed for clarification.
  ii. **Teach yourself to concentrate:** It is often easy to fix our gaze on someone who is speaking, yet think about other things at the same time. One of the reasons for this is that the thinking process is three or four times faster than a person's rate of speech; so, keeps analyzing what he or she is saying.
  iii. **Do not interrupt:** The point of anticipating and summarizing the speaker's message is to help us to concentrate on what he or she is saying, not to jump into a conclusion. Do not finish sentences for another person, as this is one of the most effective ways to breakdown communication. Apologize every time you finish a sentence for another person, as this will help to break the habit.
  iv. **Listen to what a person is saying, not how he or she is saying it:** Poor grammar, disorganized thought patterns, and slow speech can inhibit the listener from understanding the message. Instead of concentrating on delivery problems, ask yourself, "What is he saying that I need to know".

Semantics: The interpretation of messages through signs and symbols is often referred to as semantics. The importance of encoding and decoding messages with understanding has been emphasized because information, which is not clearly comprehended (misinterpretation of meaning) becomes a barrier in the communication process. Barriers to the interpretation procedure include defects in the communication skills of verbalizing, listening, telephoning, writing, and reading.

The ability to speak effectively (verbal communication) is a requisite for a nurse manager. Oral communication requires one-to-one or face-to-face exchanges, fostering a cooperative spirit, and encouraging feedback. The lower or first-level nurse manager must develop verbal skill in one-to-one relationships, keeping up with the high value placed on group or participatory decision-making. A barrier in the communication process occurs when the manager experiences difficulty in expressing verbal skills. A constant challenge in communicating is to develop a delivery that is inviting to hear the one that avoids talking too much or too little. Some members "tune out" when they hear unpleasant, confusing, or even too many messages (sensory overload). Others are left without enough information to perform well. Both extremes should be avoided. Listening is "tuning in" or giving heed to something. It involves hearing, but also includes thought processes.

Management Functions and Communications

Leaders and managers determine the work climate and influence the attitudes of staff members (authoritative people must communicate with the staff and vice-versa). There are three forms of necessary managerial communication they are (1) downward, (2) upward, and (3) horizontal.

Downward communication flows from the people at the top management levels to those at the lower levels in the organizational hierarchy. Media used for downward oral communication include instructions, speeches, meetings, telephones, loudspeakers, and the grapevine. Examples of written communication are memorandums, letters, handbooks, pamphlets, posters, policies, and procedures.

Upward communication travels from staff and lower and middle management personnel and continues up to the organizational hierarchy. Barriers can confront both sender and receiver. The dominating emotion (eagerness, anticipation, trust, lethargy, fear, and defensiveness) affects the communication process. Positive emotions indicate the process, which is open and receptive, while negative emotions indicate the presence of a barrier.

Lack of trust in the nurse leader/manager; by those governed, is a major barrier to communication. Trust is a firm reliance in the integrity and ability of another to the extent that there is confidence in that person. Team members, for example, commit guidance into the care of the nurse manager, believing that the manager will maintain that trust. Relying on a person implies a decision to accept the consequences of the actions taken, whether they are successful or failures. There are three major barriers to the development of trust.

1. Insincerity, whenever managers ask for feedback and do not value their member's opinions.
2. Time, when the demand of task accomplishment precludes devoting time on hearing what the workers want to say.
3. Defensiveness, when the manager is threatened by an open climate, which may have generated from a variety of causes such as inadequate knowledge, skill, or low self-image.

FACTORS INFLUENCING THE COMMUNICATION PROCESS

There are a variety of factors that influence the communication process. These factors may act as potential barriers to effective communication, if not considered. The assertive nurse uses these factors in order to ensure effective/therapeutic interpersonal communication techniques (communicating assertively).

Ability of the Sender and Receiver

Effective communication depends on the ability of the sender to convey the message in a logical and systematic way (responsible communication) based on facts and theoretical knowledge.

Effective communication also depends on the ability of the receiver to listen attentively to the entire message verbally or nonverbally and to maintain silence. The receiver's ability to hear, see, and comprehend to stimuli influences the communication process. The nurse should consider the ability of the patient (receiver) while communicating, e.g., using short, loud, and clear information while communicating with patients who have got difficulty of hearing.

Personal Space

Personal space is the distance people prefer in interactions with each other. There are four categories of space, distance, or zone.

1. **Intimate distance or zone (15–45 cm from the body surface)**: This is most important to an individual, who considers it as his own property. Only those who are emotionally close to the individual are allowed to enter this zone, e.g., spouse, parents, children, close friends, and relatives. Nurses in their therapeutic roles, may enter the intimate zone, e.g., when positioning patients, observing an incision, etc.
2. **Personal distance or zone (46 cm–1.2 m)**: This is approximately the distance, an individual's keep between them at friendly gathering and social functions. Most of the communication between nurses and patients occur at this distance, e.g., giving medications or starting an intravenous infusion, etc.
3. **Social distance or zone (between 1.2 and 3.6 m)**: This is the distance the individuals keep between themselves and strangers. Communication between nurses and patients is formal and is limited to seeing and hearing, e.g., nursing rounds.
4. **Public distance or zone (over 3.6 m)**: This is a comfortable distance at which an individual generally chooses to stand when he is addressing a large group of people. Public distance requires loud clear vocalizations.

Roles and Relationships

The roles and relationships between the sender and the receiver affect the communication process. A person generally feels more comfortable when communicating with another person with whom he has developed a positive and close relationship. The nurse who meets a patient for the first time will communicate differently from the nurse who has previously developed a relationship with that patient. Choice of words, sentence structure, and tone of voice vary from one role to another, e.g., roles such as nursing student and teacher, patient, and physician will affect the content and responses in the communication process.

Time

The nurses should select the appropriate time for teaching or communicating. The time factor in communication includes the events that precede and follow the interaction. For example, the hospitalized patient who is anticipating surgery will not be very receptive to the information while he is in a state of anxiety and fear.

Environment

People usually communicate most effectively in a comfortable environment. Temperature extremes, excessive noise, and a poorly ventilated environment can all interfere with communication. Also, lack of privacy may interfere with a patient's communication about the matters he considers private.

Attitudes

Attitudes convey beliefs thoughts and feelings about people and events. Attitudes such as caring, warmth, respect, and acceptance facilitate communication, whereas superior attitude, lack of interest and coldness (opposite of coring and warmth) inhibit communication. The message sent by the nurse (sender) needs to relate to the receiver's (patient/client) interest and concerns.

Sociocultural Background

Communication difficulties can arise when there is a difference in social standing or culture between individuals, the greater the difference, the lesser are the people capable of understanding the intended meaning of a message.

Education or Knowledge

Communication can be difficult when the level of education or knowledge between the two people (sender and receiver) is different. A nurse must always remember the possible barrier to communication when she is talking with patients she must be careful to express messages in words and phrases that will be understood.

Language

The sender uses simple, clear language, which is easily understood by the receiver according to his intellectual capacity. Ambiguity of language itself may create barriers to mutual understanding, e.g., a 6-year-old boy was being prepared for a surgery and the nurse told him, he would be going to the theater in 2 hours time. Imagine his surprise and distress when he arrived in the operation room for tonsillectomy, when he thought that he was being taken to see a film.

Emotions and Self-esteem

Large parts of a message may not be heard, or the message may be misinterpreted when the receiver is experiencing strong emotion. For example, a patient feeling great fear of surgery may not remember all the preoperative instructions offered by the nurse.

Self-esteem also influences communication patterns. People whose self-esteem is high communicate honestly with confidence and in conformity between verbal and nonverbal message. For example, a nurse explaining the preoperative exercise would present a sincere and serious facial expression.

Maintaining effective human relations and communication with vulnerable groups (children, women, physically and mentally challenged and elderly).

Communication with the Child and Adolescent

Perceive the child or adolescent as the unique person he/she is—not a miniature adult, an infantile being, and extension of the parents, as you focus on the parents, be respectful. Consider the developmental level of the child in your approach. Take time to establish rapport with this young person and these family members, if they are present. Acknowledge if you have cared for the child or parents before acknowledging some special event, such as birthday, school entry, club membership for the child, or progress with health care. The child tends to mirror the parents feelings and attitudes, so it is essential to establish a sense of rapport and trust with the parents to help the child become more calm and reassured.

Plan to talk with the child/adolescent alone at some point in the assessment or intervention but do not force a separation, if either party protests greatly. If parents are with the offspring, at some point, you want to ask them to wait in a separate area, so that you can speak more privately with the child. Here, confidentiality may be important; the child/adolescent may share secrets with you that will not be shared with the parents. You may need to clarify that confidential issues by saying, "Unless there is a chance of harm to you, I will keep the secrets you tell me. Or "If I feel that your health and safety depend on it. I'll tell your parents what you told me, but I'll first tell you that I'm going to do so".

If at all possible, conduct interviews, or teaching/counseling sessions when the child is comfortable, and in an environment free of distracting machines, fear-producing instruments, or uncomfortable procedures.

The principles of therapeutic communication described earlier are useful to combine with the following guidelines when giving emotional support to the child/adolescent.

Preschool or school-age child: The preschool or school-age child has a relatively short attention span, especially when ill. Simple words and direct statements or questions about concrete or tangible topics and experiences are more effective than abstractions. Since all adults are viewed as omnipotent by the young child, avoid stimulation fantasies, if possible. Speak softly and gently, but with confidence. Use of toys can help to promote relaxation, emphasize a point, encourage expression of feeling, and engage the client in an interchange. A playful attitude is helpful with the young child, for example, talking on a play telephone enables you to elicit information from a very shy child as well as help the child express fears, anxiety, anger concerns or fantasies about self, parents, and death itself.

Preadolescent and adolescent: The preadolescent and adolescent will appreciate an adult-like approach, sentence structure and words appropriate to the understanding level, focus on him/her rather than the parents and a private environment. Talk to this person first, if you are obtaining assessment information; if you talk first to the parents you may get no further response. Be observant of nonverbal behavior that indicates anxiety, embarrassment, eye contact or avoidance, shrug of shoulders, and clenched fist. Note the manner of speaking as well as interaction with the parents modifies your approach and reduce the sense of threat. If you are teaching, give information directly to the youth including the parents. If you observe that the family is very parent-centered, then you will need to re-emphasize your teaching points with the parents to ensure compliance.

Parents: The parent (s) accompanying the child should be acknowledged for their ability to add information, make decisions about the care of the child, and their ability to carry out necessary core measures. Further, determine how the parent feels about the child's health problem and what has been done and the effectiveness of the intervention to date. Take time to learn by what the parent feels to be done. This can give you clues for both assessment and intervention. Convey that it is normal to feel angry or frustrated with one's child. For example, instead of saying "Do you ever get angry at the child?" (Which may cannot disapproval) you might ask "What do you do when you feel angry at the child"? Be able to move from your informal or though respectful approach to the child or adolescent to a more formal one with the parents as indicated by their behavior manner or response. Do not continue with the child directed manners of conversation when speaking to the mother, or speak in a simple way to the mother and in a professional, adult manner to the father.

Communicating with the client who has communication difficulties

You will need to gather data from clients with sensory impairments. When you interview a person with a communication disorder, caused by hearing impairment, aphasia, inability to speak the language or visual impairment, the basic principles still apply although the specific condition will necessitate some adaptations. Develop a rapport and a trusting relationship slowly to overcome the reticence of suspicion that might be present. Introduce yourself and your purpose. Use appropriate nonverbal behavior to convey ideas. Use an intermediary such as a family member or interpreter, if available or necessary, but not to the exclusion of talking with the client.

Communication with the hearing impaired client
- When you meet a person who seems ineffective or slow to understand you, consider that hearing rather than manners or intellect may be the reason. Same hard-of-hearing person may refuse to wear a hearing aid. Others wear aids so inconspicuous that you may not see them at first glance. Others cannot be helped by a hearing aid.
- Be sure the person's hearing aid is in place, turned on, and in working order. Batteries need frequent replacement.
- The hard-of-hearing may depend to a considerable extent on reading your lips to understand what you are saying, even if they are wearing a hearing aid. No hearing aid can completely restore hearing. Always speak in a good light, face the person and the light as you speak, and do not have objects in or covering your mouth (gum, cigarettes, and hand).
- When you are in a group, which includes a hard-of-hearing person, try to carry on your conversation with others in such a way that she can watch your lips. Never take advantage of the disability by carrying on a private conversation in his/her presence in low tones that cannot be heard.
- Speak distinctly but naturally. Shouting does not clarify speech sounds, and mouthing or exaggerating your words, or speaking too slowly, makes you harder to understand. On the other hand, try not to speak too rapidly.
- Avoid excessive environmental noise, which when magnified by a hearing aid, is distracting and distressing and over-rides normal conversational tones.
- Do not start to speak to a hard-of-hearing person abruptly. Attract attention first by facing him/her and looking straight into the person's eyes. If necessary, touch the phrase, e.g., "Let us plan our week-end now".
- If the person you are speaking to has one "good" ear. Always stand or sit on that side when you address him/her. Do not be afraid to ask a person with an obvious hearing loss whether he/she has a good ear and, if so, which one it is. The person will be grateful that you care enough to find out.
- Facial expressions and gestures are important clues to meaning. Remember, that an affectionate or amused tone of voice may be lost on a hard-of-hearing person.
- In conversation with a person who is especially hard-of-hearing and hence having difficulty understanding, occasionally jot down key words on paper. The person will be grateful for the courtesy.
- Many hard-of-hearing persons, especially teenagers, who dislike being different, are unduly sensitive about their handicap and pretend to understand when they do not.
- The speech of a person who has been hard-of-hearing for years may be difficult to understand, since natural pitch is the result of initiating the speech of the other. To catch such a person's meaning more easily, watch the face while he/she talks.
- If you do not understand the person, ask him to repeat rather than ignoring the person.
- Use common sense and fact in determining which of these suggestions apply to the particular hard-of-hearing person you meet. Some persons with only a slight loss might feel embarrassed by any special attention you pay them. Others, whose loss is greater, will be profoundly grateful for it.

Communication with the visually impaired client
- Talk to the person in a normal tone of voice. Being visually impaired is no indication that he/she cannot hear well.
- Accept the normal things, which a blind person might do, such as consulting a watch for the correct time, dialing a telephone, or writing name in longhand, without calling attention to them.
- When you offer assistance, do directly. Ask, "May I be of help". Speak in a normal, friendly tone.
- Be explicit in giving verbal directions.
- Advise the person when you are leaving so that he/she will not be embarrassed by talking when no one is listening.
- There is no need to avoid the use of the word "see" when talking with a blind person.
- In guiding the person, permit him/her to take your arm. Never grab the visually impaired person's arm for he/she cannot anticipate your movement. Proceed at a normal pace. Hesitate slightly before stepping out or down.
- When assisting the person to a chair, simply place his/her hand on the back or arm of the chair. This is enough to give location.
- Never leave the person without a way to secure help. Make a call signal available.
- Never leave a blind person in an open area. Instead, lead him/her to the side of a room, to a chair, or some landmark from which direction can be undertaken.
- A half-open door, low stools, or loose cords or rugs are dangerous obstacles for the visually impaired person.
- When serving food to a visually impaired person who is eating without a sighted companion, offer to read the menu. As you place each item on the table call attention to it, food locations should be described on a plate according to the face of the clock. If the persons wants you to cut food, he/she will tell you.
- Be sure to tell who else is present in the environment.
- Encourage use of a magnifying glass, if it is helpful.
- Read mail to the person and assist him/her with business matters, if necessary.

Communication with the aphasic or mute client
- Be aware of the cause, type, and manifestations of aphasia.
- Use nonverbal behavior, including eye and facial expression, body posture, gestures and voice tone to convey messages congruent with your spoken word.

- Stand nearby or within the person's line of vision to enable better listening and response.
- Speak slowly, with a normal tone of voice.
- Use simple short sentences; ask direct questions but do not bombard with questions.
- Be prepared to use mimicking of speech, if the person is capable.
- Use visual aids, concrete objects; with your words, if appropriate.
- Give the person adequate time to respond to each question; do not supply words for the person.
- Maintain a calm, quiet, accepting environment to enhance concentration and listening, to encourage attempts at communication and speech, and to reduce person's frustration.
- Rephrase or repeat the question if the person did not understand or remember what you said.
- Give the person a pad, pencil, or flash cards with pictures or words on them, if appropriate, to answer your question.
- Realize that an answer may indicate automatic speech and not real understanding.
- Continue to converse even though the person does not appear to understand.
- Discuss topics pertinent to the person's adaptation to the setting.
- Assist family members to converse with the person.

Communication approaches for specific behaviors

Over talkativeness—interviewing the over talkative can be a special challenge. You may feel irritated because the person is describing trivial details, repeating unnecessarily, or because you cannot get relevant information within a reasonable time frame. Further you may feel defensive because of the aggressive tone of voice or dominating manner. Realize that behavior is meaningful. Try to determine what is behind the over talkativeness—anxiety, desire to keep pertinent information from you, fear of closeness, low self-esteem, or inferiority complex conveyed by this a mandatory behavior, habit, or psychopathology. Be respectful, firm, and supportive. Your own behavior can help to manage the interview.

Ask specific questions that cover only one topic at a time. Do not encourage further talking with nods of approval, a smile, or a hum. Show limited interest by facial expression or averted eyes when the person is speaking repetitively or of truly trivial details or extraneous topics. Keep the interview focused by courteously interrupting. You may need to lean forward and touch the person's arm as you interrupt to clarify a point or ask another specific question. Do not show hurry or impatience; your anxiety will trigger off more anxiety in the person and more talking will result. There are times when all you can do is sit back, relax, and accept the situation gracefully, since your efforts at focusing on time limitation will go unheeded, during this time, listen carefully (may not be unnecessary detail, but rather truly pertinent information that adds considerably to your insights about the person).

Fear of helplessness

The person who fears helplessness needs overt and active show of concern, competence, and trust worthiness. Give an adequate, but not overwhelming explanation about what you are doing or whatever is happening so that the person feels an increasing sense of worth, support, and mastery.

Fear of dependency

The person who fears dependency may act strong and independent, avoiding essential core. Reinforce a sense of strength by saying that to seek help is a sign of strength and independence.

Reinforce behavior that shows initiative, some people cannot accept or express warmth or tenderness and become brusque, distant, irritable, embarrassed, or angry when you are warm and friendly environment, people, and events surrounding the person to enrich his/her experience and understanding.

Health Promotion Implications (Nursing)

Therapeutic communication is basic to humanistic nursing in any setting with any client. You must recognize, own, and cope with personal feeling in the nurse-client-family relationship. Since the main barrier in communication is emotions, you must develop skills in building bridges over barriers. The basic bridge to effective communication is feeling. Everyone seeks warmth, security, assurance, and appreciation.

Study yourself to discover those points at which you could be responsible for blocking communication through your own shortcomings. Know your likes and dislikes and recognize them for what they are and keep them under control. For you to be accepted by another person, you must first accept yourself. You must be aware of your own needs in order to help another person's needs.

Cultivate on understanding or the part played by body language in human interactions and be aware of what you are saying with your body and be aware of what your are saying with your body movements as you are what others say with theirs. Feelings are frequently expressed by gestures, attitudes, gait and body posture, and facial expressions.

For the person to make full use of therapeutic communication, he/she must feel safe with you and feel respected and trusted by you. Revealing one's innermost thoughts and feelings to someone when help is needed and expected. Your use of communication techniques in counseling should make no attempt to influence the speed or direction of the person's problem-solving efforts; be a facilitator instead of a doer or a teller.

You are in a key position to apply an understanding of the communication process and to carry out therapeutic communication methods in all kinds of nursing while conducting routine procedures, teaching, counseling, giving support, or establishing a therapeutic milieu and working with other staff members. Thus you can enable the person and family to achieve optimum wellness and to prevent future health problems. In addition, through communication you will learn the effectiveness of the care you have given.

Principles of therapeutic communication are mentioned in **Table 2.4**.

Table 2.4: Therapeutic communication.

Communication method	Rationale
Be accepting in nonverbal and verbal behavior. (Does not mean agreement with person's words or behavior)	All behavior is motivated and purposeful. It promotes an atmosphere in which a person feels safe and respected. Indicates that you are following the person's trend of thought and encourages further talking while you remain nonjudgmental
Use thoughtful silence at intervals, while continuing to look at and focus on the person	Indicates accessibility to mute, withdraw, or depressed person. Encourages person to talk and set his own pace. Gives both you and client time to organize thoughts, gives time for completion. Conserves energy and promotes relaxation in a physically ill person
Use "I" and "We" in proper, context; call person by name and title, as preferred	Strengthens identity of the person in relation to others
State open ended, general, leading statements, or question: "Tell me about it". "What are you feeling?"	Encourages person to take the initiative in introducing topics and to think through problems. May gain pertinent information that you would not think to ask about because a client has the freedom to pursue feelings and ideas important to him/her
Ask related or peripheral questions when indicated: "And what else happened?" You have four children? How old are they?	Explores or clarifies pertinent topic. Adds to the data base. Encourages person to work through larger or related issues and to engage in problem solving
Encourage description of feelings: "Tell me how you feel"? How do you feel?	Helps person to identify fact, and resolve his own feelings. Validates your observation. Deepens your empathy and insight.
Place described events in time sequence: "What happened then"? "What did you do after that"? "And then what"?	Clarifies how event occurred or explains relationships associated with the given event

Contd...

Communication method	Rationale
State your observations about the person: "You appear ...." "I sense that you ...." "I notice that you ...."	Acknowledges client's feelings, needs, behavior, or efforts at a task. Offers content to which person can respond mutual understanding of client's behavior. Validates your impression. Helps person notice his own behavior and its effects; encourages self-awareness. Reinforces behavior. Adds to the person's self-esteem
State the implied, what client has hinted, or a feeling that may be a consequence of an event	Expresses acceptability of feeling. Clarifies information. Conveys your attention, interest, and empathy. May be used as a subtle form of suggestion for action
Paraphrase; translate into your own words the feeling, questions, ideas, keywords of the other person: "I hear you saying ..." you feel ...	Indicates careful listening and focus on client. Encourages further talking. Validates and summarizes what you think client has said
Restate or repeat main ideas expressed by client.	Conveys interest and careful listening or desire to clarify a vague point
Clarify: "Could you explain that further"? "Explain that to me again".	Indicates interest and desire to understand. Helps the person become clearer to him/herself
Suggest collaboration and a cooperative relationship	Involves person as an active partner in care. Tells the person you are available and interested. Provides reassurance
Offer information: self-disclose by sharing own thoughts and feelings briefly, if appropriate	Makes facts available whenever a client needs or asks for them. Builds trust; orients: enables decision-making. Reduces the client's anxiety, frustration or other distressing feelings that hinder comfort, recovery, or realistic action
Encourage evaluation of situation	Helps the client appraise the quality of his/her experiences and consider people and events in relation to his own and others' experiences and values
Encourage formulation of plan of action	Conveys to a person that he is expected to be an active participant in his own care. Helps the person to consider alternate courses of action. Helps the person to plan how to handle future problems.

Contd...

Contd...

Communication method	Rationale
Seek consensual validation of words; give definition or meaning when indicated	Ensures that words being used mean the same to both you and your client. Clarifies ideas for you and your client as client defines meaning for self. Avoids misunderstanding. May help to gradually reduce autistic thinking
Summarize; condense what speaker said, using speaker's own words	Synthesizes and emphasizes important points of dialogue. Helps both you and your client leave the session with the same ideas in mind. Emphasizes progress made toward self-awareness, problem solving, and personal development

Importance of Communication among Health Team Members

Written and verbal communication among health team members is vital for the quality of patient care. Generally communication can take place through:

Discussion
It is an informal oral consideration of the subject by two or more members of the health team.

Report
It is an oral or written account by one member to others in the health team, which includes the end of shift handing over report.

Record
It is always written. It is a formal, legal documentation of the patient's progress, and treatment. Therefore, records are protected legally as private record of the patient's care. Thus, access to the record is restricted to health workers.

Purposes of records
The patient's medical record is an account of health history on current health status, treatment, and progress. It is a highly confidential legal document, by which members of health care team communicate about the patient. Although the forms of the patient's record may very considerably from one hospital to another, nurses are universally required to make entries about the patient's progress. The process of making entries on the patient's record is called recording and charting.

NURSE-PATIENT RELATIONSHIP

The helping relationship between the nurse and the patient (client) is called the nurse-patient relationship. The nurse is the helper and the client is the person being helped.

Basic Characteristics of Nurse-Patient Relationship

Nurse-patient relationship is dynamic. Here both the person are active participants to the extent each is possible.
- It is focused on the achievement of client-centered goals.
- It required active presence of the nurse.
- The person providing assistance assume the dominate role.

Importance of Nurse-Patient Relationship
- It is a central to nursing
- It can be used as a therapeutic tool
- It improves patient's health
- Through this relationship the goals of nursing are achieved.

Therapeutic Relationship
- **What is meant by therapeutic relationship?**
  The relationship between the nurse and the patient (client) is called therapeutic relationship when the interaction is beneficial to patients.
- **What is the meaning of beneficial?**
  The interaction between the nurse and the patient helps the nurse and the patient to move towards common goals.

Examples of common goals (for the nurse and the patient)
- To improve the patient physical well-being
- To increase the patients independence
- To increase the feeling of worth.

Nurse's Role

The nurse selects nursing care activities (actions, measures, interventions, management, etc.), that will move the patient toward the common goal. Achieving the goal will satisfy the patient's human needs.

Steps of Nurse-patient Relationship
There are four stage of nurse-patient relationship:
1. Orientation phase
2. Identification phase
3. Working phase
4. Termination phase

Orientation phase
- The nurse and the client meet and learn to identify each other by name.
- The nurse begins to assess the patient through data gathering as part of nursing process.
- The patient also begins to assess the nurse with various questions in order to learn about the kind of person that the nurse is.
- The nurse needs to adopt a warm friendly manner, to smile appropriately, and the use of eye contact.

❖ The nurse establishes trust by being honest, consistent in his/her own behavior.

Identification phase

In this phase, the nurse and the patient become better acquainted. Trust is established, the nurse is able to explore the patients underlying needs and the problems to establish goals.

Working phase

❖ The nurse and the client work together to meet the client's needs as identified during the orientation phase. The nurse provides support to the patient and work through his problems by his physical and active presence by:
  - Listening
  - Showing understanding
  - Empathy
  - Setting limits.
❖ The nurse helps the patient toward personal growth and independence by providing support.

Termination phase

Termination of nurse-patient relationship occurs when the patient has accomplished his goals.
❖ The nurse-patient relationship is a professional relationship.
❖ Never allow your personal feelings to impede the patient progress toward independence.
❖ The preparation for termination of the relationship should begin at the initial phase relationship. Otherwise the patient may feel angry, rejected by the nurse, or depressed and helpless.

Factors that help to Promote Successful Therapeutic Nurse-patient Relationship

❖ Encourage patient to talk about his/her feelings
❖ Use simple language, which the patient can understand
❖ Explain procedures
❖ Show understanding and acceptance
❖ Convey warmth and friendly attitude—both verbal and nonverbal, e.g., greet the patient with a smile
❖ Treat each patient as an individual, worthy of respect, and even consider individual differences also
❖ Ask related questions
❖ Maintain silence
❖ Use active listening, which means:
  - More than just hearing the words spoken by the patient
  - Noting tone of voice, body movement, posture, facial expressions, the eye, etc.
  - Complete attention to understand the entire message verbally and nonverbally
  - Encourage further talk
  - Explore unexpressed feelings.
❖ Build trust
  - Trust is an essential component of nurse-patient relationship
  - It can provide the patient with a basis for learning and growth
  - The nurse must work toward developing the patient trust
  - The nurse must be a person who can be trusted.

Barrier to Therapeutic Nurse-patient Relationship

❖ Lack of self awareness.
❖ Acting out one's own conflicts, through a relationship with the patient.
❖ Giving personal information about oneself instead of focusing on him.
❖ Becoming emotionally involved where the relationship is no longer beneficial to the patient.
❖ Feeling that he/she (nurse) is the only person who can help the patient.
❖ Spending a disproportionate amount of time with the patient.
❖ Taking sides with the patient against his family.
❖ Making false promises to the patient.
❖ Labeling the patient with disease, e.g., hysteric or schizy.
❖ Avoiding the patient.
❖ Prolonging the relationship when the therapeutic need for such a relationship no longer exists.
❖ Entering the pseudochem relationship with patient.
❖ The nurse provides support to the patient and work through his problems by his physical and active presence by:
  - Listening
  - Showing understanding
  - Empathy
  - Setting limits.
❖ The nurse helps the patient toward personal growth and independence by providing support.

RECORDING AND REPORTING

Documentation is important in healthcare today. Documentation is defined as anything written or presented that is relied on as a record of proof for authorized persons. A medical record should be a comprehensive declaration of the client health status and needs, as well as the service provided for the client care. Good documentation reflects not only quality of care but also evidence of each healthcare team member accountability in providing care.

Purposes of Reports and Records

Communication

Recording is on efficient and effective method of shoring information. It allows members of different shifts to convey one another the meaningful data about the patient; therefore, record serves as the data by which different members of the health team communicate with each other.

Legal Documentation

The client's record is a legal document and is admissible in court as evidence. This record is usually considered the property of the hospital.

Research

The information in a record can be a valuable source of data for research. The treatment plans for a number of patients with the same illness can yield information helpful in treating a particular patient. Record made years earlier may also assist the member of the health team with a current problem. The patient's memory of an illness provides limited data, but a record of that illness generally reveals additional and more accurate data.

Statistics

Statistical information from a record can help the hospital to anticipate and plan for people's future needs, e.g., birth and death.

Audit

The patient's record is used to monitor the care; the patient is receiving and the competence of the people giving that care. A nursing audit is a process in which the nursing interventions are monitored and measured against established standards.

Planning Care

The entire health team uses data from the patient's record to plan care for that patient.
Physician—Prescribes antibiotics
Nurse—Nursing care plan.

Confidentiality

Confidentiality is a concept of healthcare providers maintaining all the information received during the course of treatment, meaning that the patient on daily basis share their secrete or sensitive personal information to the healthcare providers such as doctors and nurses and others, this information should be protected because it protects patients from harm, support access to healthcare and produces better health outcomes.

TYPES OF CLIENT RECORDS

Traditional Patient Record/Common Record Keeping Form

In this type of record, each healthcare worker or department keeps a separate section (e.g., admission notes, doctors order sheet, patient's history sheet, progress note, and nurses notes). In this type of record, the information about the patient is distributed throughout the record.

Source-oriented Medical Records

Source-oriented patient records generally have four components.
1. **Admission sheet:** It contains demographic data of the patient, such as name, address, date of birth, marital status, and admitting diagnosis. Patient record, doctor order sheet, patient's history sheet, progress notes, and nurses notes, this type of patient record is distributed throughout the record.
2. **Physician's order:** The doctor is expected to write the date of the order and sign each order (or sign several written orders at once). Various hospitals have different methods of indicating the nurse that there is a new order. Phone orders when the doctor phones in orders about a patient, these are written on the physician's sheet by the recipient of the call and signed by that person indicating the telephone order. Before a nurse can accept telephone calls, the hospital policy must be consulted.
3. **Medical history sheet:** This sheet is used by the physician to record the patient's history and can be used to write the progress notes and future plans.
4. **Admission records:** The most important aspects to which a nurse should pay attention include:
   - The patient's name, address, and next of kin with telephone number.
   - Accurate record for each patient's health status on admission.
   - Method of transport and arrival in wards.
   - Note who is accompanying the patient.
   - Accurate recording of all observations made, the signs and symptoms observed.
   - To what extent the patient is able to help himself/herself.
   - Any prosthesis the patient has and uses.
   - Instructions given to the patient regarding staying on bed.

Special Records and Reports

These include X-ray reports, laboratory finding, and reports of surgery. Anesthesia records, physical therapy records vital signs, and medications records.

Kardex and Nursing Care Plan

The Kardex system consists of a series of cards kept in a portable index file. Each card is for a particular patient, often Kardex data are recorded by pencil so that they can be changed and kept up-to-date. The information on Kardex may be organized into sections, e.g.,
- Information about the patient
- List of medications
- List of daily treatments and procedures.

Types of Progress Records

Nurse's Notes

It contains the following information:
- Assessment of the patients, e.g., pale or flushed skin color, dark or cloudy urine
- Independent nursing interventions, such as special skin care of health teaching carried out on the nurse's initiative
- Dependent nursing interventions, such as medications or treatments ordered by the physician
- Evaluation of the effectiveness of each nursing intervention
- Measures carried out by the physician/nurses, e.g., shortening of postoperative drainage tube
- Visits by the members of healthcare team, such as physicians, social worker.

Flow Sheets

There are graphics records, used as a quick way to reflect the patient's condition. The time parameters for flow sheets can vary from minutes to months, e.g., ICU patients.

Clinical record (also called the graphic chart or graphic observation record)

It indicates body temperature, pulse rate, respiratory rate, blood pressure readings; some charts show evp reading, 24-hours intake and output, bowel movement, glucose and acetone in urine.

24-hour fluid balance record

It may document intake and output for the duration of one shift only. The total for each shift are then recorded and then 24-hours totals are calculated for all routes of fluid loss or output must be measured and recorded.

Medication record

Medication flow sheets usually include designated areas for the date of the medication order, medication name and dose, frequency and route of administration, the doctors and nurses signature. Some records also include a place to document the client's allergies.

Daily nursing care record

Discharge note and referral summary, this is completed when the patient is transferred to another hospital or discharged to home.

Other records required are:
- Diabetic chart
- Special observation chart
- Operation procedure, consultation chart, preoperative check list, anesthesia record, and operation notes.

Census Record

The nurse in-charge is responsible for making the daily census record on each nursing unit from which the official census of the hospital is derived. The record shows the number of beds in the unit. The census of patient transfer, the discharge of a patient, or the death of the patient. Later it is sent to the concerned administrative office.

Inventory

An item record of all furniture, medical or surgical equipment, utensils, instruments, and housekeeping equipment, etc.

Formats for Writing Progress Notes

Narrative Charting

This is a description (narration) of information, and chronological charting records data in sequence as time moves forward. The major disadvantage of narrative charting is that it is difficult for a reader to find all the data about a specific problem without examining all the recorded information. For this reason certain information is documented on specific flow records.

SOAP Format

Subjective, objective data, assessment, and planning.

SOAPIE

Subjective, Objective, Assessment, Planning, Implementation, and Evaluation.

APIE

Assessment, Planning, Implementation, and Evaluation
Assessment = Subjective + Objective + Nursing diagnosis
Planning = Nursing action + Expected outcome.

Subjective data: Report what the patient perceives, and the way he/she expresses it.

Objective Data

Measurements of vital signs, observations of health team members, laboratory, and X-ray findings, and the patient's response to diagnostic and therapeutic measures.

Assessment Stage

The observer interprets and draws conclusions from subjective and objective data. At this stage, the nurse writes nursing diagnostic statements.

Common recordkeeping forms

Health record generally contains two types of data, clinical and administrative. Clinical data document, the patient's medical condition, diagnosis, and treatment as well as health care service document which includes:
- Medical record
- Nursing record/progress record
- Medication charts
- Laboratory orders and report
- Vital signs observation charts
- Handover sheet
- Admission discharge, transfer in and out forms
- Patient assessment forms, such as nutrition, pressure area care assessment
- Account record

- Legal records
- Vital signs records forms
- Physical examination form
- Consent form
- Physician record
- Mental status examination sheet
- Operation report record

METHODS/SYSTEMS OF DOCUMENTATION/RECORDING

Some methods of documentation are:
- Subjective, objective, assessment plan (SOAP)
- Problem, intervention, evaluation (PIE)
- Charting by exception
- Source-oriented record
- Case management model
- Computerized documentation

Use of data and time is essential. Time can be recorded in the conventional manner (i.e., 9.00 AM, or 2.30 PM), or according to the 24-hour clock.

Do's and don'ts of documentation/legal guidelines for documentation/recording.

Documentation should be:
- Accurate, relevant, and consistent
- Clear, concise, and complete

Legible/readable document should follow as:

Use of Ink

All entries are made in dark-colored ink (black). Hand printing or easily understood handwriting is permissible. Use of erasable ink is prohibited.

Signature

Each recording on the nurse's notes is signed by the nurse making it.

Error

When an error is made in charting, a line is drawn through it, and the word "error" is written above it, with nurse's name and initials or name, depending on the hospital policy. Errors should not be blotted out or erased.

Accuracy

The notations on records should be accurate and correct. Accurate notations consist of facts or exact observations, e.g., it is more accurate to write that the patient "refused medications" (fact), rather than "the patient was uncooperative" (opinion), e.g., the patient was crying (observation). The patient was depressed (interpretation).

Opinions or interpretations may or may not be accurate. Similarly, when the patient expresses worry about a diagnosis or problem. This should be quoted directly on the record, stating "I am worried about my leg", nurses should record what they hear and what they observe. Correct spelling is essential for accuracy and if unsure refers to a dictionary. Two decidedly different medications may have similar spelling, e.g., dioxin and digitoxin.

Appropriateness

The nurse records information that pertains only to patient's health problems and care. Any other personal information that the client conveys to the nurse is inappropriate for the record, e.g., a patient who tells the nurse that he had "venereal disease" (VD) would not be recorded on the medical record unless it has a direct effect on the patient's health problem or investigated, or laboratory test report is present.

Completeness

The information entered into the patient's record should be complete and helpful to the patient, physician, nurses, and other participants of healthcare, e.g., if a diabetic patient's record does not indicate that insulin was given and that the urine was not tested, the record could be used as evidence of negligence, e.g., a complete notation for a patient who has vomited including the time, amount and color of the vomit.

Sample Recording

Date vomited approximately 500 mL of block liquid with foul-fecal odor.

12/8/2010 C/O cramp-like pain in epigastric region immediately prior to vomiting.

The following facts may assist nurses selecting essential and complete information to record about a patient:
- Any behavior changes, e.g.,
  - Indication of strange emotions such as anxiety or fear
  - Marked changes in mood
  - Change in the level of consciousness.
- Any change in physical function, e.g.,
  - Loss of balance
  - Loss of strength
  - Difficulty in hearing or in vision.
- Any physical sign or symptom:
  - That is severe, such as severe pain
  - Tends to recur or persistent "convulsions"
  - Gets worse, such as gradual weight loss
  - Indicates a complication, such as inability to void following surgery
  - It is not relieved by prescribed measures, such as continued failure to defecate or sleep
  - Indicates faulty health habits, such as lice on the scalp
  - Indicates danger signal, such as a lump in the right breast
- Any nursing intervention provided:
  - Medications administered
  - Therapies

- Activities of daily living (ADL), if hospital policy requires
- Teaching patient's self-care.
- Visits by a physician or other members of the health team.
- Use of standard terminology: The nurse needs to use only universally known abbreviations, symbols, and terms.

Brevity

Recording needs to be brief, as well as complete to save time in communication, e.g., the nurse may write "perspiring profusely, respiration shallow".

Record information as close to the time you deliver care. Do not document in advance, leave important notation still the end of the shift. The higher the risk situation the greater the effort you should make to record.

Write notes only for patients you have cared for, do not let someone else document your assessment or intervention, eliminate bias from your notes, prejudging or labeling a patient can impair patient care and charting, e.g., nurses syndrome.

For example, in one such situation, nurses caring for a teenager with chest pain labeled her as spoiled and demanding, which made them miss the cues to her pulmonary embolism.

Do not Generalize

If the patient has a sleep problem, avoid vague terms such as "had a bad night". Be specific, patient slept from 0100 to 0400 hours. For the patient with bowel disturbance, do not write moderate distention chart the actual measurement of the girth.

Admission Records

The most important aspects to which a nurse should pay attention include:
- The patient's name, address, the next of kin with telephone number
- Accurate record of the patient health status on admission
- Method of transport and arrivals on ward
- Note who is accompanying the patient
- Accurate recording of all abnormal mode signs and symptoms observed
- To what extent the patient is able to help himself/herself
- Any prosthesis the patient has and uses
- What instructions are given to the patient regarding staying on bed.

REPORTING

"A better shift report means better nursing care".

Definition

A report is a system of communication aimed at transferring essential information necessary for safe and holistic patient care. Reports can be either oral or written. The purpose of reporting is to communicate specific information to a person or group of people. A report should be concise. A good report includes pertinent information but no extraneous details. Two common types of reports are the change of shift reports and the incident reports.

Purposes

- To communicate the patient's health status to all nurses on different shift
- To prepare staff members for their days work
- To ensure that all members of the health team have the same information
- To provide quantity and continuity core from one shift to the next.

Kinds of Reports

Oral

Report is between the head nurse and her assistant. Report is between nurses, report of a staff member to the in charge nurse or nurses, in charge report to the side nurses, etc.

Written Report

- Central report
- Incidents
- Unit report.

Example of information to be included in the report:
- Day, date, time
- Patient name, age, and diagnosis
- Nursing problem
- Physiological and psychological condition
- Test procedure surgery scheduled
- New therapies ordered
- Directory restriction teaching plan
- Patient response to nursing care measures
- Admission discharge, seriously ill patient or transfers from other unit.

Characteristics of a Good Record (or) Report

Documentation and reporting are two of the most important functions a nurse performs. The important characteristics must be followed by good documentation, which results in a good record and report.
- Timing
- Permanency
- Completeness
- Signature
- Confidentiality
- Accuracy
- Use of standard terminology.

Guidelines for Giving Report of Patients

- Follow a particular order when reporting about a series of patients, e.g., follow room numbers.

- Identify the patient by name, room number, and bed designated, e.g., Ramu bed no. 2 or bed D. This enables information immediately to the patient's care.
- Depending on the type of unit, provide the reason for admission, i.e., the patient's medical diagnosis or original complaints. This information may not be necessary in long-term patients, or newborn nurseries.
- Including diagnostic tests, results, and other therapies performed in the past 24 hours. Such as blood transfusions, surgery initiation of intravenous therapy, narcotics administered, blood gases level.
- Note any significant changes in the patient's conditions.
- When reporting about changes, present the pertinent information in this order, assessment, nursing diagnosis planning, intervention, and evaluation.
- Temperature 39.3°C orally at 16:00 hours, 500 mg paracetamol given orally, and temperature draped down to 38.1°C at 18:00 hours. But not temperature was 39 point something during the course of the shift. Given some paracetamol with good effect.
- Include unremarkable measurements, e.g., BP, pulse, temperature are within normal limits.
- Report the patient's emotional responses that need attention before other interventions can be implemented, e.g., leg is gangrenous, and is now scheduled for below knee amputation, needs time to discuss his feelings before the nurse commences preoperative teaching.

NURSING PROCESS

A process is a series of planned actions or operations directed toward a particular result. In the same way nursing process is the systematic, rational method of planning, and providing nursing care. Its goal is to identify a client's health status, actual or potential health care problem, to establish plans, to meet the identified needs, and to deliver specific nursing interventions to meet those needs. The nursing process is cyclical, i.e., the component of the nursing process follow a logical sequence, but more than one component may be involved at any given time.

The nursing process provides a framework for accountability and responsibility in nursing.

Critical Thinking Competencies

Critical thinking competencies as the intellectual process. The nurses will use their judgment while providing care to clients. Critical thinking includes:
- General thinking critically
- Specific thinking critically

In critical condition in clinical situation, using scientific thinking, problem solving critically, and make appropriate decision

Critical thinking requires not only intellectual knowledge but experience in dealing with such situations, ability to think clearly about issues, use of core critical thinking such as interpretation of data while making decisions for providing care rather than taking quick decisions carelessly making quick decisions and avoiding premature or inappropriate decisions.

Attitude for Critical Thinking

Attitude of curiosity involve the ability to recognize the problem, find the evidence, and determine how to approach making an appropriate decision while understanding your knowledge and limitations.
- Responsibility
- Confidence
- Creativity
- Humility
- Fairness
- Risk taking
- Integrity
- Specific knowledge
- Discipline
- Curiosity
- Thinking independently

Levels of Critical Thinking in Nursing

Level-3	Expert who are exposed to the critical care situation
Level-2	Involved in providing care
Level-1	Basic learner

HISTORICAL PROSPECTIVE OF NURSING

Before the nursing process was developed, nurse tended to provide care that was based on medical orders written by the physician and focused on specific disease conditions rather than on the person being cared for nursing practice that was provided independently by the physician who was often guided by intuitions and experience rather than a scientific method. The term nursing process and the framework it implies are relatively new. In 1995, Hall originated the term nursing process. In the year 1967, Yura and Walsh at the Catholic University of America proposed the four components of the nursing process, such as assessment, planning, intervention, and evaluation. The American Nurses Association in 1973 suggested that there were five components: (1) Assessment, (2) Diagnosing, (3) Planning, (4) Intervention, and (5) Evaluation. These five components were described in the ANA standards of nursing practice and they gained wide recognition and use. As the nursing process developed both theoretically and clinically, the term nursing diagnosis gained a considerable recognition in the nursing literature. In 1973, the first national conference on the classifications or nursing diagnosis was held. The participants at this conference defined the nursing diagnosis as the conclusion or judgment, which occurs as a result of nursing assessment. In 1982, the conference group accepted the name North American Nursing Diagnosis Association (NANDA). Later this group was established and accepted about 100 nursing diagnostic categories.

STEPS IN THE NURSING PROCESS

1. **Assessing:** It is collecting, verifying, and organizing data about the client's health status. Data about the physical emotional, developmental, social, cultural, intellectual, and spiritual aspects of the clients are obtained from a variety of sources and are the basic for actions and decisions taken at subsequent phases, skills of observation, communication, interviewing, and physical assessment are essential to perform this phase of the nursing process.
2. **Diagnosing:** It is a process of making a clinical judgment (nursing diagnosis) about a client's potential or actual judgment. In this phase, the nurse sorts cluster the data and analyses, what are the actual and potential health problems for which the client needs nursing assistance, and what may be the contributing factors to this problem. Responses to these question lead to diagnosis.
3. **Planning:** It involves a series of steps in which the nurse and client set priorities, formulate goals or expected outcomes and establish a written care plan for nursing interventions. The plan is designed to resolve or minimize the identified problems of the client and to coordinate the care provide by all the health team members. In collaboration with the client, the nurse develops specific interventions for each nursing diagnosis.
4. **Implementing:** It is putting the nursing care plan into action (carrying out the nursing interventions). During the implementation phase, the nurse continues to collect data and carries out the prescribed nursing activities or delegates the care to an appropriate person who validates the nursing care plan
5. **Evaluating:** It is assessing the client's response to nursing interventions and then comparing the response to predetermined standards. These standards are often referred to as outcome criteria. The nurse determines the extent to which the goals are predetermined and the outcomes of care that have been achieved, partially achieved, or not met. If the goals have not been met, reassessment may involve changes in any of the previous phases of the nursing process.

BENEFITS OF THE NURSING PROCESS

The nursing process is important to both the client and the nurse. The benefits of the process are described below.

Benefit for the Client

- **Quality clients care:** The nursing care is planned to meet the unique needs of the individual, family, or community. Continuous evaluation and reassessment of the client's changing needs ensure an appropriate level of care.
- **Continuity of care:** The written care plan is accessible to all the persons involved in the client's care and it prevents the client from repeating information and preferences to each caretaker.
- **Participation by the client in their health care:** The process can help the clients to develop skills related to their health care and to become more committed to the goals of care.

Benefit for the Nurse

- **Consistent and systematic nursing education:** The agency, which accredits nursing education programs, requires all graduates to be competent in using the nursing process.
- **Job-satisfaction:** Well-written care plans, has given the nurse to be confident about that nursing interventions, which are based on correct identification of the client's problem, thus preventing the uncoordinate -rial and -error nursing. Plans can also instill a sense of pride when the goals of care are accomplished.
- **For professional growth:** By evaluating the effectiveness of the nursing interventions, the nurse learns which interventions are most effective and which ones can be adapted to meet the need of other clients. This process enhances the skill and expertise the nurse.
- **Meet professional standards:** Learning and implementing the nursing process while providing client care is a basic, and to themselves.

A FRAMEWORK FOR ACCOUNTABILITY

Accountability is the condition of being answerable and responsible to someone for specific behaviors that are part of the nurse's professional role. The nursing process provides a framework for accountability and responsibility in nursing and maximizes accountability and responsibility for standards of care. Nurses are accountable to the client (public), to their professional statutory nursing body, to colleagues to the employing agency, and to themselves.

PROCESS OF ASSESSMENT

Assessment is the first phase of the nursing process. It involves data collection and validation and it is necessary before a nursing diagnosis can be made. "Assessment is a part of each activity the nurse does for and with the patient". Assessing is a continuous process carried out during all phases of the nursing process. It may be used during the diagnosis phase to validate a diagnosis. During the planning and implementing stages, data collection may be used before writing a nursing intervention or to obtain information about a client's response to the nursing strategies. In the evaluation phase, assessment is done to determine the outcomes of the nursing strategies and to evaluate goal achievement. All phases of then nursing process depend on the accurate and complete collection of data (information).

Types and Methods of Data

Data can be objective or subjective. Objective data are detectable by an observer or it can be tested against an assented standard. They can be seen, heard, felt, or smelled, e.g., discoloration of the skin, blood pressure reading, the act of crying, or hand tremors are known as objective data. Subjective data are apparent only to the person affected and can be described or verified only by that person. Itching, pain, and feeling worried are examples of subjective data. Subjective data are collected during the nursing health history and if includes the client's perception on personal health status and life situation. Information supplied by family members, significant others, or other health professional are also considered as subjective, if it is based on opinion rather the fact.

Objective data are sometimes called signs, and subjective data are sometimes called symptoms. Client data should include past history as well as current problems, e.g., history of an allergic reaction to penicillin is a vital piece of historical data. Past-surgical procedure and chronic diseases are also example of historical data. Current data relates to the present circumstances. Such as pain, nausea, vision changes, and sleep patterns.

Data are recorded in a factual manner and are not interpreted by the nurse, e.g., the nurse records the client's breakfast intake (objective data) as "coffee 240 mL, juice 120 mL, 1 egg, and 1 slice of toast" rather than as appetite good (a judgment). A judgments or a conclusion such as "appetite good" or "normal appetite" may have different meanings for different people. To increase accuracy, the nurse records subjective data in the client's own words.

Sources of Data

Sources of data may be primary or secondary. The client is the primary source of data. Secondary or indirect sources are significant to others, other health personnel, records and reports, and relevant literature.

Client

The chief source of data is usually the client unless the client is too ill, young, or confused to communicate clearly. The client can provide subjective data that no one else can offer. However, a stoic client may understate symptoms, while another person may exaggerate.

Significant Others

Significant others are supporting person who knows the client well and often provide data. They may supplement information or vary information provided by the client. They might convey information about the stress the client was experiencing before the illness, family attitudes to illness and health, and the client's home environment.

They are an important source of data, particularly when the client is young, unconscious, or confused. In some cases, when the client is an abused child, e.g., the person information may wish to remain anonymous.

Health Personnel

Health personnel are often the sources of information about a client's health. Nurses, social workers, physicians, and physiotherapists, e.g., they might contain information from either previous or current contact with the client. A physician who knows the client's house setting may provide valuable data about the family and the environmental stress.

Medical Records

Medical records are often a source of a client's present and past health and illness patterns. These records can provide nurses with information about a client's coping behaviors, health practices, previous illnesses, and allergies.

Other Records and Reports

Other records and reports can also provide information pertinent to health. Laboratory tests are frequently ordered as part of the physician's initial examination to aid in a medical diagnosis. Laboratory tests are also used to monitor the medical treatment, e.g., determination of blood glucose level to monitor the administration of oral hypoglycemic medications. In some cases, nurses can use the same laboratory test to monitor the effectiveness of nursing measures, such as teaching about diet and self-medications. Any laboratory data about a client must be compared to the established norms for that particular test and for the client's age, sex, and so on. Laboratory tests that vary among agencies and norms can therefore be different.

Literature

The review of nursing and related literature, such as professional journals and reference texts, can provide additional information for the database. A literature review also includes data but it is not limited to the following informations:
- ❖ Standards or norms against which the finding are compared, e.g., height and weight tables, normal developmental tasks for a particular age group.
- ❖ Cultural and social health practices.
- ❖ Spiritual belief.

- Additional required assessment data.
- Nursing interventions and evaluation criteria relative to a client's health problems. Information about medical diagnosis, treatment, and prognoses.

Organizing Data and Validating Data

Method of Data Collection

The major methods of collecting data are observing, interviewing, and examining. Although these nursing activities are often carried out during the course of implementing and evaluating phases of the nursing process, they are the main nursing activities during the assessing phase. During assessment, observation occurs whenever the nurse is in contact with the client or support persons. The primary interviewing process during the assessment phase is the method used in the physical health assessment.

Observing

To observe is to gather data by using the five senses. Although nurses observe mainly through sight, all of the senses are engaged during careful observations. Observation has two aspects (1) noticing the stimuli and (2) selecting, organizing, and interpreting the data, i.e., perceiving them. A nurse who observes that a client's face is flushed must relate that observation to, e.g., body temperature, activity environmental temperature, and blood pressure. As the process of observation involved selecting, organizing, and interpreting data, there is a possibility of error. For example, a nurse might not notice certain signs simply because they are unexpected in a certain illness. Another source is faulty organization and misinterpretation of data are when a nurse may interpret a client's wish not to talk as depression when in fact the client is very tired (or) sad. Observation is a conscious, deliberate skill that is developed only through effort, and an organized approach. Nurses often need to focus on specific stimuli in a clinical situation; otherwise they are overwhelmed by a multitude of stimuli. Observing, therefore, involves discrimination among stimuli, i.e., separating stimuli in a meaningful manner. For example, nurses caring for newborns learn to ignore the usual sound of machines in the nursery but respond quickly to an infant's cry or movement. The experienced nurse is often able to attend to an intervention, e.g., giving a bed bath or monitoring and IV infusion and at the same time make important observations, e.g., a change in respiratory status or the sudden flushing of a client's face. The simultaneous observation and task completion often needs to be learned by the beginners.

Nursing observations must be organized, so that nothing significant is missed. Most nurses develop an individual sequences for observing events, e.g., a nurse walks into a client's room and observes the following:

- Clinical signs of client distress, e.g., pallor or flushing, labored breathing, and behavior indicating, pain or emotional distress.
- Threats to the client's safety and behavior indicating pain or emotional distress.
- The presence and functioning of associated equipment, e.g., intravenous equipment and oxygen.
- The immediate environment, including the people in it.

Interviewing

Interviewing is a planned communication or conversation with a purpose. Some possible purposes are to gather data, to give information, to identify problems of mutual concern, to evaluate change, to teach, to provide support, and to provide counseling or therapy. Interviewing can be viewed as a process in the nursing health history, which is the primary tool for data collection during the assessment phase of the nursing process.

Examining

Nurses perform physical assessment to obtain the objective data needed to complete the assessment phase of the nursing process. A complete database of both subjective and objective data allows the nurse to formulate nursing diagnosis, to develop client goals, and intervene to promote health and prevent disease. Developing the skills needed for physical assessment requires knowledge, practice, and time. However, the student nurse often begin to develop assessment skills by describing the general appearance of the client, assessing skin, range of motion, and mobility often during morning care and by monitoring vital signs. To conduct the examination, the nurse uses techniques of inspection, auscultation, palpation, and percussion.

NURSING DIAGNOSIS

Diagnosis is a process of analysis and synthesis is the separation into components, i.e., breaking down the whole into its parts. Synthesis is the opposite, i.e., putting together the parts into the whole.

Steps of Diagnostic Process

Data Processing

Data processing, the first aspect of analyzing, is the act of interpreting collected data. It involves the following steps:
1. Organizing the data
2. Compare data against standard (identify significant clues)
3. Cluster data (generate tentative hypotheses)
4. Identify gaps and inconsistencies.

These activities occur continuously rather than frequently

Organizing the data: Once the data are collected, they need to be organized into a usable framework for the nurse and others, who may need them to access.

Comparing data against standards: The nurse compares the client's data into a wide range of standards, such as normal health patterns, normal vital signs, laboratory values, basic food groups, growth, and development. The nurse also use personal knowledge, e.g., physiology, psychology and sociology, and past experience when comparing the data.

Clustering data: Clustering or grouping data is a process of determining the relatedness of facts and finding patterns in the facts. This is the beginning of synthesis.

Determining the Client's Health Problems, Health Risks, and Strengths

After data are processed, the nurse and the client can together identify the strengths and problems. This is primarily a decision-making process.

Health problems and risks: During data processing, the nurse groups data according to categories and labels the clusters with tentative diagnosis. However, for health problems (existing or potential) to have a successful outcome, the client must accept the existence of the problems. The nurse by contrast, determines whether the client needs help dealing with the problem. The nurse and the client then make judgments.

Strengths: At this stage, the nurse and the client also establish the client's strengths, the resources, and abilities to cope. Generally, people have a clear perception of their problems or weakness than of their strengths and assets, which are often taken for granted. By taking inventory of strengths, the client can develop a better-rounded self concept and self-image. Strengths can be an aid to mobilizing health and regenerative processes. A client's strength might be that his sight is within the normal range of his age and height, thus enabling him to cope better with surgery. In another instance, a client's resources could be a supportive family and ability to cope. Coping is a learned pattern or response that helps an individual to deal with crisis and stressful events. Nurses must remember, however, that because of the magnitude of an event, the number of stressful events occurring at one time or the unfamiliarity for the situation, a client may be unable to cope and may require assistance of the nurse.

Formulating Nursing Diagnoses

At this final stage, the nurse formulates casual relationships between the health problems and the factors related to them. These factors may be, e.g., environmental, sociological, psychological, physiological, or spiritual. More than one factor may be related to one health problem. It is also important to determine at this time that the problem can be resolved by independent nursing interventions. If it cannot, the nurse should refer the client to the appropriate health team member. By including the cause factors in diagnostic statements, the nurse can tailor a plan of care for the client.

Nurses can refer to a list of accepted nursing diagnosis, to select a diagnostic category. The causal factors are obtained from the data. If no causal factor appears in the data, the nurse may wish to make a tentative diagnosis based on scientific nursing by knowledge and experience.

Nursing Diagnosis Format

There are three essential components of nursing diagnostic statements, they are referred to as the PES format. Nurses need to consider these components when developing new diagnostic categories and writing diagnoses for specific clients. The components are:

1. **The terms describing the problem (P):** This component, referred to the diagnostic category label or title, is a description of the client's (individual, family, community) health problem (actual or potential) for which nursing therapy is given. The state of the client is described clearly and concisely in a few words.
2. **The etiology of the problem (E) or contributing factors:** This component identifies one or more probable causes of the health problem and gives direction to the required nursing therapy. Etiology may include behaviors of the client, environmental factors, or interactions between the two.
3. **The defining characteristics or cluster of signs and symptoms (S):** The defining characteristics provide information necessary to arrive at the diagnostic category. Each nursing diagnostic category is associated with signs and symptoms that occur as a clinical entity. Major signs and symptoms are those that must be present to make a valid diagnosis. Minor characteristics may or may not be present.

Writing a diagnostic statement by using the three-part statement (using related to and manifested by), since the signs and symptoms have been identified. Several alternatives for writing the PES format have been suggested.

- ❖ Nurses learning to write diagnosis may find it helpful to list the signs and symptoms before or after the two-part diagnostic statement in a care plan format. The defining characteristics may include both objective and subjective data.
- ❖ Signs and symptoms may be written after the diagnostic statement, joined by the words manifested by or evidenced by.

Characteristics of a Diagnostic Statement

- ❖ A diagnostic statement is clear and concise
- ❖ It is specific and client centered.
- ❖ It is accurate.
- ❖ It is based on reliable and relevant assessment data.

A nursing diagnostic statement (nursing diagnosis) is a clear statement about a client's actual or potential health problem, i.e., within the scope of independent nursing intervention. It is the outcome of the diagnostic process; the second phase in the nursing process. Nursing may write diagnosis as either two-part of three-part statements.

Here are some examples of three-part statements:
1. Disturbance in self-esteem (problem) related to altered body image (loss of arm) (etiology) manifested by crying and hostility (signs and symptoms)
2. Anticipatory grieving (problem) related to husband's terminal illness (etiology) manifested by anorexia and withdrawn behavior (signs and symptoms)
3. Altered family processes (problem) related to mother's hospitalization (etiology) as manifested by son's unmet physical and emotional needs (signs and symptoms).

Potential nursing diagnosis are used when a client's responses can be predicted or when health promotion can contribute to well-being. Predictable responses are based on a client's health history, known complications of a disease process, or the nurse's experience, e.g., a client who has smoked two packets of cigarettes per day for 40 years may have a potential postoperative nursing diagnosis for potential for ineffective airway clearance (P) related to smoking (E).

The two parts are joined by the words related to or associated with "due to". The phrase due to implied a cause-and-effect relationship; one cause is responsible for another. In contrast, the phrases related to an associated with, merely imply a relationship. The phrase related to is the most commonly used.

If one part of the diagnostic statement changes, the other part may change as well. Legal hazards are thus avoided. Here are some examples of nursing diagnoses containing two parts:

The two-part nursing diagnostic statement includes:
1. **Problem (P):** Statement of the client's response.
2. **Etiology (E):** Factors contributing to or probable causes of the responses.
3. Ineffective breathing pattern (problem) related to pain (etiology)
4. Disturbance in self-esteem related to altered body image (loss of arm) etiology
5. Grieving (problem) related to anticipated loss (etiology), secondary to the husband's illness (etiology)

Guideline for writing a nursing diagnostic statement (Table 2.5).

PLANNING

Types of Planning

The six components of planning are:
1. Setting priorities.
2. Establishing client goals and outcome criteria.
3. Planning nursing strategies.

Table 2.5: Nursing diagnostic statement.

Guideline	Correct statement	Incorrect and/or ambiguous statement
State in terms of a problem, not a need	Actual fluid volume deficit (problem)	Fluid replacement (need) related to fever
State so that it is legally advisable	Impaired skin integrity related to immobility (legally acceptable)	Impaired skin integrity related to improper positioning (implies legal liability)
Use nonjudgmental statements	Spiritual distress related to inability to attend church/temple/masjid services secondary to immobility (nonjudgmental)	Spiritual distress related to strict rules necessitating church/temple/masjid attendance (judgmental)
Make sure that both elements of the statement do not say the same thing	Potential impaired skin integrity related to immobility	Impaired skin integrity related to ulceration of sacral area (response and probable cause are the same)
Make sure that the client's response precedes the contributing or cause factor	Noncompliance with diet (response related to lack of knowledge contributing factor)	Knowledge deficit (contributing factor related to noncompliance with diet response)
Use statements that provide guidance for planning independent nursing interventions	Social isolation related to loss of speech (loss of speech provides direction for planning alternative communication methods)	Social isolation related to laryngectomy (the nurse can do nothing about the laryngectomy)
Word diagnosis specifically and precisely to provide direction for planning nursing intervention	Altered oral mucous membrane related to decreased salivation secondary to radiation of neck (specific)	Altered oral mucous membrane related to noxious agent (vague)
Use nursing terminology rather than medical terminology to describe the client's response	Potential ineffective airway clearance (nursing terminology)	Potential pneumonia (medical terminology)
Use nursing terminology rather than medical terminology cause of client's response	Potential ineffective airway clearance related to accumulation of secretions in lungs (nursing terminology)	Potential ineffective airway clearance related to emphysema (medical terminology)
Do not start the nursing diagnosis with a nursing intervention	Altered nutrition. Less than body requirements related to inadequate intake of protein (directs but does not state nursing intervention)	Provide high-protein diet because of potential altered nutrition (starts with nursing intervention)

4. Writing nursing orders.
5. Writing the nursing care plan.
6. Consulting.

Setting Priorities

Priorities setting are the process of establishing a preferential order for nursing strategies. To set priorities, the nurse and the client first order the nursing diagnosis preferentially, i.e., decides which deserves attention first, second, and so on. Diagnosis can be grouped as having a high, medium, or low priority. This priority setting, however, does not mean that all the high-priority diagnosis must be resolved before any others are considered. A high-priority diagnosis may be dealt with partially, and then a diagnosis of lesser priority may be dealt with, in addition, the nurse may address more than one diagnosis at a time.

Factors for setting priorities

- **Client's health values and beliefs:** Values concerning health may be very important to the nurse but not to the client. For example, a client may see attendance at school or being at home for the children as more urgent than a health problem.
- **Client's priorities:** Offering the client the opportunity to set own priorities allows client participation in care planning and enhances cooperation between the nurse and client. Sometimes, however, the client's perception of what is important conflicts with the nurse's knowledge of potential future problems or complications. For example, an elderly female may not regard ambulation or turning and repositioning every 2 hours as important, preferring to be undisturbed. The nurse, however, being aware of the potential complications of prolonged bed rest (e.g., muscle weakness and decubitus ulcers), needs to inform the client and implement necessary interventions to prevent such debilitating effects.
- **Resources available to the nurse and client:** If there are financial constraints, then a health problem may be given a lower priority than usual. If the resources needed for specific nursing strategies are not available, the solution of that problem might need to be postponed, or the client may need referral. Client resources, such may defer dental treatment; a client whose husband is terminally ill and dependent on her may consider nutritional guidance directed toward weight loss as too much to handle.
- **Time needed for the nursing strategies:** Each client feels comfortable with a certain pace of action. Some clients may want to discuss the problem with family members or think about it overnight. Others may want "to get on with it". The nurse must allow adequate time for the necessary nursing strategies resulting from the nursing diagnosis.
- **Urgency of the health problem:** Life threatening situations require that the nurse establish priorities quickly. This also applies to situations that affect the integrity of the client, i.e., this could have a negative or destructive effect on the client. Such health problems as drug abuse and radical alteration of self-concept due to amputation can be destructive not only to the individual but also to the family. These health problems should receive high priority.
- **Medical treatment plan:** The priorities for treating health problems must be congruent **with** treatment by other health professionals. For example, a high priority for the client might be to become ambulatory; however, if the physician's therapeutic regiment calls for extended bed rest, then ambulation must assume a lower priority in the nursing strategy plan. In such a case, however, the nurse can provide or teach exercise to facilitate ambulation later.

Establishing Client Goals and Outcome Criteria

Goals: A client goal is a desired outcome or change in the client's behavior in the direction of health. Goal attainment reflects the client's concern or health problem that is specified in the nursing diagnosis.

The nursing diagnosis guides the type of goal statement; goals may reflect health restoration, health maintenance, or health promotion.

The purpose of client goals into:

1. Provide direction for planning nursing interventions that will achieve the anticipated changes in the client.
2. Provide direction for establishing evaluation criteria to measure the effectiveness of the interventions.

Examples of client goals
The client/clients will:
- Increase activity tolerance
- Maintain urinary elongation pattern
- Restore fluid volume
- Decrease potential for injury
- Develop coping abilities
- Improve nutritional pattern
- Increase parenting knowledge
- Establish change in family roles.

Long-term and short-term goals: Goals may be short-term. A short-term goal might be, "Client will raise right arm to shoulder height by Friday", in the same context, a long-term goal might be, "Client will regain full use of right arm in 6 weeks". Because a great deal of the nurse's time is focused on the immediate needs of the client. Most goals are short term. In addition, the nurse is better able to evaluate the client's progress or lack of it with short-term goals.

Long-term goals are often used for clients living at home and having chronic problems or clients in nursing homes, extended care facilities, and rehabilitation centers. Short-term goals are useful for: (1) clients who require health care for only a short time and (2) for persons who are frustrated by long-term goals that seem difficult to attain and who need the satisfaction of achieving a short-term goal.

Outcome criteria: Outcome criteria or objectives are needed to add specificity to the broad goal statements. A criterion is a standard or model that can be used in judging. Outcome criteria are statements that describe specific, observable, and measurable response of the client. They determine whether the stated goals have been achieved and are therefore essential to the evaluation phase of the nursing process.

Outcome criteria serve four purposes:
1. They provide direction for nursing interventions.
2. They provide a time span for planned activities.
3. They serve as criteria for evaluation of progress toward goal achievement.
4. They enable the client and nurse to determine when the problem has been resolved.

Relationship of outcome criteria to client goals

Outcome criteria are derived from and relate to the client goals. Client goals, as described previously, are derived from the first clause of the nursing diagnosis. For example, if the nursing diagnosis of potential impaired skin integrity is related to impose bed rest and the client goal is, "Maintain intact skin, particularly over bon prominences". The outcome criteria might be as follows. The client:
- Demonstrates correct techniques for positioning and turning, and the use of pillows to prevent pressure, within 2 days.
- Discuss two methods for reducing pressure over prominences, within 2 days.
- Has an absence of redness or irritation to skin when discharged from the hospital generally, three to six outcome criteria are needed for each goal.

Guidelines for writing goals and outcome criteria

The following guidelines can help nurses formulate goals and outcome criteria:
1. Formulate goals and outcome criteria in terms of client behavior. Begin each goal and outcome criteria with "the client". This helps to focus on what the client will be able to do when the outcome criteria are achieved. Outcome criteria should focus on what the client will accomplish, not what the nurse will do. For example, a postoperative client may have the following goals (and outcome criteria): The client will maintain clear and open airways (goal) and manifest normal breath sounds (e.g., no wheezing or rales), normal rate of respiration and absence of dyspnea and cyanosis (outcome criteria).
   Avoid statement that start with enable, facilitate, allow, let, permit, or similar verbs followed by the word client. These verbs indicate what the nurse hopes to accomplish, not what the client will do. For example, the statement "assist the client to deep breath and cough every 2 hours" is a nursing action, not an observable behavior.
2. Make sure the goal statements are appropriate for the nursing diagnosis and that the outcome criteria are appropriate for the goal. Validate the outcome. If the outcome is accomplished, the goal will be achieved. Validate the goal statement. If the goal is accomplished, will the client's nursing diagnosis be resolved?
3. Make sure that the outcome criteria are realistic for the client's capabilities, internal and external limitations, and designated time span, if it is indicated. Internal limitations refer to the person's physical and mental health status and coping mechanisms. External limitations refer to finances, equipment, family support, social services, and time. For example, the goal "The client will walk with crutches on level surfaces and on stairs" may be unrealistic for an elderly woman with a heavy leg cast. "The client will walk with crutches from bed to bathroom with assistance" may be more realistic. The goal "Measures insulin accurately" may be unrealistic for a client who has poor vision due cataracts.
4. Make sure the client considers the goals important and values them. Outcomes are value decisions. Some outcomes, such as those for problems related to self-esteem parenting and communicating, involve choices that are best made by the client or in collaboration with the client. Whenever possible, clients should be given information that will allow them to make informed choices with regard to goals. Some clients may know what they wish to accomplish with regard to their health problem. For instance, the client's goal may be "relief of pain". Other clients may not know all the outcome possibilities for their specific problem. The nurse must actively listen to the client to determine personal values, goals and desired outcomes in relation to current health concerns. Then discuss the nursing diagnosis and goals of determine if the client agrees with the stated problem and goals. Clients are usually motivated and expand the necessary energy to reach a goal, if they consider it important.
5. Ensure that goals and outcome criteria are compatible with the work and therapies of other professionals. The goal "Increase the client's activity tolerance" and the attending criterion "Will increase the time spent out of bed by 15 minutes each day" are not compatible with a physician's prescribed therapy of bed rest for 3 days.
6. Make sure that each goal is derived from only one nursing diagnosis. For example, the goal "The client will increase the amount of nutrients ingested and show progress in the ability to feed self" is derived from tow nursing diagnosis. Feeding self-care deficit related to neuromuscular impairment and altered nutrition: less than body requirements related to anorexia. Keeping the goal statement related to only one diagnosis ensures that outcome criteria and planned nursing interventions are clearly related to the diagnosis.
7. When writing outcome criteria, use observable, measurable terms; avoid words that are vague and require interpretation or judgment by the observer. For example,

such phrases as "increase daily exercise", "increase participation in social activities", and "improve knowledge of nutrition" can mean different things to different people. If used in criteria, these phrases can lead to disagreements about whether the criterion was met. These phrases may be suitable for a broad client goal but are not sufficiently clear and specific for use in outcome criteria used to evaluate the client's response.

Planning Nursing Strategies

Nursing strategies or interventions are nursing actions chosen to treat a specific nursing diagnosis in order to achieve client goals. The specific strategies chosen for actual nursing diagnosis should focus on eliminating or reducing the cause of the nursing diagnosis.

Generating alternative nursing strategies

Often, the nurse and the client can establish a number of nursing strategies for each problem statement. Too many alternatives can be confusing. Usually three out of five alternative nursing strategies for each health problem are satisfactory (**Table 2.6**).

Table 2.6: Developing alternative nursing strategies.

Diagnostic statement	Client goal	Alternative nursing strategies
Sleep pattern disturbance related to anxiety	Obtain 6–9 hours of sleep	Provide warm milk and a snack in the evening. Provide more activity during daytime. Encourage the client to decrease activity 2 hours before bedtime Assess diet for stimulants, i.e., caffeine. Provide soft music. Encourage verbalization of worries

Considering the consequences of each strategy: The next step is to consider the consequences of each action, including the risks. Often each action will have more than one consequence. For example, the strategy "provide accurate information" could result in the following client behavior:
1. Increase anxiety
2. Decreased anxiety
3. Wish to talk with the physician
4. Desire to leave hospital
5. Relaxation

Choosing nursing strategies: After considering the consequences of the alternative nursing strategies, the nurse chooses one or more, that are likely to be most effective. Although the nurse bases this decision on knowledge and experience, the client's input is very important. For example, client may say, "I know I'll sleep, if I can have that". Maintaining the client's routine may indeed help the client sleep, and this action might be the first choice as a nursing strategy. The following criteria can help the nurse choose the best nursing strategy. The planned action must be:
1. Safe and appropriate for the individual's age, health, and so on.
2. Achievable with the resources available (e.g., in the previous example, sandwiches and milk must be available)
3. Congruent the client's values and beliefs.
4. Congruent with other therapies (e.g., if the client is not permitted food, the strategy of an evening snack must be deferred until health permits).

Writing Nursing Orders

The term nursing order is preferable to the terms approaches, activities, actions, and interventions because order connotes a sense of accountability, for the nurse who gives the order and for the nurse who carries it out. Nursing orders are the specific actions the nurse takes to help the client meet established healthcare goals.

The degree of detail included in the nursing orders depends to some degree on the health personnel who will carry out the order. It is advisable, however, to be exact in writing orders.

Writing the Nursing Care Plan

The nursing care plan is a written guide that organizes information about a client's health into a meaningful whole; it focuses on the actions nurses must take to address the client's identified nursing diagnoses and meet the stated goals. It is also referred to as the client care plan, since its focus is the client.

The nurse in charge (head nurse, primary nurse, or team leader) starts the care plan as soon as a client is admitted to the healthcare agency. It is constantly updated and revised throughout the client's stay, in response to changes in the client's condition and evaluations of goal achievement.

The purposes of a written care plan are:
1. To provide direction for *individualized* care of the client. The plan is organized according to each client's unique nursing care needs.
2. To provide for continuity or care. The written plan is a means of communicating and organizing the actions of a constantly changing nursing staff. The initial plan, updated to show nursing interventions and new assessment data, is often conveyed to all nursing staff at change of shift reports, nursing rounds, and client care conferences.
3. To provide direction about what needs to be documented on the client's progress notes. The care plan specifically outlines, which observations to make, what nursing actions to carry out, and what instructions the client or family members require. In this way, recording is facilitated.
4. To serve as a guide for *assigning staff* to care for the client. Certain aspects of the client's care may need to be delegated to some one who can make necessary judgments about the client's responses.

5. To serve as a guide for reimbursement from medical insurance companies, often called third-party reimbursement. Nursing care plans carefully. Written and implemented facilitate hospital reimbursement for the professional services the nurse provides.

Format: Although formats differ from agency to agency, the plan is generally organized into four columns or categories: (1) nursing diagnoses or problem list, (2) goals, (3) nursing strategies/interventions/nursing orders, and (4) outcome evaluation criteria. Some agencies have a five column plan that includes a column for assessment data before the nursing diagnoses column. Others use three column plans that subsume the evaluation (outcome criteria) column under the goal column. To help students learn to write care plans and apply their knowledge, educators often modify this plan by adding a column headed "rationale" after the nursing intervention column. A rationale is the scientific reason for selecting a specific nursing action. Student may also be required to cite supporting literature for this stated rationale.

Consulting is seeking expert advice. Nurses consult a variety of personnel, including other nurses, throughout the nursing process. Consulting implies that the nurse involved in the care seeks advice or clarification regarding client goals. Also, the nurse may serve as a resource to provide assistance in health or client-related issues. Increasingly, nurses consult with other nurses within the agency, about a variety of specialized nursing practice areas. Nurses may also consult with other healthcare personnel including physicians, nutritionists, physical therapists, and social workers.

Guidelines for writing nursing care plans

In addition to following the earlier suggestions for writing nursing orders, the nurse can use the following guidelines when writing nursing care plans:

1. Date and sign the plan. The date in the plan written is essential for evaluation, review, and future planning. The signature of the nurse who is writing the plan demonstrates accountability to the client and the nursing profession, since the effectiveness of nursing actions can be evaluated.
2. Use the category headings "Nursing Diagnoses", Goals: Nursing Orders/Interventions, and "Evaluation" include a date for the evaluation of each goal.
3. Indicate the goals are met or revised by a signature or some other method specified by the agency.
4. List the nursing orders for each goal in order to priority. For example, the nursing orders for a client with a decubitus ulcer might include "Apply an occlusive dressing for 24 hours" and "Clean the ulcer with Betadine solution daily". The appropriate sequence is to clean the ulcer before applying the dressing and the orders in that sequence. Another example or priority listing is to explore the client's feeling about administering injectable insulin before demonstrating how to do it.
5. Use standardized medical or English symbols and keywords rather than complete sentences to communicate your ideas. For example, write "Turn and reposition q2h" rather than "Turn and reposition the client every 2 hours". Or write "Clean decubitus ulcer (H_2O_2) bid" rather than "Clean the client's decubitus ulcer with H_2O_2 twice a day, morning and evening".
6. Refer to procedure books or the sources of information rather than the steps on a written plan. Using these adjuncts for commonalities of care among clients not only saves the nurse time but also focuses the carte plan on the unique differences that individualize the care of clients.
7. Tailor the plan to the unique characteristics of the client by ensuring that the client's choices, such as preferences about the times of care and the methods used, are included. This reinforces the client's individuality and sense of control. For example, the written nursing order "Provide prune juice at breakfast rather than regular juice" indicate that the client was given the choice between beverages.
8. Ensure that the nursing plan incorporates preventive and health maintenance aspects as well as restorative. For example, carrying out the order "Provide active assistance to affected limbs q2h" prevents joint contractures and maintains muscle strength and joint mobility.
9. Include collaborative and coordination activities in the plan. For example, the nurse may write orders to ask a nutritionist or physical therapist about specific aspects of the client's care.
10. Include plans for the client's discharge and home care needs. It is often necessary to consult and make arrangements with the community health nurse, social worker, and specific agencies that supply client information and needed equipment.

Types of Nursing Actions

The terms independent, dependent, and collaborative (interdependent) are often used to describe nursing actions. An action, in this context, is an activity appropriate to a person's role. It is also called a nursing strategy.

An independent nursing action is an activity that the nurse initiates as a result of the nurse's own knowledge and skill. In this instance, the nurse determines that the client requires certain nursing interventions; either carries theses out or delegates them to other nursing personnel, and is accountable for the decision and the actions.

Dependent nursing actions are those activities carried out on the order of the physician, under the physician's supervision, or according to specified routines. An example of a dependent action is giving an antibiotic injection to a client as a result of a physician's written order. The dependent activity in nursing practice is usually directly related to the client's disease and its importance should not be minimized.

In addition to the task of carrying out the physician's order, the nurse who performs a dependent nursing action also conducts the appropriate nursing activities associated with the order. In the example above, the nurse would also monitor the client for signs of improvement, worsening infection, or toxic effects of the antibiotic.

Collaborative nursing actions are those activities performed either jointly with another member of the health care team or as a result of a joint decision by the nurse and another health care team member.

Process of Implementing

The process of implementing normally includes reassessing the client, validating the nursing care plan, determining the need for nursing assistance, implementing the nursing strategies, and communicating the nursing actions. Reassessing the nursing care plan are subprocesses that operate continuously throughout the implementing phase.

Implementing Skills

Three skills are needed to implement nursing actions: (1) cognitive, (2) interpersonal, and (3) technical skills. The necessary cognitive (intellectual) skills for implementing are problem solving, decision making, critical thinking and creativity. They are critical to safe, intelligent nursing care.

Interpersonal skills are all the activities people use when communicating directly with one another. They may be verbal and nonverbal. The effectiveness of a nursing action often depends largely on the nurse's ability to communicate with others. Even when giving a medication to a client, the nurse need to understand the client and in turn to be understood. A nurse who is delegating a nursing action also needs to be understood.

Technical skills are "hands-on" skills such as manipulating equipment, given injections and bandaging, moving, lifting, and repositioning clients. These tasks are also called procedures or psychomotor skills.

Implementing Activities

To implement nursing care, the nurse generally performs the following activities: caring, communicating, helping, teaching, counseling, acting, as a client advocate and change agent, leading, and managing. These activities are associated with nursing roles and include: (1) assigning and delegating care to other nursing personnel, and (2) supervising and evaluating the nursing activities of others.

Process of Evaluating

The evaluation process has six components
1. Identifying the outcomes (standard for measuring success) that will be used to measure achievement of the goals.
2. Collecting data related to the identified criteria
3. Comparing the data collected with the identified criteria
4. Relating nursing actions to clients outcomes
5. Re-examining the clients care plan
6. Modifying the care plan.

Evaluating the Quality of Nursing Care

Over the past 30 years, there has been considerable work on the evaluation of the quality of nursing care to determine what good care is, whether the care nurses give, is appropriate and effective, and whether the quality of care provided is good. Evaluating the quality of nursing care is an essential part of professional accountability. Other terms used for this measurement are quality assessment and quality assurance. Quality assessment is an examination of services only; quality assurance implies that effort is made to evaluate and ensure quality healthcare.

Guidelines for Implementing Nursing Strategies

❖ Nursing actions are based on scientific knowledge and nursing research, the nurse must be aware of the scientific rationale for all interventions and any possible side effects or complication of the activities.
❖ Nursing actions resulting from a physician's order must be understood by the nurse. The nurse is responsible for intelligent implementation of these orders. This requires knowledge of the activity, procedure, or dedication its purpose in the client's plan of care, and any contraindication (e.g., allergies) or changes in the client's condition that may be applicable. If the nurse has any question regarding prescribed nursing actions, the nurse's manager or supervisor and/or physician must be consulted.
❖ Nursing actions are adapted to the individual. A client's belief's values, age, health status, and environment are factors that can effect a nursing action.
❖ Nursing actions should always be safe. Nurses and client's need to take precautions to prevent injury. For example, when changing a sterile dressing, the nurse practices sterile technique to prevent infection; when turning a client, the nurse protects the client's skin from abrasions, which could also lead to infection.
❖ Nursing actions often require teaching, supportive, and comfort components. These independent nursing activities can often enhance the effectiveness of a specific nursing action.
❖ Nursing actions should also be holistic. The nurse must always the client's self-esteem. Providing privacy. Active participation enhances the client's sense of independence and control. Clients vary in the degree of participation they desire. Some clients want total involvement in their care, while others prefer little involvement. The amount of involvement desired is often related to the severity of the illness and the number of stressor, as well as the client's energy, fear, understanding of the illness, and understanding of the intervention.

Patient Assessment Format

Name of the Training Institute_____

Student Name_____Date_____

Assessment_____Week_____

Patient Identification Date

Patient Name_____ Age_____Sex _____ I.P. no _____

Address_____

Religion_____Language Known_____ Marital Status Single/Married/Widow/

Divorced Date of Admission _____ History of Present illness Chief complaint _____

Present History of Illness_____Duration _____

Provisional Diagnosis _____

Pastmedical History _____

Past history of illness _____History of Hospitalization_____Diagnosis_____

Treatment Postsurgical History _____

History of any Surgery _____ if yes, Name of the surgery _____

Postoperative Duration _____ H/O accidents of blood transfusion _____

Health History of the Family _____

Sl. No	Name	Relationship with patient	Age and sex	Education status	Occupation	Health status

Any family history of diabetics/heart diseases/hypertension/tuberculosis, etc.

Socioeconomic Data: Occupation _____ Salary _____ Type of House _____

Water Supply_____ Pet and Domestic Animals _____

Physical Assessment: General appearance, well-built/thin/obese/alert/active/dull semiconscious/disoriented/unconscious

Skin: Color-Normal/Pale/Cyanosed/Turgor-Normal/Rashes/Purpura spots

Head: Scalp clear: Yes _____ No _____ Any abnormalities: Yes/No

Face: Puffiness/wrinkles/scar

Eyes: Last examination, Good: Yes/No; Surgery: Yes/No; Blurring/Burning: Yes/No; Inflammation: Yes/No; Color conjunctive/sclera/Visual acuity-Normal/Biot's Spot/Squint/Cataract

Ear: Hearing ability: Good: Yes/No; Ear discharge: Yes/No

Nose: Septal deviation: Yes/No; Discharge: Yes/No; Allergic rhinitis: Yes/No, if yes-relief measure

Nose bleeding: Yes/No; Sense of smell good: Yes/No; Sinus inflammation: Yes/No

Throat and Mouth: Last dental checkup: Yes/No; difficulty in swallowing: Yes/No; Condition of the Lips/Tongue coated: Yes/No; Sense of taste good: Yes/No; Bad odor: Yes/No; Stomatitis: Yes/No

Neck: Color symmetry _____ range of motion any enlargement, Yes/No

Respiratory System: Cough: Yes/No. If yes when _____ Productive/nonproductive _____ dyspnea: Yes/No; If yes specify, how relieved-Activity tolerance-Chest pain: Yes/No If yes describe; Hemoptysis: Yes/No (Stridor/Crepitus/Rhonchi) Flaring of nostrils Air entry—Respiratory rate

Abdomen: Distended: Yes/No; Abdominal Girth. Ascites: Yes/No; Peristalsis—Present/Absent Palpable mass: Yes/No; Umbilicus-Normal/Protruded.

Liver: Palpable: Yes/No; Tenderness Yes/No

Cardiovascular System: Chest pain, Yes/No. Describe if Yes _____
History of cardiac diseases, Yes/No. Medication. Yes/No. BP _____ mm/Hg, Heart rate, S1 _____
S2 _____ S3 murmur _____ Nails. Normal/Pale/Clubbing? Spoon-Shaped/Edema _____ Yes/No.
Numbness, Yes/No. Cyanosis, Yes/No. Varicose vein, Yes/No Extremities. Cold and Clammy/Cyanosed

Nutrition

Veg/Non-veg/Mixed presence of Anemia: Yes/No; Appetite, good: Yes/No Usual time for meals_kind, and amount of food/day _____ Kind and amount of fluid/day. Anorexia: Yes/No; Vomiting: Yes/No. Weight loss: Yes/No; Weight gain: Yes/No; Weight loss: Yes/No

Elimination (bowel)

No. of stool in the day Use of laxative: Yes/No; Constipation: Yes/No; Diarrhea: Yes/No; Melina: Yes/No; Ostomies: Yes/No/ Hemorrhoids: Yes/No

Elimination

(Urine) _____ **Incontinence:** Yes/No; Retention: Yes/No; No of voiding per day _____ Night, Catheter: Yes/No; Hematuria: Yes/No; Burning: Yes/No

Reproduction

Pregnancies: Yes/No; Children: Yes/No; Number
Last Pap smear test: Yes/No; If yes result Bleeding: Yes/No
Vaginal discharge: Yes/No; Breast self-examination: Yes/No
Prostate enlargement (In male) Yes/No

Neurological

Syncope: Yes/No; Confusion: Yes/No; Convulsion: Yes/No; Incoordination: Yes/No; Headache: Yes/No (Describe if yes) touch and feeling of cold and hot

Musculoskeletal

Pain: Yes/No; Stiffness: Yes/No; Describe if yes limitation
Exercise pattern/specify Adaptive response
Injuries: Yes/No. Swelling. Yes/No; Difficulty in working: Yes/No

Investigations

Sl. No.	Name of test	Patient value	Nominal value	Remarks

Medical Diagnosis: (Final Diagnosis)_____

Drugs prescribed

Sl. No	Name of the drug	Dose	Route	Side effect	Nursing responsibilities

Diet Plan:_____

Assessment	Nursing diagnosis	Expected outcome	Interventions	Rational	Evaluation
• Subjective data • Objective data	Problem statements • Actual • High risk/potential	• Short-term outcomes • Long-term outcomes	Detailed nursing interventions aim of causes to achieve goals and objective stating. • What need to be done? • Where is to be done? • Who is to carry it out?	Rational for interventions indicated; why certain specific nursing interventions are planned, i.e., the principles underlying the order?	Evaluation should be done on the basis of interventions

UNIT 3

Meeting the Basic Needs of a Patient

LEARNING OBJECTIVES

After completing this unit, learner will be able to:

- Discuss physical needs
  - Comfort, rest, sleep, and exercise
  - Importance and its promotion
  - Body mechanics: Moving, lifting and transferring
  - Position and posture maintenance
  - Comfort devices
  - Beds and bed making: Principles of bed making, types, and care of bed linen
  - Safety devices, restrains and splints
  - Exercise: Active and passive
- Explain hygienic needs
  - Personal and environmental hygiene personal
  - Nurses note in maintaining personal and environmental hygiene
  - Care of eyes, nose, ears, hands, and feet
  - Care of mouth, skin, hair, and genitalia care of pressure areas, bed sores
- Describe elimination needs
  - Health and sickness
  - Problems: Constipation and diarrhea, retention and incontinence of urine
  - Nurses role in meeting elimination needs
  - Offering bedpan and urinals
  - Observing and recording abnormalities
  - Preparing and giving of laxative, suppositories, enemas, bowel wash, and flatus tube
  - Perineal care, care of patient with urinary catheter, diapers
  - Maintenance of intake and output records
- Explain nutritional needs
  - Diet in health and disease
  - Factors affecting nutrition in illness
  - Nurses role in meeting patient nutritional need
  - Modification of diet in illness
  - Diet planning and serving
  - Feeding helpless patients including artificial method of feeding
- Discuss psychological and spiritual needs
  - Importance
  - Nurses role: Diversional and recreational therapy
  - Care of terminally ill and dying patient
  - Dying patient's sign and symptoms, need of dying patient and family
  - Nursing care of dying patient: Special considerations, advance directives, euthanasia, will dying declaration, organ donation, etc.

- Medicolegal issues
- Care of the dead body
- Care of unit
- Autopsy
- Embalming

COMFORT, REST, AND SLEEP

Comfort, rest, and sleep are essential for health. People who are ill frequently require more rest and sleep than normal. Often, debilitated people expend unusual amounts of energy just to regain health or maintain activities of daily living. As a result, such people experience increased and frequent fatigue and thus, need more rest than usual.

Comfort

Comfort is a concept that is inherently linked to the practice of nursing care in a health context. It is characterized by the satisfaction of one's needs and by the person feeling strong, safe, supported, and cared for.

Factors Influencing Comfort

- Pain
- Immobility
- Delayed in meeting personal needs
- Extreme weather
- Stress
- Illness

Nurses provide and facilitate comfort with patients and their families through comfort measures. For example, bathing, providing skin care, repositioning, dressing, linen change, etc.

Importance of Rest

Rest: Implies calmness, relaxation without emotional stress, and freedom from anxiety. Providing a restful environment for the patient is an important function of the nurse. She needs to assess the patient's need for rest and evaluate how effectively, this need is met. The nurse needs to consider a condition that promotes rest.

Condition that promote rest: Feeling that things are under control.

To rest, the patient needs to feel that their personal care and their health condition are under control and that they are receiving competent healthcare. By providing competent care the nurse gives peace of mind and helps the patient to relax.

Understanding What is Going on

The unknown things generate a varying degree of anxiety and interfere with rest. The nurse can help by offering explanations about diagnostic tests, surgery, hospital policies or routines, and the patient's progress.

Freedom from Irritation and Discomfort

Irritation and discomfort have both physical and emotional aspects. Generally, the nurse easily detects physical discomforts, such as pain, insufficient support for body positions, damp bed clothes, and loud noise. Emotional discomforts include having too many or too few visitors, feeling a lack of privacy, being alone, or being concerned about the life problems of your own or others.

Having Satisfying Amount of Purposeful Activity

Purposeful activity can be relaxing and often provides a sense of self worth. Such activity often promotes rest throughout the day and undisturbed sleep at night, knowing one will receive help when needed. The patient who feels isolated and helpless cannot rest properly. Friends and family members can promote rest by helping the patient with daily tasks and difficult decisions. Nurses can help by anticipating and meeting the patient needs.

Sleep

According to Maslow, sleep is a basic human need. Sleep is defined as "a state of consciousness in which the individual's perception and reaction to the environment are decreased". Sleep is characterized by minimal physical activity, variable levels of consciousness, changes in the body's physiological processes, and decreased responsiveness to external stimuli.

Factors Affecting Normal Sleep

Both the quality and quantity are affected by several factors. Quality of sleep is the total time for which the individual sleeps.

Illness

People, who are ill, require more sleep than normal and normal rhythm of sleep and wakefulness is also disturbed.

Pain can affect sleep

Either preventing sleep or awakening the sleeper, pain associated with certain diseases such as arthritis, or migraine can also affect normal sleep.

Respiratory condition

It can disturb an individual's sleep, shortness of breath often makes sleep difficult, and people who have nasal congestion may have trouble breathing and have a difficult sleep. Certain endocrine disturbances can also affect sleep (e.g., hyperthyroidism); the need to urinate during the night also disturb sleep and people who awake at night to urinate some time have difficulty in getting back to sleep.

Environment

Environment can promote or hinder sleep. The absence of usual stimuli or presence of unfamiliar stimuli can keep people from sleeping.

Lifestyle

It is thought that a person who is moderately fatigued usually has a restful sleep. Fatigue can also affect a sleep pattern.

Psychological stress

Anxiety and depression frequently disturb sleep. A person preoccupied with personal problems may be unable to relax sufficiently, so as to fall asleep.

Medications

Medication, especially hypnotics and sedatives, affect the sleep pattern, even though they may increase total sleep time. Amphetamines and antidepressants decrease sleep abnormally.

Alcohol and stimulants

People who drink an excessive amount of alcohol often find their sleep disturbed.

Caffeine

Containing beverages act as stimulants of the central nervous system, thus interfere with sleep.

Diet

The amino acid L-tryptophan is thought to affect sleep. Dietary L-tryptophan found in cabbage, cheese, milk, beef, and canned tuna may be sleep inducing, a fact that might explain why milk help some people get to sleep.

Promoting rest and sleep these may include:
- Reducing environmental distraction
- Promoting bed time rituals
- Providing comfort measures
- Scheduling nursing care
- Teaching stress reduction, relaxation techniques.

Implementation

For hospitalized patients, sleep problems are often related to hospital environment and their illness. Assisting the patient to sleep in such instances can be challenging for a nurse, often involving scheduling activities, administering analgesics, and providing supportive environment. Explanations and a supportive relationship are essential for the fearful or anxious patient. Some of the interventions that may promote a patient's sleep are listed below:

- **Reducing environmental distractions:**
  - Provide a calm and comfortable environment
  - Close the door of the patient's room or pull curtains around the patient's bed
  - Reduce or eliminate lighting
  - Decrease the amount and type of stimuli, e.g., staff conversation, television
  - Place the patient with a compatible (other) patient
  - Avoid visitors during sleep
- **Schedule nursing interventions, so that the patient has the minimum possible interruptions while resting or sleeping.** For example, if a patient requires an intramuscular injection during the night, other interventions may be carried out at the same time, such as assessing vital signs or changing position.
- **Creating a safe environment:**
  - Use night light
  - Place the bed in a low position
  - Rise side rails
  - Place the call bell within easy reach
  - Instruct the patient on how to obtain assistance move about
- **Supporting bedtime rituals:**
  - Assist with bedtime activities/hygienic routine (common prebedtime activities of adult include listening to music, taking a soothing bath, praying, and hygienic routines such as washing the face and hands, brushing the teeth, and voiding).
  - Assist with bedtime snacks/drink.
  - Avoidance of excessive physical exercise and mental stimulation.
  - Adherence to consistent time for sleep and walking.
- **Promoting comfort and relaxation:**
  - Show a concern and caring attitude. Assist patient with hygienic routine.
  - Make sure bed linen is smooth/clean and dry, provide additional blankets for warmth.
  - Assist or encourage the patient to void before bedtime.
  - Offer back massage before sleep.
  - Position dependent patient appropriately to aid muscle relaxation, and provide supportive devices to protect pressure areas.
  - Encourage relaxation technique.

Sleep rarely occurs until a person is relaxed. Relaxation techniques can be encouraged as part of the nightly routine. Slow deep breathing for a few minutes followed by slow, rhythmic contraction, and relaxation of muscle can alleviate tension and induce calm.

Common Sleep Disorders

Knowledge about common sleep disorders assists the nurse to obtain and to recognize pertinent data. Insomnia, the most common sleep disorders, is the inability to obtain an adequate amount or quality of sleep.

There are three type of insomnia:
1. Difficulty in falling asleep (initial insomnia)
2. Difficulty in staying asleep because of frequent or prolonged waking (intermittent insomnia)

3. Early morning or premature awakening (terminal insomnia). Insomnia can result from physical discomfort but more often is a result of mental over stimulation due to anxiety. Treatment of insomnia frequently requires the patient to develop new behavior patterns that induce sleep. The usefulness of sleeping medications is questionable. Such medications do not deal with the cause of the problem; instead their prolonged use creates drug dependences.

Sleep apnea

It is the periodic cessation of breathing during sleep. The periods of apnea lasts from 10 seconds to 2 minutes occurs during sleep. Frequency ranges from 50 to 600 per night. These apneic episodes drain the person's energy and lead to excessive day time sleepiness. Sleep apnea profoundly affects a person's work or school performance. In addition, prolonged sleep apnea can cause a sharp rise in blood pressure and may also lead to cardiac arrest.

Parasomnias

Refers to a cluster of walking behaviors that appear during sleep and interfere with sleep. Parasomnias include:
- Somnambulism (sleep walking)
- Night terrors (horrifying dream)
- Nocturnal enuresis (bed wetting)

BODY MECHANICS

Body mechanics is the efficient use of the body as a machine. As a means of locomotion, it is directly related to the function of bones, joints, muscles, nerves, and brains to maintain posture balance. The nurse must understand and use correct body mechanics. Every activity in which the nurse engages needs understanding and use of these principles. It is important for the nurses to understand body mechanics and alignment, balance, and coordinated movement, which means optional musculoskeletal balance.

Balance

A body, in correct alignment, is balanced and objects are balanced when its center of gravity is close to its base of support. Later, when the line of gravity goes through the base of support, the object that as a wide base of support. The center of gravity of an object is the point at which its mass is centered. In humans, the center of gravity when standing is located in the center of pelvis about midway between the umbilicus and the symphysis pubis. Wider the base of support, the lower the center of gravity.

Nurses can increase body balance when working, by spreading their feet, further apart (broadening the base of support) and by flexing their hips and knees (lowering the center of gravity). These two simple maneuvers are important principles in body mechanics, by which nurses can decrease musculoskeletal strain. The nurses providing direct client, care must frequently use the body to assist the positioning, turning, lifting. Both clients and equipment, it is important to do this knowledgeably, to avoid musculoskeletal strain and injury.

Develop a habit of erect posture, begin activity by broadening the base of support and lowering the center of gravity. Use the strongest and longest muscle of the arms and the legs to help and provide the power needed in strenuous activities. Work as closely as possible to the object that is to be lifted or moved. This brings the body center of gravity close to that object being move. The nurse can demonstrate to others the proper way of using the musculoskeletal system, if good habit is developed.

RANGE OF MOTIONS

Definition

Range of motions, exercises help prevent contractures and joint stiffness by moving all the patient's joints through their complete range of motions is not very appropriate.

Purposes

- To prevent or rest or normal motion for joints.
- To prevent contractures.
- To stimulate circulation.
- To help maintain muscle strength.
- To help maintain/restore coordination.

Moving, Lifting, and Transferring

See **Figure 3.1**.

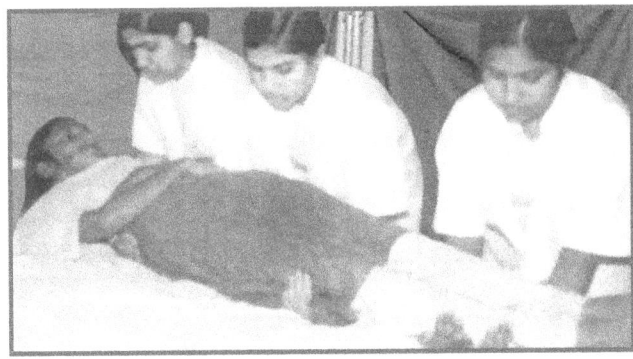

Fig. 3.1: Shifting and lifting of patient.

Types

1. **Passive:** No assistance from the patient (**Table 3.1**).
2. **Active:** Patient does without assistance.
3. **Active assisted:** Patient needs some assistance to perform motion.

Passive Movement Exercise

Table 3.1: Passive movement exercise.

Nursing action	Rationale
1. Check the physician's order, progress notes, and care plan.	To obtain specific instructions/information.

Contd...

Contd...

Nursing action	Rationale
2. Identify the patient.	To ensure that the right procedure is to be performed on the right patient.
3. Explain the procedure to the patient. Allow him to ask questions. Allow the patient to participate in the procedure as much as possible.	To allay fears and gain patient's confidence and cooperation.
4. Ensure patient's privacy.	To avoid unnecessary embarrassment to the patient during the procedure.
5. Reassure the patient during the procedure.	To gain cooperation for effective performance of the procedure.
6. Wash and dry hands.	To prevent cross-contamination.
7. Adjust height of the bed of possible.	To prevent injury and make maneuvers easier.
8. Position the patient in a comfortable position, near the side of bed where you will be working.	
9. Support the extremity or the part to be moved above and below joint. Do not hold the joint.	
10. Move joint through full range of motion. Perform all movements smoothly and slowly.	To prevent pain and damage to the joint.
11. If pain or strong resistance is present, do not force movement.	Forceful motion may cause damage to the joint.
12. Perform each movement three times during exercise periods per day. Exercise period may be incorporated to an activity such as bed bath.	
13. Move all joints of the body during the exercise period.	
14. When the exercise period is completed, assist the patient to a comfortable position.	
15. Place call bell within easy reach.	To assure that patient that help may be summoned if needed.
16. Wash and dry hands.	
17. Document the procedure appropriately. Note: a. Type of motion performed b. Patient's tolerance	

Ambulation (Table 3.2)

Table 3.2: Ambulation of patient.

Nursing action	Rationale
1. Explain the procedure to the patient.	To allay fears and gain patient's confidence and cooperation
2. Wash and dry hands.	To prevent cross-contamination.
3. Ensure privacy.	To avoid unnecessary embarrassment to the patient during the procedure.
4. Perform procedure on the patient by making him sit on/in chair/wheelchair. See transfer from bed to chair procedure.	
5. Stand at the patient's side. The assistant should hold the hand of the patient by his similar hand (right hand by right hand or left hand by left hand). The other hand goes round back to hold opposite hip.	
6. Observe patient when walking. Allow time for rest. Let the patient sit down at short intervals. Note patient's tolerance of the procedure.	
7. Position the patient on the bed. Ensure that he/she is in a safe and comfortable position.	
8. Wash and dry hands.	
9. Document the procedure appropriately. Note: a. Patient's tolerance. b. Length of the procedure c. Adverse effects.	

Position and Posture Maintenance

Body alignment refers to the relationship of body parts to each other. Alignment is effected by the condition of the joints, tendons, ligament, and muscles in various body positions. When the body is aligned, whether standing, sitting, or lying, no excessive strain is put on these structures. Body alignment contributes to body balance. Without this balance, the center of gravity is displaced, which increases the force of gravity. The person is consequently at risk of falling and receiving an injury. Good body alignment is important for the patient and the nurse.

Body balance is achieved when a wide base of support exists, the center of gravity falls within the base of support, and a vertical line can be drawn from the center of gravity through the base of support. Body balance is also enhanced by posture. The more aligned the posture, the greater the balance. Clinical nursing activities require the nurse to maintain body alignment. It is essential for the nurse to provide an opportunity for the client to observe posture and to identify the client's learning needs for maintaining body alignment. In addition, the nurse needs to identify trauma, muscle damage, or nerve dysfunction in the client (**Table 3.3**).

Table 3.3: Position and posture maintenance.

Steps	Rationale
Assessment	
Observe alignment of client in standing, sitting, or lying position	Determines if client assumes body alignment.
Standing	
a. Head is erect and at midline	Maintains body alignment in relation to body's normal center of gravity.
b. Shoulders and hips are straight and parallel.	
c. Vertebral column appears straight when viewed posteriorly.	
d. Lateral observation indicates head is erect and spinal curves are aligned in reverse pattern.	In reverse S-pattern, cervical vertebrae are anteriorly convex, thoracic vertebrae are posteriorly convex, and lumber vertebrae are anteriorly convex.
e. Lateral observation documents that abdomen is comfortably tucked in and knees and ankles are flexed.	Maintains abdomen and trunk directly over body's center of gravity
f. Arms are comfortably positioned at each side.	
g. Feet are placed slightly apart, with toes pointed forward.	Produces good/broad base of support and improves balance.
h. Center of gravity is located midline and forms vertical line from middle of forehead to midpoint between feet.	Laterally, line of gravity runs vertically from middle of skull to posterior one third of foot
Note: A pregnant woman's center of gravity is more anterior to adapt to normal weight gain, and growing fetus. Thus, she leans slightly backward and spinal column is slightly sway-backed.	

Contd...

Steps	Rationale
Sitting:	
a. Head is erect, and vertebrae are in straight alignment.	Prevents stress on intervertebral joints.
b. Body weight is evenly distributed on buttocks and thighs.	Prevents increased pressure over bony prominences and reduces damage to underlying musculoskeletal system.
c. Thighs are parallel and in horizontal plane.	Maintains flexion of hips and provides broad base of support.
d. Both feet are supported on the floor, and ankles are comfortably flexed.	Maintains plantar flexion and reduces risk of foot-drop.
e. If client is unable to flex one or both knees, nurse should make sure that elevated legs are supported and ankle is flexed.	
f. A 2.5–5 cm (1–2 inch) space is maintained between edge of seat and popliteal space on posterior surface of knee.	Ensures that no excessive pressure is put on popliteal artery or nerve, which could decrease circulation or impair nerve function.
g. Client's forearms should be supported on the armrest, in the lap, or on the table in front of the chair.	Reduces force of gravity on shoulder joint and chance of accidental shoulder dislocation.
Implementation	
1. Instruct the client or the family on proper body alignment for standing, sitting, or lying.	Provides client or family with necessary knowledge to identify potential altered body alignments.
2. Demonstrate to the client or family correct body alignment for standing, sitting, or lying.	Demonstration is a reliable technique for teaching psychomotor skill and enables client or family to ask questions.
3. Discuss with the client or the family hazards of prolonged immobility on body alignment and mobility.	Alerts the client or the family to early assessment factors associated with incorrect body alignment or impaired mobility.
4. Provide the client or the family with resources (community health agency, physician) to contact when mobility or body alignment is impaired.	Alerts the resource persons to assist with minor problems of body alignment before severe, irreversible problems occur.
Evaluation	
1. Inspect skin surfaces.	Reveals pressure sites.
2. Have the client demonstrate body alignment standing, sitting, and lying.	Return demonstration reveals, if learning occurred.
3. Ask the client to describe the benefits of body alignment.	Evaluates cognitive learning.

Contd...

Contd...

Steps	Rationale
4. Unexpected outcomes that may occur include: ➢ Incorrect body alignment is indicated by poor posture or decreased joint mobility. ➢ Damage to skin and musculoskeletal system (e.g., pressure sore, contracture) occurs.	Indicates need for follow-up learning activities.

Recording and Reporting

1. Record information presented to the client and progress toward learning selected knowledge.	Documents client teaching with plan of care.
2. Report information taught to the client at change of shift.	Alerts oncoming nursing personnel to information already presented.

Key Points

- ❖ Clients with lower extremity weakness, paralysis, or immobilization are at risk for musculoskeletal trauma because of uneven or prolonged distribution of body weight.
- ❖ Clients with upper extremity weakness or paralysis are at risk for shoulder dislocation, if their forearms are unsupported.
- ❖ Clients with impaired mobility, decreased sensation, or lack of voluntary muscle control are at risk for musculoskeletal damage and must have their positions changed frequently.

Lifting and Moving Techniques

General Procedure of Lifting and Moving (Table 3.4)

Table 3.4: Procedure lifting and moving.

Activities	Supporting figure
1. **Position yourself:** Correct foot position is essential to maintain balance. Keep feet at least one his breadth apart. Point one foot in the direction in which you will be moving; keep this foot ahead of the other, if possible.	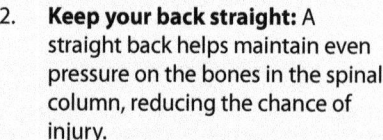
2. **Keep your back straight:** A straight back helps maintain even pressure on the bones in the spinal column, reducing the chance of injury.	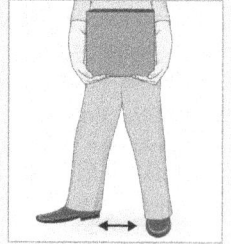
3. **Lift with leg muscles:** Leg muscles are much stronger than lower muscles. By squatting, bending your knees, keeping your back straight and lifting with your legs, you can avoid strain on back muscles and lift more weight.	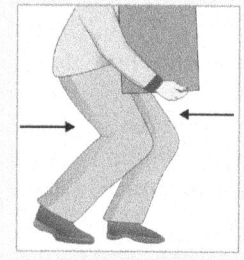
4. **Select a suitable grasp:** Using the correct grip minimize the strain on filters because they do not have to make muscles overwork to maintain their hold.	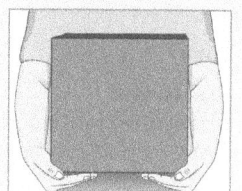
5. **Tuck your chin:** The act of tucking the chin may reduce the need for spinal muscles to contract, so there is less chance of muscle straining the back.	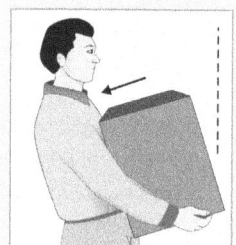
6. **Use rocking movements:** Rocking an object builds momentum, which can aid the lifting process.	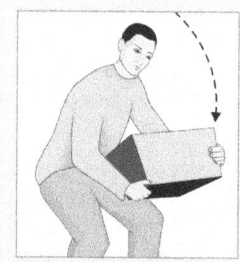
7. **Hold the load close:** If you hold the load as close to you as possible, you will cut down on the stress exerted on your arms and back.	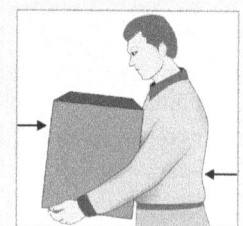
8. **Do not twist or bend:** Moving your feet instead of your upper body can help balance the load and minimize the strain your back and abdominal muscles.	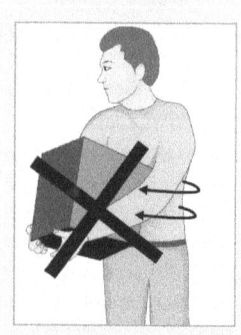

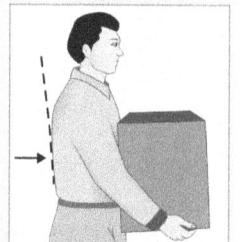

Contd...

How to Apply the Technique of Lifting and Moving? (Table 3.5)

Table 3.5: Technique of lifting and moving.

Activities	Supporting figure
1. **Evaluate the situation:** Make sure you are aware of what you have to do, and make sure you have the necessary equipment and personnel.	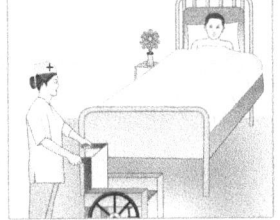
2. **Inform patient:** Explain to the patient exactly what you are going to-do. An informed patient will be more relaxed and be able to cooperate. Many patients can help partly lifting themselves. Always encourage the patient to help with the move whenever possible.	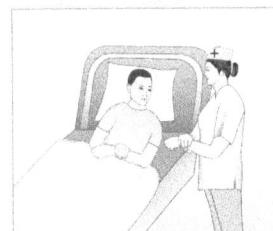
3. **Position the equipment:** Provide equipment (e.g., ladder), which may help the patient assist in the move. Prepare lifting aids and hoists, if used, position wheelchairs or stretchers as close to the patient as possible.	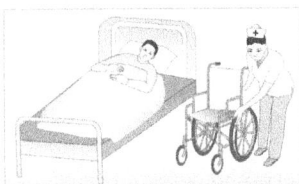
4. **Make necessary adjustments:** Adjust the chair, stretcher, etc., to the bed level or vice-versa, and lower any hand rill or side rail. This will minimize the amount of lifting or lowering required, be sure to lock the wheels on the chair or bed.	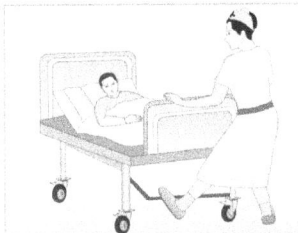
5. **Hold the patient close:** This will help keep your balance strain on your arms and back.	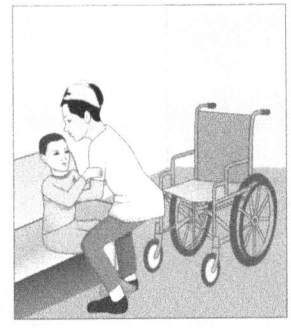 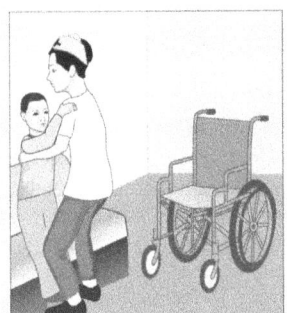
6. **Keep your feet apart:** This will provide a stable base, help you maintain your balance and leave you more energy for the lift. Put one foot close to the patient and one foot facing in the direction of the move, so as to take the weight off the patient.	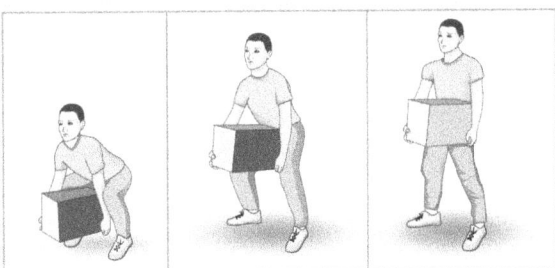

Contd...

Contd...

Activities	Supporting figure
7. **Use of rocking motion:** With special training, it is possible to lighten the load of lifting by using gentle rocking movements to assist the initial movement of the patient.	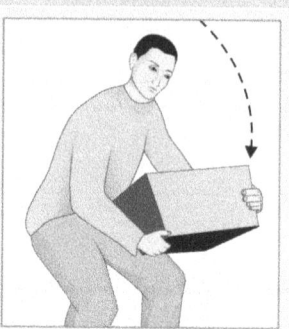
8. **Use your arms and legs:** Remember the importance of lifting your legs. Bend our elbows to hold the patient close and make the lift easier.	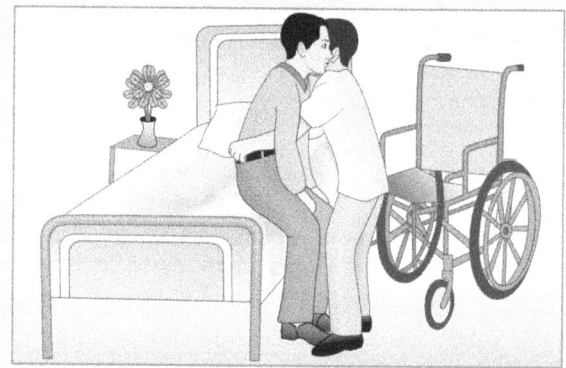
9. **Lift unison:** When working with others, make sure everyone knows what to do in advance and move at the same time. Also make sure everyone knows who is the leader and listens to and follows his/her commands. Avoid sudden jerky movements.	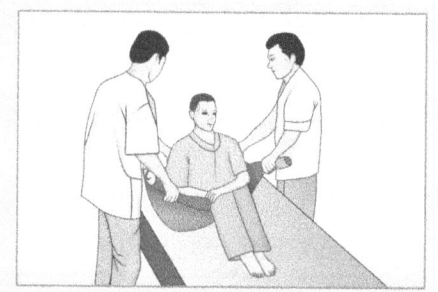

Other Basic Guidelines (Table 3.6)

Table 3.6: Basic guidelines.

1. **Do not take chance:** Use only those procedures with which you are familiar. Guessing the correct procedure, improvising, or failing to exercise proper caution when lifting or moving a patient may men danger to both the patient and you.	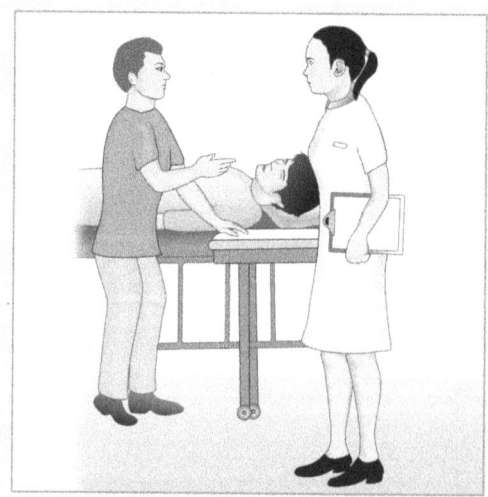

Contd...

Contd...

2. **Get help, if you need it:** Do not hesitate to ask questions or seek help, if you are unsure of which procedure to use, or if you don't think you can handle the lift or carry without strain. It is better to be safe than to be sorry.

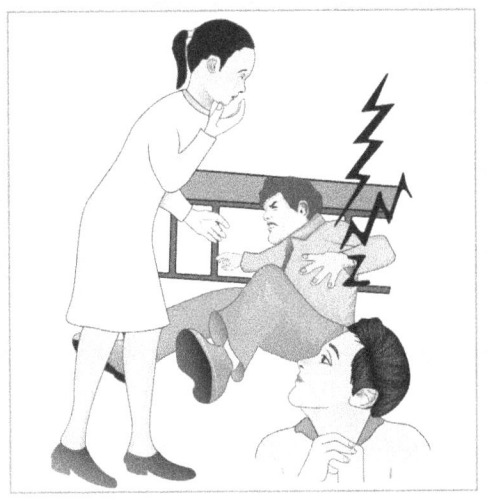

Correct Grasp or Correct Grasp Technique (Table 3.7)

Table 3.7: Correct grasp technique.

Activities	Supporting figure
1. **Two lifter** **Double wrist grasp** To use this grasp without causing pain to the patient, one lifter must turn his/her palm fully up; the other must turn his/her palm fully down.	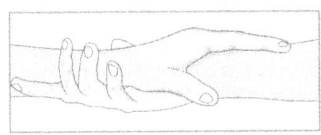
Single wrist grasp One lifter positions palm upward while the other lifter grasps the wrist of the first lifter.	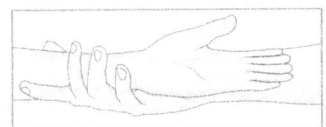
2. **One lifter** **Through arm grasp** Lifter carefully pushes on back of the patient's head or shoulders. Standing behind the patient, the lifter inserts his/her hands between patient's chest and arms to grasp the forearms. The patient helps by grasping the forearms. The patient helps by grasping his own wrist with his own hand.	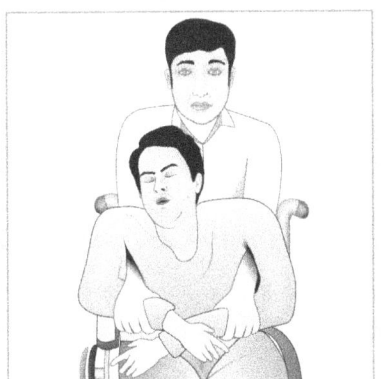
Elbow grasp The lifter stands in front with one side beside the sitting patient. One foot is beside the patient while the other blocks his/her knees. The patient places his head near the shoulder against the lifter's elbows. Lifter uses his/her arm to lock patient's far shoulder.	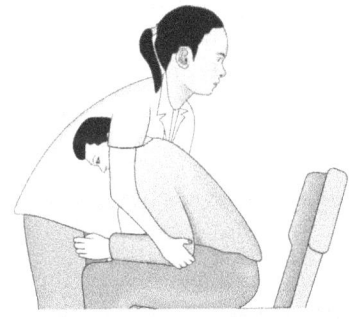

Whenever you lift or move a patient remember to:
1. Keep your grasp firm but relaxed.
2. Take care that you don't drag or pinch the patient's skin.

Changing Position

Note: This procedure does not apply to spinal injury cases.

Definition
Changing position of the patient in bed.

Purposes
- To provide comfort to the patient.
- To prevent contractures.
- To stimulate circulation and to help thrombophlebitis, pressure sores, and edema of the extremities.
- To facilitate activities of living.
- To relieve pressure.

Equipment
- One person, if the patient is light and able to assist.
- Two persons, if the patient is helpless and heavy.
- Lift the sheet, if required.
- Pillows as needed.

Procedure: Changing Position (Table 3.8)

Table 3.8: Changing position procedure.

Nursing action	Rationale
1. Check the physician's order, progress notes, and core plan.	To obtain specific instructions and/or information (e.g., changing position schedule).
2. Identify the patient.	To ensure that the right procedure is to be performed on the right patient.
3. Explain the procedure to the patient, allow him to ask questions. Encourage him to participate in the procedure as much as possible.	To allay fears and gain the patient's confidence and cooperation. To promote the patient's education.
4. Ensure patient's privacy.	To avoid unnecessary embarrassment to the patient during the procedure.
5. Wash and dry hands (refer to Hand Washing procedure)	Prevent cross-contamination.
6. Adjust height of bed, if possible. Adhere to lifting and moving instruction.	To prevent injury.
7. Move patient to the side of bed, apposite to which the patient is to be turned. Move shoulders and head first then hips and legs at the end.	To maintain body alignment.

Contd...

Contd...

Nursing action	Rationale
8. Flex the nearest arm across chest and flex the near by leg. Place a pillow under the flexed arm and leg.	To promote comfort to the patient.
9. Raise side-rails before going to the other side.	To prevent injury.
10. Standing on the opposite side, place one hand under the patient's shoulder and the other hand under the hip. At one time, move patient upward to the side of bed.	
11. Rearrange pillows and covers.	To provide comfort and ensures privacy.
12. If the sheet is to be lifted, place it folded under the patient. The sheet should be extended from the shoulders to the thigh.	To follow orderly steps of procedure
13. Pull the patient to the side of the bed opposite to which the patient is to be turned.	To ensure safe placement of the patient
14. Perform step 7 and 8.	
15. Standing on the opposite side, grasp the far side of the turned sheet and pull slowly rolling the patient toward you.	To ensure safety
16. Place pillow between legs, and under the flexed arm.	To maintain body alignment and promote comfort.
17. Arrange covers.	To make patient comfortable
18. Raise side-rails of the bed.	To prevent fall
19. Wash and dry hands (refer to hand washing procedure)	To prevent infection
20. Documents the procedure appropriately. Note: a. Position changed b. Patient's tolerance c. Adverse effects.	Timely documentation ensure accurate intervention

Transfer from Bed to Chair and Vice Versa

Definition
Transfer patient from bed to chair and vice versa.

Purposes
- To restore normal functions of the body.
- To prevent of control postoperative complications.
- To promote activities of daily living.
- To encourage independence.

Equipment

- One person, if the patient is light and able to assist.
- Two persons, if the patient is helpless and heavy.
- Lift the sheet, if required.
- Pillows as needed.

Procedure: Transfer from Bed to Chair and Vice Versa (Table 3.9)

Table 3.9: Transfer from bed to chair and vice versa procedure.

Nursing action	Rationale
1. Check the physician's order, progress notes, and care plan.	To obtain specific instructions and information.
2. Identify the patient.	To ensure that the right procedure is to be performed on the right patient.
3. Explain the procedure to the patient. Allow him to ask questions. Encourage to participate in the procedure as much as possible.	To allay fears and gain the patient's confidence and cooperation. To promote the patient's education.
4. Wash and dry hands (refer to hand washing procedure).	To prevent cross-contamination.
5. Ensure patient's privacy.	To avoid unnecessary embarrassment to the patient.
6. Position the chair.	To allow minimal turning and carrying.
7. Lock wheels of the bed and wheelchair. Lower the entire bed and raise the head part of bed to sitting position.	To prevent injury during transfer.
8. Assist the patient to put on appropriate dress and footwear.	To ensure privacy during transfer.
9. Assist the patient to bring legs over the side of the bed. Allows patient to sit for a few minutes.	To prevent fainting.
10. Assist the patient to slide to edge of the bed.	To prevent fall
11. Ask the patient to put his/her hand on the arm of the chair.	To prevent injury.
12. The assistant stand on the patient's left hand side. Bring the right hand a round back to hold right hip. Left hand holds left hand. Patient pushes up with right hand to stand or vice versa.	To provide comfort to the patient.
13. Turn patient until back of legs touches the chair.	To provide safety

Contd...

Nursing action	Rationale
14. Lower the patient into the chair while holding securely.	To prevent accident
15. Reassure and observe the patient during the procedure.	Psychological support
16. Arranges covers.	To ensure privacy.
17. Place call button or bell within easy reach.	To assure that he/she may summon help when needed.
18. Wash and dry hands (refer to hand washing procedure).	To prevent infection
19. Document the procedure appropriately Note: a. Patient's tolerance. b. Adverse effect such as weakness, dizziness, diaphoresis, cold or clammy skin, change in color, pain.	To ensure procedure done safely

BEDS AND BED MAKING

In hospital, bed linens need to be changed frequently as clients spend much of their time on bed, patting, bathing, urinating and undergoing many therapeutic procedures. It is essential that nurses be able to make beds in different ways for specific purposes.

Clinical Guidelines for Bed Making

- Wash hands before and after bed making to prevent cross-infection.
- Soiled linen is placed directly in a portable linen hamper.
- Soiled linen is never shaken in the air because shaking can discriminate secretions and excretions.
- Hold soiled linen away from uniform.
- Maintain good body mechanics to prevent fatigue.
- Make the bed firm, smooth, and unwrinkled.
- Conserve time and energy by collecting all needed linen before starting procedure and working on onside completely before working on the other side.

Making an Unoccupied Bed

Purposes

- To promote comfort of the clients.
- To give a neat appearance to the unit.
- To promote clean linen
- To establish an effective nurse patient relationship.

Equipment

- Two large sheets
- Draw sheet

- Blankets
- Bed spread
- Pillow cases
- Waterproof sheet or rubber mackintosh
- Linen hamper
- Bedside table or chair
- Disposable gloves (optional)

Procedure: Making an Unoccupied Bed (Table 3.10)

Table 3.10: Procedure of making an unoccupied bed.

Action	Rationale
1. Wash hands	Hand washing reduces spread of microorganisms.
2. Wear disposable gloves.	Wearing gloves prevents cross-infection.
3. Assemble and arrange equipment on a bedside table.	Organizations save time and energy.
4. Adjust the bed height to a comfortable working position and lower the side rail.	Provides easy access to bed and reduces strain on back.
5. Loosen all linen from head to foot on the side near to you. Move to the other side of bed, lower side rail, and loosen all linen.	Allows easy removal of linen and prevent tearing of sheets.
6. Fold and keep reversible linens such as blanket or bedspread on bedside table.	Folding saves time and energy.
7. Bundle all soiled linen in bottom sheet and directly place into the laundry bog.	Prevents spread of microorganisms.
8. Bring mattress toward the head of bed.	Allows more foot room for client.
9. Place the bottom sheet with its center fold in the center of bed and toward the top to have sufficient sheet to tuck under the head of the mattress.	Keeps the bed firm.
10. Unfold the bottom sheet, spread it over the mattress and tuck in severely with mitered corner.	Wrinkle free bed reduces discomfort.
11. Spread the mackintosh at the center of the bed and tuck it along the side.	Protects the bottom sheet from soiling.
12. Place the draw sheet over the mackintosh and tuck it along the side.	Protects the skin of the client from direct contact irritation.
13. Move to the opposite side and tuck the sheets	Saves time and energy. Wrinkles can cause irritation

Contd...

Action	Rationale
14. In the same manner pull the sheets tightly while tucking excess linen under mattress. Return to the side of the bed first made. Place the top sheet with its centerfold in the center of bed. Unfold it with the top edge even with the top of the mattress. Spread excess sheet over the bottom edge of the mattress.	
15. Place the blanket over the top sheet about 6 inches below the top of the sheet.	
16. If the bed spread is used place it over the blanket.	
17. Tuck the top sheet, blanket and bed spread under the foot of the bed on the side close to you and miter the corners.	Keeps the top linen in place.
18. Fold the upper 6 inches of the top sheet down over the spread and make a cuff.	Makes it easier for the client to get in and pull the covers up.
19. Move to the other side of the bed and follow the same procedure for screening top sheets.	Saves time and energy.
20. Put the pillow case and place the pillow at the head end with the open end away from the entrance.	Provides neat appearance.
21. Fanfold or pie fold top linens.	Makes it easier for client to get in.
22. Rearrange furniture and place personal items within easy reach.	Promotes sense of well-being.
23. Adjust the bed to a comfortable height for the client.	Provides for client safety.
24. Dispose off soiled linen and wash hands.	Reduces spread of microorganisms.

An unoccupied bed can be either closed or open. To open beds the top covers are folded back to receive the client just before the admission. In closed bed, the top covers are drawn up to the top of the bed and under the pillow.

Making an Occupied Bed

Purposes

- To conserve client's energy and maintain current health status.

- To promote client's comfort.
- To provide a clean, neat environment for the client.
- To prevent bedsore.
- To observe the client, e.g., pressure of bed sore, or a hygiene, self-care ability, etc.
- To establish an effective nurse-client relationship.
- To provide active and passive exercise.

Procedure: Making an Occupied Bed (Table 3.11)

Table 3.11: Procedure for making an occupied bed.

	Action	Rationale
1.	Explain the procedure to the client and identify the client's physical ability.	Facilitates client cooperation and determines the level of activity.
2.	Wash hands and put on gloves.	Reduces transmission of microorganisms.
3.	Assemble equipment and arrange on the bedside chair in proper order and remove unnecessary equipment.	Organization facilitates performance of tack and saves energy and time.
4.	Close door or draw bedside curtain.	Maintains client's privacy.
5.	Adjust the bed's height to a comfortable working position.	Reduces strain on the back.
6.	Place the bed in a flat position if the client can tolerate it.	Facilitates easy removal and applying of bed linen evenly.
7.	Lower the side rail on one side of bed.	Provides easy access to bed.
8.	Loosen all top linen and remove bedspread and blanket separately.	Reduces spread of microorganisms and maintains client's privacy.
9.	Fold and place on the bed side table, if bed spread and blanket to be reused.	Facilitates replacement and prevents wrinkles.
10.	With assistance shift mattress up to the head of bed.	Allows more foot room for client.
11.	Assist the client to turn toward the opposite side and reposition the pillow under the client's head.	Provide space for placement of clean linen.
12.	Loosen all bottom linens and fanfold soiled linens as far from the client as possible.	Facilitate removal of linens.
13.	Place the clean bottom sheet lengthwise making sure that middle fold is in the middle of the bed and vertically fanfold the half toward the center of the bed.	Allows making one side of bed.
14.	Tuck the head end, miter corners, and tuck sides.	Mitered corner cannot be loosened easily.

Contd...

Contd...

	Action	Rationale
15.	Bring the rubber mackintosh back into place and tuck, if tightly under the mattress. (If rubber mackintosh is to be reused).	Rubber mackintosh protects bottom sheet from soiling.
16.	Plan the clean draw sheet on the mackintosh with center fold at the center of bed. Fanfold upper half vertically toward the center of bed Tuck the side edge under the mattress.	Provides comfort to the client.
17.	Raise side rail on working side and go to the other side.	Maintains client's safety during turning.
18.	Lower side rail. Assist the client to roll slowly on to the other side over folds of linen. Reposition the pillow and top sheet.	Allows making the other side of bed.
19.	Loosen and remove all bottom linen. Place them in a linen bag on a hamper.	Proper disposal of soiled linen prevents spread of microorganisms.
20.	Spread clean, fanfold linen smoothly over the edge of the mattress and tuck, if from head to foot.	Helps to make wrinkle-free bed.
21.	Assist the client to turn on the back and reposition the pillow.	Maintains the client's comfort.
22.	Place a clean top sheet over the client with center fold lengthwise down middle of bed. Unfold over-client and ask the client to hold clean top sheet or tuck the sheet around the client's shoulders. Remove the soiled top sheet and discord in a linen bog.	Prevents exposure of body parts and encourages participation in client core.
23.	Place blanket over the top sheet and unfold to cover the client making sure that the top edge should be parallel to the edge of top sheet and 6–8 inches from the edge of top sheet.	Provides adequate warmth.
24.	Place and unfold bedspread over blanket extending top edge of spread about 2 inches above blanket edge. Tuck top edge of spread over and under top edge of blanket.	Provides extra warmth and a neat appearance.
25.	Turn the edge of top sheet down over the top edge of blanket and spread.	Protects client's face from rubbing against blanket or spread.

Contd...

Contd...

Action	Rationale
26. Tuck the foot end of top linen under mattress giving enough freedom for movement.	Provides a neat appearance and prevents pressure sore.
27. Raise side rail lower the bed height to a comfortable position. Reattach call bell and drainage tubes, if any.	Maintains the client's safety.
28. Change pillow cases and place them in position. Replace the comfort devices in place. Rearrange furniture and open bedside curtain.	Promotes sense of well-being.
29. Dispose of soiled linens according to the hospital policy and wash hands.	Prevents spread of microorganisms.

Different Kinds of Beds to Meet the Special Needs of Clients

Postoperative Bed or Postanesthetic Bed or Recovery Bed

It is one which is prepared for a client who is recovering from the effects of anesthesia following a surgical operation.

Purposes
- To meet any emergency
- To provide warmth
- To protect the mattress and pillows from soiling by vomitus.
- To transfer the client quickly from the trolley to the bed.

Procedures
- The foundation of the bed is prepared as in an open bed.
- Head end of the bed is protected with water-proof sheet or rubber mackintosh and draw sheet.
- The top linen at the bed is left untucked and folded back even with mattress.
- The top linen is fan-folded to one side.
- Pillow is not kept at the head end. It may be used to protect the head of the client against the bars of the bed.
- Extra rubber mackintosh and draw sheet may be used according to the site of operation to protect the bed from soiling with blood.
- All items needed for the immediate core of the client such as infusion stand, blocks, post anesthetic tray, oxygen cylinder, hot water bottles, suction apparatus, etc., must be kept ready.

Cardiac Bed

It is used to relieve dyspnea caused by cardiac diseases.

Procedures
- Place the back rest and arrange the pillows in such a position, so that back is well-supported.
- Arrange the pillows one it her sides that arms are well-supported.
- Keep the cardiac table with pillow in front of the client, so that client can lean forward and rest on it.

Fracture Bed

It is used for a client with fracture of trunk or extremities provide firms support.

Procedures
- Fracture boards are arranged to give firm support to the fractured area.
- A basket frame may be fitted to support pulleys and weights, if traction is needed.
- A divided mattress may be used for giving bed pan, if lifting the hips of client is contraindicated.

Amputation Bed or Stump Bed or Divided Bed

Purposes
- To take off the weight of bed linen after amputation of the leg.
- To keep the stump in good position.
- To avoid disturbing the client when constant observations or repeated treatments are necessary for abdomen or legs.

Procedures
- The foundation of bed is made as an open bed.
- The top linen is folded back toward the head end at the level of the stump or the part that is to be observed.
- Another set of the top linen starts from the level of the stump by overlapping the first set while the excess is tucked under the mattress at the foot end.
- Both sets of top linen are fan-folded toward one side to receive the client.
- A small pillow with a water proof cover issued to elevate the stump.
- Sandbags are placed on either side of the stump to prevent the jerking movements of the stump.
- Bed cradle may be used to take off the weight of the top linen.

Safety Devices: Restraints, Splints; Exercises: Passive and Active Exercises

Restraints

Restraints are devices that limit a patient's movement; restraint can help keep a person from getting hurt or doing harm to others. They are used as a last resort.

Following are some of the different kinds of physical restraints:
- Belts placed around the waist and connected to a bed or chair
- Cloth vests or poesy's placed around your chest
- Lapboard hooked to chairs that limit ability to move
- Mittens placed in the hands.

Chemical restraints: They are medicine used to calm down and relax.

Seclusion
- A patient is held in a room involuntarily and prevented from leaving.
- Many emergency department and psychiatric department have seclusion room.
- Seclusion is used only for patient who are behaving violently or self-destructive manner.

Indication for restraints
- To prevent pulling out by patient
- To keep person in proper placement
- Avoid physically combative and immediate danger

Determining when to use a restraints
The patient current behavior determines, if and when a restraints is needed. A history of violence or previous fall alone is not enough to support using a restraints thorough medical and psychological nursing assessment, sometimes, addressing the issues that is underlying a patient disruptive behavior may eliminate the need for a restraint.

Hazards of restraints
Strangulation and restricted breathing, bedsores/pressure sores, infections

Principles of restraints
- Maintain safety, well-being, and dignity of patient is essential
- Physical restraints should only be used for the minimum period of time
- Restraints required physician order and patient's consent.

Nurses responsibility
Before applying restraints, the nurse must exhaust alternative measures to restraints such as bed alarm, distraction and a sitter, if the nurse determines that a restraint is necessary, its use is discussed with the client and family and taken physician order and patient consent.

Splints

Splints are a supportive device that protects a broken bone or injury. A splint keeps the injured part of the body.

Casts and splints are orthopedic devices that are used to protect and support fractured or injured bones and joints. They help to immobilize the injured limbs to keep the bone in place until it fully heals.

Types of splints
- Finger splints, hand tape splint
- Long arm posterior splint
- Radial splint
- Thumb spica splint
- Ulnar gutter splint
- Long-leg posterior splint
- Posterior ankle splint

Exercises: Passive and active exercises.

Hygienic Needs
- Personal and environmental hygiene personal
- Nurses note in maintaining personal and environmental hygiene
- Care of eyes, nose, ears, hands, and feet
- Care of mouth, skin, hair, and genitalia care of pressure areas, bed sores.

Personal and Environmental Hygiene

Care of skin and mucous membrane

Skin
While assessing skin and hygiene practice, the nurse carefully, its color, texture, thickness, turgor, temperature, and hydration. The skin should be smooth, warm, and supple with good turgor. Hygienic practice includes:
- Nursing history to determine the patient
- Skin care practices
- Self-care abilities
- Pat or present skin problems.

Common skin problems
- **Abrasion:** Superficial layer of the skin are scrapped or rubbed away. Area is reddened and may have localized bleeding or serous weeping
- **Excessive dryness:** Skin can appear flaky and rough
- **Ammonia dermatitis (Diaper rash):** Caused by skin bacteria resulting with urea in the urine. The skin become reddened and is sore.
- **Erythema:** Redness associated with a variety of conditions, e.g., rashes, exposure to sun, elevated body temperature.

Identifying patients at risk
The nurse should be especially observant in noticing any redness, which might indicate increased pressure over a bony prominence or pallor, which is indicative of inadequate circulation to the skin tissues.

A number of conditions place patient at risk of developing skin impairment as follows:

Alteration in nutritional status
Emaciation is a wasted appearance due to extreme weight loss. In emaciated individuals, subcutaneous fat is insufficient to provide padding or support over bony prominence to withstand normal stress or pressure. Individual with inadequate protein intake are also prone to skin breakdown. Since, protein is essential for the building, maintenance, and repair of all tissues.

Immobility

Normally people change position frequently, even during sleep. When position cannot be altered, e.g., due to paralysis or unconsciousness, blood circulation, which carries essential nutrients to the skin is reduce, in turn skin become weak and eventually takes place.

Altered hydration

In dehydrated individuals, the skin become excessively dry and skin turgor is diminished. Both conditions make the skin less resistance to injury.

Altered sensation

Loss of sensation in body part may be the result of paralysis or other neurologic diseases reduces person ability to sense the heat, cold, or pricks. This loss makes the person prone to skin damage.

Presence of secretions or excretions on the skin

An accumulation of secretion such as perspiration. Excretions such as urine or feces are irritating to skin and it harbor microorganisms and make an individual prone to skin breakdown and infection.

Mechanical devices

The presence of restraints, casts, or devices, which creates pressure or a sheering force, can alter skin integrity considerably.

Altered venous circulation

Stasis of venous blood in the lower extremities, which is associated with varicose vein, can cause stasis dermatitis (inflammation of the skin), on the feet and around the ankles. This dermatitis is characterized by redness, dryness, and swelling. Ultimately skin tissue becomes ischemic and necrotic, which leads to ulceration.

Hygienic Activities

The hygienic activities, that the nurse carry out or assist the patient to meet the hygienic needs are:
- Bed bath.
- Care of hair/shampooing the hair.
- Care of eyes, ear, and teeth.
- Perineal care.
- Performing nail and foot care.

Bathing a Patient

Nursing provide two categories of baths: Cleansing and therapeutic.

Cleansing baths

Cleansing baths are usually given early in the morning before scheduled tests or procedures. However, patients may prefer bathing in the evening, if this is their routine at home. In addition to cleansing the skin, the bath stimulates circulation and reduces body odor by removing secretions, perspiration, and bacteria from the skin. Therefore, self-image is restored. While bathing the patient, the nurse can get to know the patient better and interact therapeutically. Further assessment can be made, and range of motion (ROM) exercises to the joint can be made.

The type of cleansing bath a nurse provides depends on the patient's physical capabilities and the degree of hygiene required. The nurse is responsible for assessing what type of bath is most appropriate for the patient's needs.

Types of cleansing baths include:

- **Complete bed bath:** Administered to patients who are totally dependent, the nurse gives the bath to the patient in bed.
- **Partial bed bath:** Consist of bathing only body parts that would cause discomfort, if left unbathed such as hands face, axillae, and perineal area. Dependent patients in need of partial hygiene or self-sufficient bedridden patients who are unable to reach all body part, receives a partial bed bath.
- **Tub bath:** Patient is immersed into a tub of water. The tub bath allows more thorough washing and rinsing than a bed bath. Patient may still require the nurse's assistance. Tubs are available that facilitates lifting dependent patients into the water.
- **Shower:** Patient sits or stands under a continuous stream of water. The shower provides more thorough cleansing than a bed bath.

Therapeutic baths

Therapeutic baths are generally ordered by physicians for a specific therapeutic effect, in order to remove crusts, scales, and old medications or to relive inflammation and itching. Soaks are an easy way to treat a variety of skin disorders involving large areas of the skin. They relive general aches and pains and can ease dry or oily, inflamed or itchy skin. Hot baths are relaxing and stimulating; cool baths can reduce inflammation.

Types of therapeutic baths include:

- **Colloidal oatmeal**—coats, soothes, stops itch and does not dry out the skin.
- **Potassium permanganate**—makes a good disinfectant.
- **Bath oils**—are used as an emollient to ease itchy skin and eczema.
- **Corn starch**—is a soothing, drying bath for itchy skin.
- **Sodium bicarbonate**—can be cooling for hot, dry skin conditions.
- **Saline (salt) water baths**—are used to treat lesions scattered over the body.

Bed Bath

Definition

Bed bath is assisting a bedridden patient to maintain his personal hygiene during the period of bed rest.

Purposes
- To clean and refresh the patient.
- To promote comfort.
- To stimulate blood circulation.

Equipment
- Basin.
- Jug of hot water at 35–40°C.
- Lotion thermometer.
- Soap and soap dish.
- Tooth brush and paste.
- Patient's own toiletries (soap, scrubs, etc.).
- Bathtowels-2.
- Washcloth-2.
- Bathing blanket/draw sheet (optional).
- Patient's brush and comb.
- Nail scissors.
- Disposable gloves for oral and perineal care.
- Clean patient cloths.
- Clean bed lines.
- Bed pan or urinal (if required).
- Bathing trolley.
- Equipment for catheter care, if required.
- Equipment for mouth care, if required.
- Receptacle for soiled bed linen.
- Receptacle for soiled disposables.
- Additional bed screen, if required.
- Talcum powder.

Procedure: Bed bath (Table 3.12)

Table 3.12: Procedure of bed bath.

Sl. No.	Nursing action	Rationale
1.	Explain the procedure to the patient. Encourage the patient to participate in the procedure as much as possible	To allay fears and gain the patients cooperation, confidence and his consent. To promote health education.
2.	Collect and prepare the equipment	
3.	Ensure the patient privacy	To avoid unnecessary embarrassment to the patient during the procedure
4.	Ensure that the bed brakes are locked	
5.	Offer bed pan or urinal, if required	
6.	Wash and dry hands	To prevent cross-infection
7.	Assist patient into a comfortable position as medically indicated	To promote comfort during the procedure

Contd...

Sl. No.	Nursing action	Rationale
8.	Remove excess bed linen and bed appliances, if in use, but leaving the patient covered with bed sheet.	
9.	Assist the patient to remove clothing. If intravenous infusion is in progress, remove clothing from the unaffected arm first, then lower the intravenous fluid container, remove the clothing, and then rehang the container	
10.	Check the temperature of the water and pour into basin. (Change water frequently throughout the procedure)	
11.	If possible ask the patient to test the water temperature by placing hand into basin	To ensure comfortable temperature
12.	Check with the patient, if the uses soap on his face	To prevent discomfort
13.	Using the wash cloth (without soap), wipe one eye from inner canthus to outer canthus. Rinse the wash cloth and clean the other eye	
14.	Wash the patient's face, ears and neck. Rinse wash cloth and remove excess soap from the face. Dry the area. When possible assist the patient to do this by himself.	
15.	Expose the arm opposite to you, place towel lengthwise under it. Wash arm, axilla using firm strokes, rinse and dry the area. Observe the bony prominences carefully for any discoloration and pressure symptoms.	Washing the patient's limbs, farthest away from you will allow your assistant to dry that limb as the other limb is washed, thus, avoiding other the long exposure of limb to the cooling effect of the environment. Careful observations alert the nurse to the potential problem of bedsore.
16.	Place towel on the bed next to the patient's hand. Place and immerse hand in basin and wash, rinse and dry.	It avoids unnecessary movement for the nurse. She can reach it easily. Immersing the hands softens the nails, and helps in easy removal of the nails and hidden dirt from finger beds.

Contd...

Contd...

Sl. No.	Nursing action	Rationale
17.	Repeat steps 15 and 16 for the other arm also.	
18.	Spread towel across the chest, fold bed sheet, bathing blanket down to the umbilicus level. Wash rinse and dry the chest, keep the chest covered with a towel in between washing and rinsing. Pay special attention to skin folds under the breasts of female patients.	To protect the privacy of the patient. It avoids unnecessary exposure of the chest to atmosphere cold. It helps to remove the hidden dirt.
19.	Lower the sheet, blanket down to the level. Place towel over the chest, wash, rinse, and dry the abdomen.	To aid in step-by-step cleaning, without leaving any part of the trunk.
20.	Spread the sheet/bath blanket and expose the leg opposite to you. Place towel under the leg. Wash, rinse, and dry the leg from ankle to knee, and knee to groin.	Placing towel under the leg protect the bed linen. It avoids contaminating the cleanest area and it also helps in maintaining proper cleaning.
21.	Place a towel near the foot, put basin on it. Place patient's foot in the basin. Support the ankle and heel in your hand and the leg on your arm. Repeat steps 18–20 for the other leg.	Proper support avoids foot drop, and gives comfort the patient
22.	Change water, place the patient on side position exposing back and buttocks. Assistant support the patient.	Proper positioning aids in cleaning. Support from the assistant ease the work, and it gives comfort to the patient
23.	Wash, rinse, and dry the back and buttocks. Pay attention to the Gluteal folds and inspect for any redness or skin odors	Proper washing and drying keeps the skin healthy. Proper inspection helps to identify the potential problem of bedsore
24.	Change the water and discard the wash cloth and towel as you have washed the Gluteal (anal) area	To avoid infection to other area
25.	Assist the patient to wash, rinse, dry his pubic area, and wash from the front of the perineal area to the back	To prevent cross-infection from the anal region
26.	Carry out catheter care, if required	To prevent ascending infection

Contd...

Contd...

Sl. No.	Nursing action	Rationale
27.	Assist patient into a clean gown	
28.	Protect the pillow with a towel and comb the hair	
29.	Change bed linen	
30.	Ensure that the patient is left with feeling as comfortable as possible	
31.	Clean and dispose off equipment	
32.	Wash and dry hands	
33.	Record procedure in appropriate charts.	Any procedure needs proper documentation for further follow-up and communication among care takers.

Care of Hair

The hair growth, distribution, and pattern can indicate a person's general health status, hormonal changes, emotional and physical stress, aging infection, and certain illness. However, change in its color or condition are caused by hormonal and nutrients deficiencies.

Hair and scalp problems

1. **Dandruff:** Scaling of scalp is accompanied by itching. In severe cases, dandruff, if found in eye brows.
   Management: Shampoo regularly with medicated shampoo, in severe cases.
2. **Pediculosis (lice):** Tiny, grayish, white parasites, infest mammals.
   * **Pediculosis capitis (head lice):** Parasite, if found in scalp attached to hair strands, eggs look like oval particles, similar to dandruff, bites, or pustules may be observed behind ears, and at hairlines.
     Management: Check entire scalp, use medicated shampoo of eliminating lice. Repeat 12–24 hours later.
   * **Pediculosis corporis (body lice):** Parasites tend to cling to clothing, so they may not be easily seen. Body lice suck blood and lay eggs on clothing.
     Management: Bath or shower thoroughly. After skin is dried, apply recommended pediculicide lotion. After 12–24 hours take another bath or shower. Infested cloth or linen should be soaked in hot water before washing.
   * **Pediculosis pubis (crab lice):** Parasites are found in pubic hair. Crab lice are grayish white with red legs.
     Management: Shave hair off in the affected area. Cleanse as per body lice.

Shampooing the hair of a bedridden patient

Frequency of shampooing depends on condition of the hairs and the person's daily routines. Hair condition may have gender and racial variations. Dry hair, which commonly results from aging and protein deficiency, requires less frequent shampooing than hairs of people who exercise actively. Hospitalized client who stay in bed with excess perspiration or treatments that leave solutions in the hairs may require more frequents shampooing. If the client is allowed to sit in a chair, shampooing can be done in front of a sink. If the client is unable to sit in a chair or be transferred to a stretcher, shampooing must be done along with a bed bath or later as a separate procedure.

Contraindications for hair shampooing
- The clients with increased intracranial pressure.
- For clients with cerebrospinal fluid leakage.
- Clients having open lesions or incision of face, head, or neck.
- Cervical neck injuries.
- Presence of tracheostomy.
- Severe facial edema.
- Respiratory distress.

Equipment
- Shampoo.
- Hair conditioner (optional)
- Water pitcher.
- Plastic shampoo through
- Bucket.
- Bath blanket, two bath towels, face towel, or wash cloth.
- Water-proof pad.
- Comb and brush.
- Hair dryer (optional).
- Bottle of hydrogen peroxide and saline (optional), nonabsorbent cotton balls to plug the ears.

Procedure: Shampooing the hair of a bedridden patient (Table 3.13)

Table 3.13: Procedure of shampooing hair of bedridden patient.

Sl. No.	Nursing action	Rationale
1.	Wash hands	Reduces transmission of prior organism
2.	Arrange the equipment in a convenient place and lower side rails	Easy access to bath client and equipment prevents interruptions
3.	Place water-proof pad under client's shoulders, neck, and head. Position client with head and shoulders at the top edge of bed. Place plastic trough under client's head and bucket at the end of trough.	Prevents soiling bed linen
4.	Placed rolled towel under client's neck and bath towel across client's shoulders	Hyperextension of neck minimizes problems of water draining down at the back of the neck.

Contd...

Contd...

Sl. No.	Nursing action	Rationale
5.	Plug the ears with nonabsorbent cotton	Prevent water entering into ears.
6.	Brush and comb client's hair	Removing tangles results in more thorough cleansing
7.	Obtain water at about 43–44°C (110°F)	Proper water temperature prevents burns to face and scalp.
8.	Put the face towel over eyes	Prevents shampoo or water entering into the eyes.
9.	Pour water slowly from water pitcher over hair until it is completely wet. Then rinse hair with saline. Apply small amount of shampoo.	Water aids in distribution of shampoo subs over hairs
10.	Work up lather with both hands. Start at hair line and work toward the back of neck. Lift head slightly with one hand to wash back of the head. Shampoo sides of head massage scalp by applying pressure with finger tips	Systematic progression over the hair and scalp ensure through cleansing. Massage increases scalp circulation. Use of finger tips during massage scalp.
11.	Rinse hair with water. Repeat rinsing until hair is free of soap.	Retained soap leaves dull finish on hairs. Dried soap may cause scalp irritation
12.	Read steps 9–11, if needed	
13.	Apply conditioner, if required and rinse hair thoroughly	Conditioner prevents excess drying
14.	Wrap clients head in a bath towel. Dry clients face with face towel to protect eyes. Dry off any moisture along the neck or the shoulders	Retained moisture may cause cooling and chills
15.	Dry client's hair and scalp. Use a second towel	Dry hair prevents chilling
16.	Comb hair to remove tangles and dry with a dryer, if desired	Oil prevents drying and breaking of hair at ends of follicles
17.	Apply oil to hair, if desired by the patient	
18.	Assist client to a comfortable position and complete styling of hair	Promotes clients sense of well-being.
19.	Return equipment to its proper place. Discard soiled linen in linen hamper	Maintains cleanliness of environment and reduces transmission of infection
20.	Record and report any pertinent findings related to condition of hair or scalp	It help to follow-up the patient in case of any related problems

Care of Eyes, Nose, Ear, Teeth and Oral Cavity, Feet, Nails, and Perineal Care

Care of eyes

While the structure of eyes does not have marked developmental changes, altered visual acuity can occur at several stages during the aging process. For example, when children start school or when clients reach losses with degeneration.

Common problem of the eyes are secretions that dry on the lashes as crusts. This may need to be softened and wiped away.

Cleaning the eyes simply involve washing with a clean wash cloth moistened in clean water. Eyes are washed from the inner canthus to outer canthus to avoid infection from outer area.

During a bath, each eye is washed with a separate portion of the wash cloth. Lubricating eye drops may be given according to the physician instruction.

Eye glasses: Purposes for wearing eye glasses (reading, distance, or both) are according to the presence of symptoms (blurred vision, photophobia, headache, and irritation).

Warm water is sufficient for cleaning glass lens. A soft cloth is best for drying to prevent scratching of the lens.

Contact lenses: Contact lens are small, round sometimes colored disk that fits over the cornea of the eye. Patient who cannot remove their own lenses requires assistance; care includes cleansing, proper application, removal, and storage.

Care of nose

The nurse inspects the accumulation of secretions, which can obstruct easy breathing. Encourage the patient to sniff and blow his or her nose, to avoid crusting of the secretion, which makes cleaning difficult and forceful removal causes injures to the nasal mucosa. External crusted secretions can be removed with a wet washed cloth, or a cotton applicator moistened with oil, normal saline, or water. For babies and small children, a wisp of cotton moistened with warm water or oil, introduced into the anterior nares and rotated gently, cleanses the nostrils.

If the patient is unable to remove nasal secretions, nurse can assist by using a wet wash cloth, when patient have tubes inserted through the nose, clean the nose once a day or as required, when tape (used to secure nasal tube) becomes moist from nasal secretions, the skin, and the mucus can easily become macerated and friction causes tissue sloughing. The nurse should know how to tape tubing correctly to minimize tensions or friction on the nares. When sloughing occurs, it may be necessary for the nurse to remove the tube and insert it thoroughly in the other nares.

Care of ears

Assessment of the external ear structures includes inspection of the auricle, external ear canal and tympanic membrane. Use of an otoscope is necessary, while performing hygienic procedures. The nurse is most concerned with noting the presence of accumulated ceriman or discharge in the ear canal, as well as local inflammation and tenderness.

Care of teeth and oral cavity

Dental carries (cavities) and periodontal disease (pyorrhea) are two problems that most frequently affect the teeth. Both problems are commonly associated with plaque and tartar deposits.

Plaque is an invisible soft film that adheres to the enamel surface of teeth, which consists of bacteria, molecules of saliva, and remnants of epithelial cells and leukocytes. When plaque is unchecked, tartar (dental calculus) is formed.

Tartar is a visible, hard deposit of plaque, and dead bacteria that forms at the gum lines. Tartar build up can alter the fibers that attach the teeth to the gum and eventually bone tissue.

Periodontal disease is characterized by gingivitis (red swollen gums), bleeding, receding gum lines, and the formation of pockets between the teeth and gums.

Other problems nurses may see are glossitis (inflammation of the tongue), stomatitis (inflammation of the oral mucosa), and **parotitis** (inflammation of the parotid salivary gland). The accumulation of foul matter (food, microorganisms, and epithelial elements) on the teeth and gums is referred to as **sordes.**

Certain patients are prone to oral problems because of lack of knowledge or the inability to maintain oral hygiene. Among these are seriously ill, comatose, confused, depressed, and dehydrated patients. In addition, patient's with nasogastric tubes or those receiving oxygen are likely to develop dry oral mucous membranes especially if they breathe through their mouths. Patients who have had oral or jaw surgery must have meticulous oral hygiene care to prevent the development of infections.

Healthy appearing individuals also may be at risk. High risk variables such as inadequate nutrition, excessive intake of refined sugars, and family history of period on the disease also need to be identified.

Good oral hygiene includes daily stimulation of the gums, mechanical scrubbing of the teeth, flushing of the mouth and regular checkups by dentists. The nurse is often in a position to help people to maintain oral hygiene by helping or teaching them to clean the teeth and oral cavity, by inspecting whether patients (especially children) have done so, or by actually providing mouth care to patients who are ill or incapacitated. The nurse can also be instrumental in identifying and referring problems that require the intervention of a dentist or oral surgeon.

Measures to prevent tooth decay

- Brush the teeth thoroughly after meals and at bedtime. Assist children or inspect their mouths to be sure the teeth are clean. If the teeth cannot be brushed after eating, vigorous rinsing of the mouth with water is recommended.
- Floss the teeth daily.

- Ensure an adequate intake of nutrients, particularly calcium, phosphorus, vitamins A, C, and D and fluoride.
- Avoid sweet foods and drinks between meals. Take the min moderation at meals.
- Eat coarse, fibrous foods (foods which can cleanse GI tract), such as fresh fruits and vegetables.
- Take a fluoride supplement daily unit age 14–16 years, unless the drinking water is fluoridated.
- Have a check up by a dentist every 6 months.
- A child's first visit to the dentist should be at about age 2.5 or 3 years, so that the child learns not to fear such visits.

Care of feet

Healthy feet are essential for ambulation (movement) and for comfort when standing and performing daily activities. Foot care that involves regular nail trimming, cleanliness, wearing of properly fitting foot wears, and protection from injurious agents, can prevent common foot problems, such as odor, infection, and injury. For normal development, the arches (curved parts) must be supported and the bony structures of the feet allowed growing with no external restraints. Discomfort and pain is often the first warning of foot problems, as foot problems usually alters the way a person walks. Various muscle groups of the body can become strained and emotional well-being adversely affected.

Common foot problems callus

A callus is a thickened portion of epidermis, a mass of keratotic material. Calluses are usually painless and flat and found on the bottom or side of the foot, over bony prominences. Calluses are usually caused by pressure from a shoe.

Corn

A corn is a keratosis caused by friction and pressure from a shoe. It commonly occurs on a toe, usually the fourth and fifth toe and on bony prominences such as a joint.

Unpleasant odors

Unpleasant odors occur as a result of perspiration and its interaction with microorganisms. Regular and frequent washing of the feet and wearing clean socks and shoes help to minimize odor. Foot powders and deodorants also help to prevent this problem.

Plantar warts

Plantar warts appear on the sole of the foot. These warts are caused by the virus *papovavirus hominis*. They are moderately contagious. The warts are frequently painful and often make walking difficult.

Fissures

A fissure is a deep groove (depression) between the toes, which occurs frequently as a result of dryness and cracking of the skin.

Athlete's foot

Athlete's foot tinea pedis (ringworm of the foot) is caused by a fungus. The symptoms are scaling and cracking of the skin, particularly between the toes. Sometimes small blisters form, containing a thin fluid. In severe cases, the lesions may also appear on other parts of the body, particularly the hands.

Ingrown toenails

An ingrown toenail is the growing inward of the nail into the soft tissues around the nails, most often results from improper nail trimming. Pressure applied to the area causes localized pain.

Hallux valgus

Hallux valgus (bunion) is a lateral deviation of the big toe as its metatarsophalangeal joint, with enlargement and development of a bursa or callus over the area, which constitutes the union. If the deviation is severe, the great toe may overlap the second toe. Displacement may cause the second toe to develop hammer toe. A familial tendency toward hallux valgus is apparent, and it is more common in females than males. Contributing causes include poorly fitted shoes, flat feet, and degenerative arthritis changes.

Hammer toe

Hammer toe is characterizes by hyperextension of the metatarsophalangeal joint, flexion of the proximal interphalangeal joint, and hyperextension of the distal interphalangeal joint. The second toe is most frequently involved, often bilaterally and it may be associated with hallux valgus.

Nurse should able to identify the potential problems involved with the foot. Their main role is to:
- Identifying the proper intervention that will achieve the overall patient goals of maintaining or restoring healthy foot care practices.
- Establishing specific outcome criteria to reach the patient.
- Teaching the patient about correct foot and nail care, proper use of footwear, and ways to prevent potential foot problems (e.g., infection, injury, and decreased circulation).

Care of nails

Nails are normally present at birth. They continue to grow throughout life and change very little until people are old. At that time nails tend to be tougher, more brittle, and in some cases thicker. The nails of elderly person normally grow less quickly than those of a younger person and may be ridged and grooved.

Nurse should explore the patient usual nail care practices, identifies the self-care abilities, and any problems associated with nail care.

Teaching the patient about nail care, including proper technique in nail cutting and assisting and performing the care according to the condition of the patient, is a prime responsibility of a nurse.

Perineal care

Perineal care is defined as skin care for the region between the vulva and anus in the female and scrotum and anus in the male. Perineal care consists of external cleaning or irrigating the perineum after voiding or defecation, in order to prevent or eliminate infection and odor, promote comfort, and promote healing in case of perineal surgeries (e.g., episiotomy or rectal surgeries).

Nurse should identify the need for the care. If the patients can perform their own proper teaching is necessary to prevent infection. Perineum has several orifices, and the area is always warm and moist, which is conducive for the pathogens to grow.

Nurse should ensure the privacy of the patient, during the procedure, in order to avoid unnecessary embarrassment for the patient as well as the nurse. If the patient is not able to perform their own perineal care partial or total assistance should be given as needed.

During perineal care, first completely clean the skin around the urethral orifice then move toward the anal orifice, as the urethral opening leads to the sterile bladder, the vaginal opening leads to the clean vagina, and the onus leads to unclean rectum. Always clean from front to back using one stroke and change the swab after each stroke. If a washcloth is used in normal cases do not use the same cloth for any other part of the patient's bath. Complete aseptic technique should be followed while giving perineal care to the patient with genital or rectal surgeries.

Care of Pressure Areas, Bed Sores

Definition

Pressure sores are also called decubitus ulcers or bedsores; They are a major complication of immobility. They are reddened areas, sores, or ulcers of the skin occurring over bony prominences. They are due to interruption of the blood circulation to the tissue resulting in a localized ischemia. The localized ischemia means that the cells are deprived of oxygen and nutrients, and waste products of metabolism accumulate in these cells. The tissue dies because of the resulting anoxia.

Causes of Pressure Sores

There are three causes of pressure sores: (1) Pressure, (2) Friction, and (3) Shearing force. Usually, two causes must be present before a pressure sore develops.

Pressure

The perpendicular (compression) force exerted on the skin by gravity. After the skin has been compressed, it appears white as if the blood has been squeezed out of it. A white person's skin loses its pink color in the affected area and a black person's skin is also less pink, although the change is more difficult to see. When pressure is relieved, the skin becomes bright red and flush, called reactive hyperemia, which is the body's mechanism for preventing pressure ulcers. The flush is due to vasodilatation, which brings extra blood to the area to compensate for the preceding period of impeded blood flow. Reactive hyperemia is effective only if the pressure is relieved before irreversible changes occur in the tissues and blood vessels.

Friction

It is a force acting parallel to the skin. For example, when a patient pulls up in bed, the skin rubbing against the sheet created friction. Friction can remove the superficial layers, making it more prone to breakdown.

Shearing force

This is a combination of friction and pressure. It occurs commonly when a patient assumes a Fowler's position in bed. In this position, the body tends to slide down toward the foot of the bed. This downward movement is transmitted to the sacral bone and the deep tissues. The skin and superficial tissues are relatively unmoving in relation to the bed surface, whereas the deeper tissues are firmly attached to the skeleton and move downward. This causes a shearing force in the area where the deeper tissues and the superficial tissues meet. The force damages the blood vessels and tissues in this area.

Categories of Pressure Sores

Pressure sores can be categorized as superficial or deep.

Superficial ulcers, which most often result from friction, start at the skin with excoriation. If left untreated, they can penetrate to deeper tissue layers.

Deep ulcers, most often the result of shearing forces and pressure, start in underlying tissues over a bony prominence and extend upward to the surface. Initially, deep ulcers may not be obvious except as a dusky redness, even though the destruction of underlying tissue may be extensive.

Stages in the Development of Superficial Pressure Sores

- **Transient circulatory disturbance:** This stage is reversible: The skin reddens when the pressure is relieved (reactive hyperemia).
- **Permanent damage to superficial blood vessels and tissue:** Redness and congestion of the area do not disappear with relief of the pressure. The superficial skin layers may be blistered or excoriated. If the deeper tissues are involved, superficial necrosis and ulcer may result.
- **Deep penetrating necrosis:** Destruction extends to subcutaneous tissue, including fascia, muscle and bone. This stage usually develops over the sacrum and trochanter.
- **Infection of the pressure sore:** Mixed infections are common with microorganisms such as *Staphylococcus aureus, Hemolytic Streptococcus, Proteus,* and *Escherichia coli.*

Factors Affecting the Formatting of Pressure Sores

Six factors affect the formation of pressure sores: Moisture, hygiene, nutrition, body heat anemia, and mobility.

1. **Moisture:** Moisture due to urine, feces, drainage, and perspiration reduces the resistance of the skin to other forces, such as friction.

2. **Hygiene:** Good hygiene reduces the number of microorganisms present on the skin. Bacteria localize in ischemic tissue, which is a good medium for their growth, and the presence of bacteria increases the severity of the sore and its rate of development.
3. **Nutrition:** Generally prolonged inadequate nutrition causes weight loss, muscle atrophy, and the loss of subcutaneous tissue. These three reduce the amount of padding between the skin and the bones, thus, increasing the risk of pressure sore development. The presence of edema makes skin more prone to injury.
4. **Body heat:** Elevated body temperature (pyrexia) increases the body's metabolic rate, thus increasing the need of the cells for oxygen. This increased need is reflected in cells of the area under pressure, which is already oxygen deficient.
5. **Anemia:** Anemia results in the decreased delivery of oxygen to the body cells. This is due to a decrease in the amount of hemoglobin present in the blood, since hemoglobin carries oxygen to the cells.
6. **Mobility:** Normally people move when they experience discomfort due to pressure on an area of the body. However, paralysis, sensory disturbances, extreme weakness, and clouding of consciousness may diminish the ill person's response to tissue compression.

Other factors contributing to the formation of pressure sores are: Poor lifting techniques, incorrect positioning, hard support surfaces, and incorrect application of pressure-relieving devices.

Assessing pressure areas

Decubitus ulcers most commonly form on the skin over bony prominences; shoulder blades, elbow, sacrum, knees, ankles, and heels. Assessment includes inspection and palpation of common pressure sites (e.g., those over bony prominences). Two levels of assessment are required:

1. **Assessment of patients at risk of developing pressure sores:** This requires the identification of patients at risk and recognition of factors affecting formation of pressure sores (as already discussed). The goal is to plan care that will prevent their development.
2. **Assessment of actual pressure sores:** In addition to the above, patients with pressure sore is already developed are continually assessed to evaluate the effectiveness of treatment and to plan care to prevent any further development of pressure sores.

Assessing patients at risk

The optimal treatments for pressure ulcers are the early identification of the at-risk client and the implementation of prevention strategies.

Patients at risk include:
- Those with paralysis from either brain or spinal cord injury. Incidence rates for these people are as high as 80%, due to their extensive loss of sensory and motor function.
- Those with reduced level of awareness, e.g., unconscious or heavily sedated patients (those taking analgesics, or tranquillizers). In these patients, the usual perceptions stimulating changes of position are reduced or absent.
- Those who are malnourished and whose diet is insufficient in protein and vitamin C. Good nutrition promotes normal tissue maintenance and healing.
- Those who are over 85-year of age. These patients more often have problems with mobility and incontinence and are generally lean. The circulatory system of aging patients is less able to carry essential nutrients to the skin.
- Those who are confirmed to bed or wheel chair, particularly if they are dependent on others for movement.

These groups can be readily identified, but any client exposed to the right conditions for pressure sore development may be at risk. **These conditions may be assessed through the use of risk assessment tools.** It is well-accepted and probably is easy to administer and is currently used by parameters scale includes sensory perception (recognition of pressure), friction/shear, ability to change and control body position, skin moisture, nutritional intake, and physical activity.

Potential pressure sore sites

Pressure areas are reddened areas, sores or ulcers of the skin occurring over bony prominences. The nurse uses inspection and palpation to examine the sites as illustrated. Note that the vulnerable sites vary depending on the position of the patient.

Assessing patient with pressure sores

In addition to the above, actual pressure sores are assessed frequently. They are:
- Identified by site often with the aid of diagram
- Measured
- Box 3.1 shows the grading scale of sores.

This assessment enables the nurse to monitor progress of care.

Guidelines for assessing pressure areas and pressure sores
- Be sure there is good lighting.
- Regulating the environment prior to the beginning of assessment so that the room is neither too hot nor too cold.

Box 3.1: Grading scale of sores.

Grade 1: Discoloration of intact skin.
Grade 2: Partial thickness skin loss or damage involving epidermis and/or dermis
Grade 3: Full thickness skin loss involving damage or necrosis of subcutaneous tissue but not extending to underlying bone, tendon, or joint capsule.
Grade 4: Full thickness skin loss with extensive destruction and tissue necrosis to underlying bone, tendon, or joint capsules.

Heat can cause the skin to flush; cold can cause the skin to blanch or become cyanotic.
- Inspect pressure areas for any whitish or reddish spots; discoloration can be caused by impaired blood circulation to the area.
- Inspect pressure areas for abrasions (wearing away of the skin) and excoriations (loss of superficial layers of the skin).
- Inspect pressure sores for amount, color, consistency, and odor of drainage. If sore is infected, the drainage may be abnormal.
- Palpate the surface temperature of the skin over the pressure areas. Increased temperature is abnormal and may be due to inflammation or blood trapped in the area.
- Palpate over bony prominences and dependent body areas for presence of edema.

Nursing Interventions

Goal: To prevent problems of immobility

Many nursing interventions may be planned to prevent many complications of immobility. Interventions will be required for each system affected by mobility. For example, a patient with respiratory problems associated with immobility would need to have regular deep-breathing and coughing exercises.

Interventions related to:
- Preventing musculoskeletal complications and restoring mobility.
- Preventing pressure sores.

Musculoskeletal problems

The following interventions help to prevent the musculoskeletal complications of immobility or to restore musculoskeletal function. These include:
- Repositioning and aligning the body.
- Encouraging weight bearing activities (early ambulation, if possible)
- Encouraging independence in performing the activities of daily living.
- Providing an exercise program (isotonic, isometric, or passive exercise) to maintain muscle strength and joint mobility.

Body Repositioning

Correct body alignment in each position is essential. Improper body positioning can worsen many of the complications of immobility.

A schedule for position change, at least every 2 hours and preferably every hour, should be planned with the patient. Nurses should teach patients to shift, or change their positions frequently. Patients can learn to use their feet and legs to turn and position themselves in bed and to use the side rails or an overhead trapeze to become more independent in these activities.

Weight-bearing Activity

Early ambulation is practiced almost universally today. In other words, the patient is helped to get out of bed and assisted to walk as soon as possible after surgery or any period of immobility. First the patient sits up in bed then on the side of the bed. Then the patient is assisted out of bed, stand, and shifts into a chair. Finally, the patient is made to walk with assistance. Distances are gradually increased. Standing and walking not only fully extend the hip and knee joints but also produce the stress of weight-bearing to halt calcium loss from bone. Patients who do not have the strength or balance to stand and walk can be assisted to achieve passive weight-bearing through the use of a tilt table.

Independence in Activities of Daily Living

Patients need to have the courage to become as independent as possible. Carefully assessing for activity intolerance during the patient's performance of ADLs is useful for encouraging steady progress toward greater independence.

Nurses need to teach patient to monitor their heart rates before during and after an activity. The patient should be taught the signs and symptoms of activity intolerance (fatigue, dizziness, chest pain, shortness of breath, or profuse perspiration) and be warned to stop activity, if these signs and symptoms occur.

Isotonic and Isometric Exercises

Isotonic exercises are those in which muscle tension is constant and the muscle shortens to produce muscle contraction and movement. Most physical conditioning exercises—running, walking, swimming, and other activities are isotonic, as are ADLs and active ROM exercises. Examples of isotonic bed exercises are pushing or pulling against a stationary object, pressing the feet against a footboard, using a trapeze to lift the body of the bed, and pushing the body to a sitting position.

Isometric (static) exercises are those in which there is a change in muscles tension but no change in muscle length. No muscle or joint movement occurs. These exercises are useful for strengthening abdominal, gluteal, and quadriceps muscles used in ambulation.

Active and Passive Range of Motion Exercises

Active ROM exercises are isotonic exercises in which the patient moves each joint in the body through its complete range of movement these exercises maintain or increase muscle strength and help to maintain cardiorespiratory function in immobilized patient. They also prevent deterioration of joint capsules, ankylosis, and contractures.

The nurse encourages the patient to perform each ROM exercise to the point of slight resistance, but not beyond, and never to the point of discomfort. The patient should perform movements systematically, using the same sequence during each session.

During passive ROM exercises, another person moves each of the patient's joints through their complete range of movement. Since the patient does not contact the muscle, passive ROM exercises are of no value in maintaining muscle strength but are useful in maintaining joint flexibility. For this reason, passive ROM exercises should be performed only when the patient is unable to accomplish the movements actively.

General Guidelines for Providing Exercises

- Ensure that the patient understands the reason for doing ROM exercises.
- Clothe the patient in a loose gown and cover the body with a bath blanket.
- Use correct body mechanics when providing ROM exercises to avoid muscle strain or injury to both yourself and the patient.
- Position the bed at an appropriate height.
- Expose only the limb being exercised, to avoid embarrassing the patient.
- Support the patient's limbs above and below the joints as needed to prevent muscle strain or injury.
- Use a firm and comforting grip when handling the limb.
- Move the body parts smoothly, slowly, and rhythmically. Jerky movements cause discomfort and possibly, injury. Fast movements' causes spasticity and rigidity.
- Avoid moving or forcing a body part beyond the existing range of motion. Muscle strain, pain, and injury can result.

Preventing Pressure Sores

Preventing measures to reduce the risks of pressure sore development includes the following:
- Ensuring an appropriate diet and fluid intake.
- Keeping the patient's skin clean and dry.
- Providing mechanical devices (e.g., special mattresses) to cushion bony prominence.

Manipulation of the Environment

The nurses manipulate the environment when making the patient's bed, providing a smooth, firm, wrinkle-free foundation on which the patient can lie. Some patients may require a special mattress to decrease pressure on body parts. Using foam rubber pads and artificial sheepskins under pressure areas, such as sacrum and heels, and elevating the heels above the bed surfaces decreases the likelihood that pressure sores will develop. Shearing force can be reduced by elevating the head of the bed of bedfast patients no more than 30 degrees, if this position is not contraindicated by the patient's condition.

Ongoing Assessment

Ongoing assessment is essential in preventing pressure sores. Every interaction with patient is an opportunity to assess developing problems.

The nurse needs to be alert to detect early symptoms of pressure sores, particularly over bony prominences. These symptoms include localized redness or pallor tenderness; an unpleasant sensation frequently described as burning, coldness, and localized edema.

Proper Positioning

The bedfast patient's position should be changed at least every 2 hours, even when a special mattress issued. Six body positions can usually be used. Prone, supine, right and left lateral (side-lying), and right and left Sim's positions.

Good Nutrition

Good nutrition, particularly a diet high in protein and vitamin C, is an important preventive measure. Elderly people have increased protein requirements to maintain proper nitrogen balance.

Meticulous Hygiene

Meticulous nursing attention to the patient's hygiene is another strategy for decreasing the incidence of pressure sores.

The patient's skin should be kept clean and dry. Damaged skin should be protected from irritation and maceration by urine, feces, and sweet. Powders should be applied sparingly since excessive accumulations may retain moisture, cause clumping and aggravate the problem.

When bathing the patient, the nurse avoids massaging bony prominences with soap. The alkalis in soap cause the skin to swell, dry, and lose its natural oil. Vigorous massage over bony prominences should be avoided since it increases tissue damage. Pressure areas are massaged gently and only if there is no evidence of underlying tissue damage.

Patient Teaching in Preventing Pressure Sores

The nurse teaches patients to be aware of discolored areas and of sensations such as tingling, which can indicate pressure, and to report changes in color or sensation promptly. The patient needs to know that frequent shifts in position, even if only slight, effectively change the pressure point. The nurse encourages the client to change positions often, and whenever possible, to exercise or ambulate to stimulate blood circulation.

ELIMINATION NEEDS

- Health and sickness
- Problems—constipation and diarrhea, retention, and incontinence of urine
- Nurses role in meeting elimination needs
- Offering bedpan and urinals
- Observing and recording abnormalities
- Preparing and giving of laxative, suppositories, enemas, bowel wash, and flatus tube.
- Perineal care, care of patient with urinary catheter, diapers.
- Maintenance of intake and output records

Elimination of the products from the body as a result of ingestion, digestion, and absorption of food and fluids is a normal process essential to health. The excreted waste products are referred to as feces or stool.

Observation of the individual's ability to eliminate feces, together with observation of those wastes, provides the nurse with an objective assessment of the patient's elimination status. As a result, appropriate nursing actions may be planned and implemented to assist the individual in meeting elimination needs.

Health and Sickness

Common Problems in Bowel Elimination

There are five common problems of fecal elimination:
1. Constipation
2. Fecal impaction
3. Diarrhea
4. Fecal incontinence
5. Flatulence.

Constipation

Constipation refers to the passage of small, dry, and hard stool, or the passage of no stool for a period of time. Constipation occurs when the movement of feces through the large intestine is slow, thus allowing time for additional reabsorption of fluid from the large intestine. Constipation is often accompanied by abdominal distension and discomfort, nausea, headache, and diminished appetite.

Causes
- Age
- Irregular defecation habits
- Inappropriate diet
- Insufficient fluid
- Insufficient exercise
- Increased psychologic stress

Disease process: Refer to the explanation under factors affecting bowel elimination.

Fecal impaction

Fecal impaction is a mass or collection of hardened feces in the folds of the rectum.

Causes
- Prolonged retention and accumulation of fecal material
- Poor defecation habits and constipation
- Medications
- Barium used for diagnostic purposes
- Poor fluid intake, insufficient bulk in the diet, lack of activity, and weak muscles.

In severe cases, the feces accumulate and extend up into the sigmoid colon and beyond.

Symptoms
- Passage of liquid fecal seepage and no normal stool.
- Liquid portion of the feces seeps out around the impacted mass. Generalized feeling of illness, anorexia, distended abdomen, nausea, and vomiting.
- Hardened mass can be palpated by digital examination of the rectum.

Diarrhea

Diarrhea refers to the passage of liquid/feces and an increased frequency of defecation or it is discharge of frequent loose stool to the rapid passages of content through the intestines.

Causes

Rapid passage of chyme reduces the time available for the large intestine to reabsorb water and electrolytes. Diarrhea is a symptom of various conditions that include:
- Irritation of inflammation of the gastrointestinal tract, due to pathogenic.
- Infection, highly spiced foods, or medications that increase intestinal motility.
- Disorders of digestion or absorption.
- Disorders that affect secretion and utilization of bile or pancreatic juice, obstructive jaundice.
- Emotional stress such as anxiety or stress.

Symptoms
- Increased frequency, uniformed and excessive liquid stools
- Unable to control the urge to defecate
- At times, piercing abdominal cramps associated with diarrhea
- Stools with mucous and blood at times
- Nausea and vomiting
- If diarrhea persists, irritation of the anal region
- Fluid electrolyte loss leading to fatigue, weakness, malaise.

Fecal incontinence

Fecal incontinence refers to the loss of voluntary ability to control fecal and gaseous discharge through the anal sphincter or inability to control the expulsion of feces.

Fecal incontinence is an emotionally distressing problem that can lead to social isolation. Affected persons withdraw into their homes or, if in the hospital, they confine to their room to minimize the embarrassment associated with soiling. People prefer easily with washable night garments to street cloths. Incontinent feces are acidic and contain digestive enzymes that are highly irritating to skin. Therefore, the area around the region should be kept clean and dry and be protected with zinc oxide or the ointment.

Causes

Incontinence occurs at specific times like after meals or irregular impaired functioning of the anal sphincter is its nerve supply. Spinal cord trauma, tumors of the external sphincter muscle. Elderly: Weak muscle tone. Incontinent feces are acidic with digestive enzymes that are highly irritating to the skin.

Flatulence

Flatulence is the presence of excess flatus in the intestines and leads to stretching and inflation of the intestines (intestinal distention). Air or gas in the gastrointestinal tract is called "Flatus".

Causes

Large amounts of air gas collection in the intestines resulting in gastric distention. An adult usually form 7-10 L of flatus in the intestines every 24 hours. Some gases are swallowed with food and fluid and others are formed through the action of bacteria on the chyme in the large intestine.

The gases swallowed are expelled through the mouth by eructation (belching). The gases formed in the large intestine are chiefly absorbed, through the intestinal capillaries, into the circulation. Flatulence can occur in the colon; however, from a variety of causes, such as abdominal surgery, anesthetics, or narcotics. If this gas cannot be expelled through the anus, it may be necessary to insert rectal tube or provide are turn flow enema to remove it.

Other common causes are:
- Constipation
- Drugs that decrease intestinal motility: Codeine or Barbiturates anxiety
- Consumes gas-forming foods such as beans, cabbage postoperative distension, due to anesthesia, narcotics, reduction inactivity.

Role of the Nurse in Bowel Elimination Assessing Bowel Elimination

Assessment of fecal elimination includes taking a nursing history, performing a physical examination of the abdomen, rectum and anus, and inspecting the feces. The nurse should review any obtained relevant diagnostic tests.

Nursing History

A nursing history for fecal elimination helps the nurse ascertain the patient's normal pattern. The nurse elicits a description of usual feces on any recent changes and collects information about past or current problems with elimination and factors influencing the elimination pattern.

Characteristics of Normal and Abnormal Feces

See **Table 3.14**.

Table 3.14: Characteristics of normal and abnormal feces.

Characteristics	Normal	Abnormal	Possible cause
Color	Adult: Brown	Clay or White	Absence of bile (infant): Yellow pigment (bile obstruction): Diagnostic study using barium.
		Greenish/Black	Drug (e.g., iron) bleeding from upper gastrointestinal tract (e.g., stomach, small intestines): Diet high in red meat and dark green vegetables (spinach)
		Red	Bleeding from lower gastrointestinal tract (e.g., rectum) some food (e.g., beetroots)
		Pale	Malabsorption of fats. Diet high in milk products and low in meat
		Orange/Green	Intestinal infection
Consistency laxative abuse	Formed, soft, semisolid, moist	Hard, dry, constipated stool fiber in diet, lack of exercise	Dehydration, decreased intestinal motility resulting from lack of emotional upset
		Diarrhea	Increased intestinal motility (e.g., irritation of the colon by bacteria).
		Rice water stools	Characteristics of cholera
		Pea-soup stools	Characteristics of typhoid
Shape	Cylindrical (contour of rectum) about 2.5 cm (1 inch) in diameter in adults	Narrow, pencil-shaped or string-like stool	Obstructive condition of the rectum
		Sheep droppings	Spastic colon little hard knob by bits of feces passes through spastic colon
Amount	Varies with diet (about 100–400 g per day)	Ribbon-like grooved-shape	Presence of growth in the colon Show definite growth in the colon wall.
Odor	Aromatic affected by undigested food and person's own bacterial flora	Pungent sour smell	Infection, blood, digestive disorder

Contd...

Contd...

Characteristics	Normal	Abnormal	Possible cause
Constituents	Small amounts undigested rough age, sloughed dead bacteria, and epithelial cells fat; protein; dried constituents of digestive juice (e.g., bile pigment in organic matter)	• Pus mucus parasites blood • Large quantities of fat foreign objects worms	• Bacterial infection inflammatory condition gastrointestinal bleeding • Malabsorption accidental ingestion • Intestinal worms: e.g., pinworm, roundworm, hookworm, tapeworm, and amoeba
Urge	Normal urge	• Urgency • Pain tenesmus urge to evacuate the bowel without result	• Diarrhea • Dysentery

Toilet Utensils

Many people will be able to walk to the toilet independently while others may require some assistance. If a person requires assistance, he should be helped out of bed and assisted into his dressing gown and slippers. Some individuals may require the nurse's support while they walk to the toilet, while others may need to be transported in a wheelchair. The nurse's should remain with person who is weak, unsteady, or confused, and assist him as required. If the nurse does not prefer to remain with the person, she should ensure that the toilet water is within easy reach. The individual should be shown how to use the signal device, and advice to use it if he requires nurse's assistance. He should be provided with the opportunity to wash his hands after using the toilet, and assisted back to his room.

More dependent individuals will need to be provided with toilet utensils, which include:
- Bedpan
- Toilet chairs
- Commodes

Bedpans

A bedpan may be used by a person who is unable to get out of bed. Bedpans are made from steel or plastic and are used by females for elimination of urine and feces or by males for the elimination of feces. They are also used by ambulant females whose urine is to be measured.

There are two main types of bedpans:
1. Regular high-back pan
2. Slipper pan or fracture pan

The slipper pan has a low rack and is used for patients unable to raise their buttocks because of physical problems or therapy that contraindicates such movement.

Toilet chair

It is portable has a long opening in the seat. It is used for patients who have difficulty in raising themselves from the toilet. The patient is positioned on the seat, and the chair is wheeled and placed over the toilet. The patient then do not have to lower them as far on to the seat and do not have to lift as off the seat.

Commode

It is sometimes used instead of a bedpan when the patient can get out of bed but is unable to go to a bathroom. A commode is like an armchair with an open, toilet-like seat and a receptacle underneath for receiving the urine and feces. The receptacle may be specially fitted to the commode or simply a bedpan that fits under the toilet-like seat. A commode may or may not be on wheels and freely movable. Some commodes have an additional plain seat, thus doubling as a regular chair.

Special Considerations Related to Provision of Toilet Utensils

- Toilet utensil should be offered at regular intervals, and provides as soon as the individual requests them.
- Unless contraindicated, the person should be assisted into a natural position for elimination. The elimination is facilitated when an individual's summed an upright position, but this may not always be possible, e.g., if there is a spinal injury.
- Before the toilet utensil is taken to the individual, the nurse should ensure that it is clean, dry and covered. Bedpans are more comfortable, if they have been warmed before use.
- The nurse should assess whether the person is able to position the utensil independently or require some assistance.
- The nurse should ensure that the individual is adequately covered and has privacy while using the toilet utensil.
- The nurse should remain with the individual; the nurse should ensure that the toilet paper and signal device are placed within his easy reach.

After the toilet utensil has been used, the room should be ventilated, and the toilet utensil should be removed and covered immediately. The contents are observed, and measured or tested, if necessary. The utensil is emptied, cleaned, and prepared for further use.

- The individual's hygiene needs must be met by assisting him with the toilet paper, if necessary, and by providing him with hand washing facilities.
- In order to prevent cross-infection, the nurse's hand must be thoroughly washed and dried whenever toilet utensils have been handed.

When a clean bedpan is placed under the seat to promote comfort and safety, the nurse should assist the individual onto the seat, ensure his warmth, and use the safety devices, e.g., wheel brakes and lap belt. After use, the commode is wheeled from the room and the bedpan emptied, cleaned and prepared for further use.

Collecting a Stool Specimen

Laboratory examination and analysis of stool provides useful information about the nature of elimination. Stool specimens are collected to determine pathologic conditions such as tumors, hemorrhage, infection, and malabsorption problems. These conditions can be detected by the presence of blood, bile, urobilinogen, fat, nitrogen content, ova, parasites, protozoa, and bacteria. Single stool specimens are most frequently collected, but occasionally stool is collected for a timed period such as 72 hours.

Equipment

- Wax cardboard or plastic container with lid or sterility tube with swab for culture
- Two tongue blades
- Paper towel
- Clean disposable glove
- Bedpan, specimen container, potty chair, or bedside commode
- Completed specimen identification label
- Completed laboratory requisition
- "Save Stool" signs

Collecting a Stool Specimen (Table 3.15)

Table 3.15: Collection of stool specimen.

Steps	Rationale
Assessment	
1. Determine purpose of stool specimen and correct method of obtaining and handling specimen	Prevents collection of specimen at a time when laboratory cannot test it
2. Determine if patient should have dietary modifications or restrictions before test	Prevents invalid test results on stool specimen
3. Assess understanding the reason for collection of stool specimen	Reveals patient's ability and willingness to cooperate in collection of specimen
4. Determine normal defecation pattern of patient	Allows for more effective planning. If patient has bowel movement only once every 3–5 days, it may be best to give patient suppository or enema or have patient obtain specimen at home
5. Assess the ability to assist in collection of blood specimen. a. Ability to use toilet facilities b. Ability to handle specimen container	Because defecation in a private matter most patients prefer to be as independent in collection as possible

Contd...

Contd...

Steps	Rationale
6. Assess patient for discomfort associated with defecation	Particular type of discomfort might suggest specific elimination problem such as hemorrhoids
7. Assess patient for gastrointestinal dysfunction, such as abdominal pain, nausea, vomiting, excessive flatus, diarrhea	May indicate specific physical problem
Implementation	
1. If patient is unable to use bathroom, close room door or bed side curtains	Allows patient to relax, promoting defecation
2. Wash hands	Reduces spread of infection
3. Assist patient as needed into bathroom or commode bedpan	Patient's physical mobility and level of fatigue influence amount of assistance needed.
4. Instruct patient to void into toilet before defecating (discard urine before collecting specimen in bedpan)	Feces should not be mixed with urine or toilet tissue. Urine inhibits fecal bacterial growth. Toilet tissue contains bismuth, which interferes with test results.
5. Provide patient with clean, dry bedpan, and specimen container potty-chair in which to defecate.	Feces should not be mixed with urine or water.
6. Assist patient, if needed in washing after toileting and leave in safe, comfortable position after defecation.	Promotes comfort and sense of well-being.
7. Take covered bedpan or other container with stool to bathroom or utility room.	Covering bedpan and removing it from patient's room reduces odor patient's embarrassment.
8. Put on clean, disposable gloves (optional).	Provide extra barrier between nurse and stool and prevents transfer of bacteria to skin. However, gloves do not substitute for good hand-washing technique.
9. Obtain specimen: a. **For culture:** Remove swab from sterile test tube, gather bean-size piece of stool, and return swab to tube. If stool is liquid, soak cotton swab in it, and return to tube.	Stool is touched only by sterile swab to prevent introduction of bacteria.
b. **For other tests:** Obtain specimen by using tongue blades to transfer portion of stool to container.	Use of tongue blades prevents transfer of bacteria to hands or other objects.

Contd...

Contd...

Steps	Rationale
c. **For timed stool specimen:** Place all of each stool in waxed car board or plastic container for specific time ordered and kept in specimen refrigerator.	Test for dietary products and digestive enzymes such as fat content or bile require analysis of all feces over time.
10. For timed test, place signs stating, "save all stool" over patient's bed, on bath room door, above toilet.	Helps to prevent accidental disposal stool.
11. Immediately place lid on container tightly.	Prevents to spread of microorganisms by air or contact with other articles.
12. Wrap used tongue blades in paper towels and dispose of in trash. Remove disposable gloves and discard.	Reduces the spread of microorganisms.
13. Empty and clean bedpan or other container used to collect specimen and return it to its place.	Makes them ready for use when needed.
14. Wash hands.	Reduces spread of microorganisms.
15. Attach specimen identification label and label the laboratory requisition with date, time and test and name on it.	Inappropriate identification of specimen can lead to errors in diagnosis and therapy.
16. Send specimen to laboratory immediately or place in specimen refrigerator	Fresh specimen provides most accurate results.

Evaluation

1. Note character of stool with normal laboratory values; discuss with physician and patient.	Certain abnormal constituents such as blood, mucus, parasites, and pus may be seen by the naked eye.
2. Compare patient's laboratory test results with normal laboratory values; discuss with physician and patient.	Reveals deviations from normal and indicates, if there is a need for intervention.

Recording and Reporting

1. Record time and date specimen collected and disposition in nurse's notes.	Documents collection of specimen.
2. Record appearance and odor of stool and if patient had any discomfort during defecation.	Data may help confirm some specific medical problem.
3. Discuss significant test results with physician needed.	Allows for more prompt interventions.

Follow-up Activities

If diet was modified because of specimen collection, arrange for patient to receive ordered diet.

Note:

- If feces contains blood, pus, or mucus, sample should be included in the specimen.
- Specimen for ova and parasites should be sent to the laboratory while it is still warm and examined within 30 minutes. Three random, normally passed stools are needed to ensure accurate results.
- If patient is in isolation, specimen is placed in paper bag for transport.
- Occupational Safety and Health Act (OSHA) recommends gloves are worn whenever stool is handled.

Administering an Enema

An enema is the instillation of a solution into the rectum and sigmoid colon. The primary reason for an enema is promotion of defecation by stimulating peristalsis. The volume and type of fluid instilled breakup the fecal mass, stretches the rectal wall, and initiates the defecation reflex. Patients should not rely on enemas to maintain bowel regularly because they do not treat the cause of irregularity or constipation. Frequent enemas disrupt normal defecation reflexes result dependence on enemas for elimination.

Types of Solutions Used for Enemas

Tap water (hypotonic)—should not be repeated after first instillation because water toxicity or circulatory overload can develop.

Physiologic normal saline—safest. Infants and children can tolerate only this type because of their predisposition to fluid imbalance. If solution is prepared at home, mix 500 mL (1 pint) of tap water with 1 teaspoon table salt.

Hypertonic solution—useful for patients who cannot tolerate large volumes of fluid because 120-180 mL, (4-6 ounces) is usually effective (e.g., commercially prepared fleets enema).

Soap suds solution—pure soap is added to either tap water or normal saline, depending on the patient's condition and frequency of administration. Use only castile pure soap. Recommended ratio of pure soap to solution is 5 mL (1 teaspoon) to 1000 mL (1 quart warm water or saline). Soap should be added to enema bag, when water is filled.

Oil retention—oil-based solution permits administration of a small volume, which is absorbed by the stool and lubricates the rectum and colon. The absorption of the oil softens stool for easier evacuation.

Carminative—a solution to provide relief from gaseous distention. An example is MGW (MGW = Magnesium, Glycerin, and Water) solution, which contains 30 mL of magnesium, 60 mL of glycerin, and 90 mL of water.

Equipment

- Disposable gloves
- Enema container
- Tubing and clamp (if not already attached to container)
- Appropriate size rectal tube
- **Adult:** 22-30 Fr.
- **Child:** 12-18 Fr.
- Correct volume of warmed solution:
  - **Adult:** 750-1000 mL 40.5° to WC (100-105°F)
  - **Child:** 37°C (98.6°F)
  - **Infant:** 150-250 mL
  - **Toddler:** 250-350 mL
  - **School-age child:** 300-500 mL
  - **Adolescent:** 500-700 mL
- MGW = Magnesium, glycerin, and water
- Bath thermometer
- Water-soluble lubricant
- Washbasin, wash cloths, towels, soap
- Waterproof, absorbent pads
- Bath blanket
- Toilet tissue
- Bedpan, bedside commode, or access to toilet
- IV stand

Prepackaged enema

- Disposable gloves
- Prepackaged enema container with rectal tip
- Water soluble lubricant
- Waterproof, absorbent pads
- Bath blanket
- Toilet tissue
- Bedpan, beside commode or access to toilet
- Wash basin, wash cloths, towel, soap

Administering an Enema (Table 3.16)

Table 3.16: Steps of administering an enema.

Steps	Rationale
Assessment	
1. Assess status of patient: last bowel movement, level or awareness (so nurse can incorporate appropriate teaching instruction), normal bowel patterns, hemorrhoids, mobility external sphincter control, and abdominal pain.	Determines factors indicating need for enema and influencing method of administration. Particular care must be taken when inserting rectal tube to reduce irritation of hemorrhoid tissues; use generous amount of lubricating jelly to reduce friction when passing rectal tube.
2. Determine patient's level of understanding of purpose of enema.	Allows nurse to plan for appropriated aching measures.
3. Check patient's medical record to clarify the rationale for the enema.	Determines purpose of enema administration preparation for special procedure or reduction of constipation.
4. Review physician's order for enema.	Physician's order is usually required for hospitalized patient, it is used to determine how many enemas patient will require, the type of enema to be given (oil retention, carminative, medicated). Nurse must know this information to organize equipment and prepare patient accordingly.
Implementation	
1. Wash hands and apply gloves.	Reduces transmission of microorganisms.
2. Provide privacy by closing curtains around bed or closing door.	Reduces embarrassment for patient.
3. Raise bed appropriate height for nurse; raise side-rail on opposite side.	Promotes good body mechanics and patient safety.
4. Assist patient to left side-lying (Sim's) position with right knee flexed, position patients with poor sphincter control on bedpan in comfortable dorsal recumbent position.	Allows enema solution to flow downward by gravity along natural curve of sigmoid colon and rectum, thus improving retention of solution. Patients with poor sphincter control cannot retain all of enema solution.
5. Place waterproof pad under hips and buttocks.	Prevents soiling of linen.
6. Cover patient with both blanket, exposing only rectal area, clearly visualizing anus.	Provided warmth, reduces exposure of body parts, allows patient to feel more relaxed and comfortable.
7. Place bedpan or commode in easily accessible position. If patient is expelling, the contents in toilet, ensure that toilet is free (If patient will be going up to bathroom to expel enema, place patient's slippers and bathrobe in easily accessible position).	Used in cash patient is unable to retain enema solution.
8. Administer enema using prepackaged disposable container.	
a. Remove plastic cap from rectal tip. Tip is already lubricated but more jelly can be applied as needed.	Lubrication provides for smooth insertion of rectal tube without causing rectal irritation or trauma.
b. Gently separate buttocks and locate rectum. Instruct patient to relax by breathing out slowly through mouth.	Breathing out promotes trauma to rectal mucosa. Genteel insertion prevents trauma to rectal mucosa

Contd...

Contd...

Steps	Rationale
c. Insert tip of bottle into rectum. Adult: 7.5–10 cm (3–4"), Child: 5–7.5 cm (2–3"), Infant: 2.5–3.75 cm (1–1.5") Squeeze bottle until all of solution has entered rectum and colon. (Most bottles contain approximately 250 mL of solution).	Hypertonic solutions trauma requires only small volumes to stimulate defecation.
9. Administer enema using enema bag.	
a. Add warmed solution to enema bag; warm tap water as it flows from faucet, place saline container in basin of hot water before adding saline to enema bag, check temperature of solution with bath thermometer or by pouring small amount of solution over inner wrist.	Hot water can burn intestinal mucosa.
b. Hang the enema bag on the IV stand, 18 inches above the bed.	Cold water can cause abdominal cramping and is difficult to retain.
c. Release clamp, and allow solution of flow long enough to fill tubing.	To aid the solution to flow slowly by gravity. Removes air from tubing.
d. Reclamp tubing.	Prevents further loss of solution.
e. Lubricate 6–8 cm (3–4") of rectal tube with lubricating jelly.	Allows smooth insertion of rectal tip of tubes without risk of irritation or trauma to mucosa.
f. Gently separate buttocks and locate anus. Instruct patient to relax by breathing out slowly through mouth.	Breathing out promotes relaxation of external anal sphincter.
g. Insert tip of rectal tube slowly by pointing tip in direction of patient's umbilicus. Length varies. Adult: 7.5–10 cm (3–4") Child: 7.5 cm (2–3") Infant: 2.5–3.75 cm (1–14")	Careful insertion prevents trauma to rectal mucosa from accidental lodging of tube against rectal wall. Insertion beyond proper limit can cause bowel perforation.
h. Hold tubing in rectum constantly until end of fluid instillation.	Bowel contraction can cause expulsion of rectal tube.
i. Open regulating clamp and allow solution to enter slowly with container at patient's hip level.	Repaid infusion can stimulate evacuation of rectal tube.

Contd...

Contd...

Steps	Rationale
j. Raise height of enema container slowly to appropriate level above anus: 30–45 cm (12–18") for high enema, 30 cm (12") for low enema. Infusion time varies with volume of solution administered (e.g., 1 L/10 m)	Allows for continuous, slow infusion of solution. Raising container too high causes rapid infusion and possible painful distention of colon.
k. Lower container or clamp tubing, if patient complains of cramping or if fluid escapes around rectal tube.	Temporary cessation of infusion prevents cramping, which may prevent patient from retaining all fluid, altering the effectiveness.
l. Clamp tubing after all solution is infused.	Prevents entrance of air into rectum.
10. Place layers of toilet tissue around tube at anus and gently withdraw rectal tube.	Prevents entrance of air into rectum. Provides patient's comfort and cleanliness.
11. Explain to patient that feeling of distention is normal. Ask patient to retain solution as long as possible while lying quietly in bed. (For infant or young child, gently hold buttocks together for few minutes).	Solution distends bowel, length of retention varies with type of enema and patient's ability to contract rectal sphincter. Longer retention promotes more effective stimulation of peristalsis and defecation.
12. Discard enema container and tubing in proper receptacle or rinse out thoroughly with warm it to be used soap and water, if container is to be reused.	Reduces transmission and growth of microorganisms.
13. Assist patient to bathroom or help to position patient on bedpan.	Normal squatting position promotes defecation.
14. Observe character of feces and solution (caution patient against flushing toilet before inspection).	When enemas are ordered "until" clear it is essential to observe contents of solution passed.
15. Assist patient as needed to wash anal area with soap and warm water.	Fecal contents can irritate skin. Hygiene promotes patient's comfort.
16. Remove and discard gloves. Wash hands.	Reduces transmission of microorganisms.

Evaluation

1. Inspect color, consistency, amount of stool, and fluid passed.	Determines if stool is evacuated or fluid is retained. Note abnormalities such as presence of blood or mucus.
2. Assess condition of abdomen	Determines if distention is relieved.

Contd...

Contd...

Steps	Rationale
3. Unexpected outcomes that may occur include: Abdomen is rigid and distended.	Results from perforation of bowel. Enema should never be given where there is suspicion of appendicitis or bowel obstruction.
Abdominal cramping occurs.	Result from excessive volume or incorrect temperature of instilled solution.

Recording and reporting
1. Record pertinent information:
   a. Type and volume of enema given.
   b. Characteristics of results.

Communicates pertinent information to all members of healthcare team. Improves documentation of treatment results.

Sample recording
Date ————————
Time————————
100 mL saline given. Returned large amount of hard, brown stool, and large amount of flatus-tolerated, odorless, abdomen soft, and less distended.

2. Report failure of patient to defecate to physician

May indicate need for further therapies.

Note:
- If patient cannot control external sphincter, such as a patient with paralysis, then the patient must be placed on bed pan because enema solution cannot be retained.
- Administering enema with patient sitting on toilet is unsafe because curved rectal tubing can abrade rectal wall.
- "Enema until clear" order means that enemas are repeated until patient passes fluid that is clear and contains no fecal matter. But usually patient should receive only three consecutive enemas to avoid disruption of fluid and electrolytes balance.
- Some commercial enema kits come with a rectal tube, so ensure that size is appropriate.
- Some disposable kits come with are rectal tube, so ensure that size is appropriate.
- Some disposable kits come with prelubricated tip. Add additional lubricant as needed.
- Patient should be instructed that enemas should not be given to treat cause of constipation.
- For self-administration, patient should be instructed to lie in dorsal recumbent position with knees and hips flexed toward chest.

Urinary Elimination

Elimination from the urinary tract helps to remove the waste products from body. It is essential to the body's physical well-being to life itself, and to the individuals' general sense of well-being.

Definition

Urinary elimination is the expulsion of waste products from the body through the urinary system.

Common Alterations in Urinary Elimination

a. Altered urine production

Polyuria

Polyuria or diuresis refers to the production of abnormally large amounts of urine by the kidneys, about 2,500 mL or more/day. Polyuria can be the result of (1) Excessive fluid intake, (2) The ingestion of substances containing caffeine and alcohol, (3) Diabetes mellitus, (4) Hormone imbalances, (e.g., deficiency of antidiuretic hormone, or ADH), or (5) Chronic kidney disease.

Oliguria

It refers to voiding scanty amount of urine such as 100–500 mL/day. Oliguria may result from (1) extremely low fluid intake, (2) Excessive fluid loss-example burns, diarrhea, etc., (3) Renal failure. Oliguria may also accompany fever and heavy perspiration.

Anuria

It refers to voiding less than 100 mL/day. The terms complete kidney shutdown. Renal failure, and urinary suppression have the same meaning. Anuria can result from (1) kidney diseases, (2) severe heart disease, (3) burns, and (4) shock.

b. Altered voiding pattern

Frequency

It refers to voiding at frequent intervals, i.e., more often than usual. Normally with an increased intake of fluid there is some increase in the frequency with which a person voids. Frequency without an increase in fluid intake may be the result of (1) cystitis, (2) stress and (3) pressure on the bladder, e.g., in pregnancy.

In frequency, the total amount of urine voided may be normal. This is because the amount of urine voided each time is usually about 50–100 mL only.

Nocturia

It is an increased frequency at night that is not the result of an increase in fluid intake. It is expressed in terms of the number of times the person gets out of bed to void. For example, "Nocturia × 4".

Urgency

Urgency is the feeling of urge to void at once. There may or may not be a great deal of urine in the bladder, but the person feels a need to void immediately. Often the person hurries to the toilet with the fear of being incontinent. Urgency accompanies psychologic stress and irritation of the trigone and urethra.

Dysuria

It means voiding that is either painful or difficult. It can be caused by: (1) stricture of the urethra, (2) urinary infection and (3) injury to the bladder or urethra.

Enuresis

It is defined as repeated involuntary urination in children beyond 4 or 5 years of age, when voluntary bladder control is normally acquired. Enuresis can be nocturnal (night time) and diurnal (day time) or both.

Hesitancy

It is defined as delay or difficulty in initiating voiding. It may be due to:
- Urethral stricture
- Prostatic enlargement
- Surgical procedures in perineal area
- Post catheterization
- Cystitis/Urethritis.

Urinary incontinence

It is inability to control the passage of urine. Incontinence is a symptom, not a disease. Incontinence may be caused by stress, neurological impairment, injury to urethra sphincter, and physical mobility.

Urinary retention

Urinary retention is the accumulation of urine in the bladder associated with inability of the bladder to empty itself. Because urine production continues, retention distends the bladder. An adult urinary bladder normally holds 250–450 mL of urine when the urination reflex is triggered. With urinary retention, some adult bladders may distend to hold 3,000 mL of urine. Prolonged retention leads to stasis (a slowing of the flow of urine) and stagnation of urine, which increases the possibility of urinary tract infection. Distention also causes reduce blood flow to the bladder, making it less resistant to invading gram-positive organisms and thereby increases the chances of urinary tract infections.

Retention may occur due to several factors:
- After surgical procedures on perineal and anal regions.
- Prostatic enlargement and urethral strictures.
- Acute illness or chronic bedridden state.
- Anxiety and aging process.
- Drugs such as atropine, phenothiazines, actifed, and propranolol.

Assessing urinary elimination

Assessment of urinary elimination includes (1) taking a nursing history, (2) performing a physical examination of the kidneys, bladder, urethral meatus, skin integrity, and hydration, (3) examination of the urine. The nurse also should (4) review any data obtained relevant diagnostic tests and procedures.

Nursing History

The nurse determines the client's normal voiding pattern and amount, frequency, appearance of the urine and to any recent changes, any past or current problems with urination, the presence of an ostomy, and factors influencing the elimination pattern.

Examples of interview questions to elicit this information are shown below. The number of questions asked depends on the individual and the responses to the first three categories.

Examples of Interview Questions

Voiding pattern
- How many times do you void during a 24-hour period?
- Has this pattern changed recently?
- Do you need to get out of bed to void at night? How often?

Description of urine and any changes
How would you describe your urine in terms of color, clarity (clear, transparent, or cloudy), and odor (faint or strong)?

Urinary elimination problems
What problems have you had or do you now have with passing your urine, passage of large amounts of urine? Passage of small amounts of urine, voiding at more frequent intervals, trouble in getting to the bathroom in time, or feeling of urgency to void, painful voiding?

Difficulty in starting urine stream: Frequent dribbling of urine or feeling of bladder fullness associated with voiding small amount of urine.

Reduced force of stream

Accidental leakage of urine: If so, when does this occur (e.g., when coughing, laughing, or sneezing; at night; during the day).

Pasturinary tract illness such as urinary tract infection of the kidney, bladder, or urethra; urinary calculi; urinary tract surgery of kidney, ureters, or bladder.

Presence and management of urinary diversion/ostomy
- What is your usual routine with colostomy?
- What problems, if any do you have with it?
- How can the nurse help you manage it?

Factors Influencing Urinary Elimination

- **Medications:** Have you taken any medications that could increase urinary output (e.g., diuretic) or cause retention of urine (e.g., Anticholinergic—antispasmodic, antidepressant, and antihistamines, antihypertensive)? Note specific medication and dosage.

- **Fluid intake:** What amount and kind of fluid do you take each day (e.g., 6 glasses of water, 5 cups of coffee, 3 cola drinks with or without caffeine)
- **Environmental factors:** Do you have any problem with toileting (mobility, toilet seat tool low, facility without grab bar)
- **Presence of long-term catheter:** How do you care for your catheter? Do you have any discomfort with it or other problems? How can the nurse help you manage it?
- **Stress:** Are you experiencing any long-term or short-term stress. If so, what are the stressors? Do you think these affect your urinary pattern?
- **Disease:** Have you had or do you have any illnesses other than urinary tract disease that may affect urinary function, such as hypertension, heart disease, neurologic disease (e.g., multiple sclerosis), cancer, prostatic enlargement, diabetes mellitus, or diabetes insipidus?
- **Diagnostic procedures:** Have you recently had a cystoscopy or spinal anesthesia?

Examination of Urine

Normal urine consists of 96% water and 4% solutes. Organic solutes include urea, ammonia, creatinine, and uric acid. Urea is the chief organic solute. Inorganic solutes include sodium, chloride, potassium sulfate, magnesium, and phosphorus. Sodium chloride is the most abundant inorganic salt. Assessment of urine involves measuring the volume of urine; comparing the output of the client's intake; inspecting the urine for color, clarity, and odor; testing urine for specific gravity, glucose, ketones bodies, blood and pH; and reviewing of data obtained from diagnostic tests.

Maintaining Normal Voiding Habits

Positioning

- Assist the client to a normal position for voiding; standing for males, for females, squatting or leaning slightly forward when sitting. These positions enhance movement of urine through the tract by gravity.
- Use bedside commodes as necessary for females and urinals for males standing at the bedside.
- Encourage the client to push over the pubic area with the hands or lean forward to increase intra-abdominal pressure and external pressure on the bladder. Elevate the head of the client's bed to Fowler's position, place a small pillow, or rolled towel at the back to increase physical support and comfort, and have the client flex the hips and knees. This position stimulates the normal voiding position as closely as possible.

Relaxation

- Provide privacy for the client. Many people cannot void in the presence of another person.
- Allow the client sufficient time to void.
- Suggest the client to read or listen to music.
- Provide sensory stimuli that may help the client relax. Pour warm water over the perineum of a female or have the client sit in a warm bath to promote muscle relaxation. Applying of hot-water bottle to the lower abdomen of both men and women may also faster muscle relaxation.
- Turn on running water within hearing distance of the client to mask the sound of voiding for persons who find this embarrassing.

Implementing

Most interventions to maintain normal urinary elimination are independent nursing functions. These include:
- Promoting fluid intake
- Maintaining normal voiding habits
- Strengthening muscle tone
- Assisting with toileting

Promoting Fluid Intake

- Increasing fluid intake increases urine production, which in turn stimulates the urination reflex. A normal, average daily intake of 1200–1500 mL of measurable fluids is adequate for most clients.
- Additional amounts are required for clients whose fluid demands are great, such as those who have abnormal fluid losses other routes (e.g., excessive perspiration, vomiting, diarrhea, wound drainage, and burns).
- Immobilized clients who are susceptible to calculi (kidney stone) formatting require daily intakes of 2000–3000 mL per day (unless medically contraindicated). Dilute urine helps prevent urinary tract stones and infection.
- Fluid intake can also be increased by encouraging the client to eat plenty of raw fruits and vegetables, which have high-water content.
- Increased fluid intake as contraindicated in clients who require fluid restrictions, such as those with renal impairment or congestive heart failure.

Assisting a Client to Use a Urinal

The client's ability to void depends on feeling the urge to urinate and on being able to control the urethral sphincter. One factor that can interfere with micturition is bed rest or immobility, which does not allow the client to assume the normal position for emptying the bladder. The female client is accustomed to squatting, which promotes contraction of the pelvis and intra-abdominal muscles that assist in sphincter control and bladder contraction. The nurse assists the bedridden woman to use a bedpan for voiding. A man voids more easily in the standing position. If a man cannot reach the toilet facilities, he may stand at the bedside and void into a urinal (a plastic or metal receptacle for urine). If he is unable to stand at the bedside, the nurse needs to assist him to use the urinal in bed.

Equipment

- Urinal
- Disposable gloves
- Graduated cylinder (for measuring volume)
- Supplies for diagnostic urine tests specimen collection.

Procedure: Assisting a Client to Use a Urinal (Table 3.17)

Table 3.17: Procedure of assisting a client to use a urinal.

Steps	Rationale
Assessment	
1. Assess client's normal elimination habits.	Identifies normal pattern of urination helps nurse to recognize when client may required use of urinal.
2. Assess for periods of incontinence.	Recognize when client may require use of urinal.
3. Palpate for distended bladder.	Indicates if bladder is full and client needs to void.
Implementation	
1. Wash hands and apply gloves	Reduces transmission of microorganisms.
2. Provide privacy by closing bedside curtain or room door.	Promotes relaxation.
3. Assist client into appropriate position; position on side, back or sitting with head of bed elevated, or assist to the standing position.	Men find it easier to void and empty bladder while standing.
4. If possible, client should hold urinal and position penis in urinal. If client needs assistance, position penis completely within urinal and hold urinal in place of assistance or client to hold urinal.	Penis is placed completely within urinal to avoid spillage of urine on bed linen.
5. Once client has finished voiding, remove urinal, wash and dry penis, cleanse urinal, and return it to client for future use.	Avoids spilling and reduces odors. Prevents growth of microorganisms. Prevent skin breakdown.
6. Allow client to wash hands after voiding.	Reduces spread of microorganisms.
7. Remove and dispose of gloves; wash hands.	Reduces spread of microorganisms.
Evaluation	
1. Reassess client to determine ability to use urinal.	Promotes modification of nursing care plan to include more assistance or increased frequency to assist client to use urinal.

Contd...

Steps	Rationale
2. Note amount and characteristics of urine.	Indicates abnormalities.
3. Unexpected outcomes that may occur include: ➢ Client is incontinent. ➢ Client is unable to use urinal.	Increased anxiety and contributes to body image disturbance. Increases risk of skin breakdown. Increased risk of incontinence or urinary retention.
Recording and reporting	
1. Record and report client's ability to use urinal and characteristics of urinary output.	Communicates pertinent information to all health care personnel.
2. If client is on 1 and 0, include output data on flow sheet.	Monitors fluid balance.
3. Report frequency of client's voiding patterns.	Promotes normal urinary elimination, prevents incontinence.

Incontinence:

- Offer urinal more frequently
- Place urinal near client
- Provide frequent skincare
- Assess type of incontinence (overflow, stress, urge, etc.)

Inability to void using a urinal:

- Attempt to place client in standing position
- Provide privacy
- Provide relaxing environment.

Persistent urge, stress, or overflow incontinence may indicate a serious medical problem; referral for urologic evaluation may be appropriate.

Nurse must consider client's social and cultural habit. Men are accustomed to sharing public urinals and privacy may not be major concern. Nurse must consider possibility of orthostatic hypotension occurring in clients who are immobilized or who have been recumbent for prolonged period. If client is allowed privacy while voiding, ensure that call bell is within easy access, so that the nurse can be summoned to empty and, if necessary, remove urinal.

Home Care Considerations

- Assess client, primary care giver to determine ability and willingness to use urinal.
- Assess level of assistance required by client to determine if additional medical equipment is necessary (e.g., over bed trapeze, bedside commode).
- Consider referral to home care agency to follow up and reinforce teaching concepts.

Development Considerations

Aging process impairs micturition; elderly men required urinal more frequently to avoid urinary incontinence.

Collecting a Random Urine Specimen

Urine is the most frequently collected specimen because its examination provides valuable clues about the functioning of the human body. A urinalysis can provide information about the status of kidney function, nutrition, metabolic function a certain systemic diseases. Urine collection is part of every client's testing when admitted to an acute healthcare facility.

Many procedures can be used collect urine and many tests are performed for urine analysis. The method of urine collection depends on the types of test to be performed and the client's age, medical condition and ability to void voluntarily. The three major types of urine specimens are single random routine specimens, timed urine collections, and specimens for culture and sensitivity. A random routine urine specimen can be obtained with a client voiding or through a Foley catheter or Urostomy collection bag. The specimen should be clean, but it need not be sterile. The specimen is generally tested for the type and amount of routine constituents such as white and red blood cells. The laboratory also performs routine screening on random specimens for constituent that normally should not be present in urine, such as protein and bacteria. The findings from a random specimen analysis may lead to additional urine testing or other types of diagnostic testing.

Before performing this procedure, the nurse should know the signs and symptoms of urinary elimination alterations and the normal characteristics of urine. The nurse should also know how to properly assist a client to use a bedpan or urinal.

Equipment

- Wash cloths, towel, soap and water.
- Clean disposable gloves.
- Clean collection container bed pan or urinal.
- Wide-mouth specimen container with lid.
- Complete specimen identification label.
- Completed laboratory requisition with date and time of collection.

Procedure: Collecting a Random Urine Specimen (Table 3.18)

Table 3.18: Procedure of collecting random urine specimen.

Steps	Rationale
Assessment	
1. Assess client's ability to independently provide specimen: able to position self; hold container, stand or sit to void.	Determines ability to cooperate and level of assistance required.
2. Assess client's understanding of need for specimen.	Determines need for health teaching. Client understands of purpose and promotes cooperation.

Contd...

Contd...

Steps	Rationale
3. Assess for signs and symptoms of urinary tract infection: frequency, urgency, dysuria, hematuria, flank pain, fever, and cloudy urine with sediment, foul odor.	Suggests bacteria in urine.
Implementation	
1. Wash hands and prepare equipment at bed side	Reduces transfer of microorganisms.
2. Provide privacy for client who will give specimen in bed by drawing curtain around bed or closing room door.	Privacy allows client to relax and produce specimen more quickly.
3. Give client or family member towel, wash cloth, soap to cleanse perineal area, or assist client to cleanse perineum.	Client prefers to wash their own perineal area when possible. Cleansing prevents contamination of specimen as urines passes from urethra.
4. Given male client specimen container and direct to bathroom; give female client specimen hat and direct to bathroom; assist client as needed to void into bedpan or urinal.	Maintains as much independence in client as possible.
5. Put on gloves before assisting client in collection of specimen or handling urine.	Reduce risk of exposure to pathogens.
6. If client did not void directly into specimen container, transfer 4 oz. of urine into it.	Nurse should handle transfer of urine to specimen cup to avoid contamination of specimen. Proper volume of specimen ensures test can be completed.
7. Place lid tightly on container without touching inside of lid.	Prevents contamination of specimen by other substances and loss from spillage.
8. If urine has been splashed on outside of container, wash if off.	Prevents spread of bacteria.
9. If bedpan or urinal was used to collect specimen cleanse and return to bedside.	Reduces transfer of microorganisms.
10. Remove and discard gloves and wash hands.	Reduces transfer of microorganisms.
11. Securely attach properly completed identification label and laboratory requisition to specimens.	Incorrect identification can result in diagnostic or therapeutic errors.
12. Send specimen to laboratory immediately.	Bacteria grow quickly in urine; therefore it should be analyzed immediately.

Contd...

Contd...

Steps	Rationale
Evaluation	
1. Compare results of client's urinalysis with normal laboratory values.	Identifies deviations from normal and indicates need for further testing.
2. Unexpected outcomes that may occur include ➢ Urine specimen is accidentally discarded. ➢ Urine specimen is contaminated with feces or toilet paper. ➢ Client is unable to urinate on demand.	Requires repeat of specimen collection procedure. Urine collection should be repeated. May require more time or more fluids to drink.
Recording and reporting	
1. Record collection of specimen in nurses' notes. Note time, date, purpose, appearance, and odor of urine, and abnormal signs or symptoms.	Verifies collection of specimen if report is slow to return from laboratory.
2. Notify physician of significant abnormalities.	May indicate need for therapy.

Note:
- Varying degrees of assistance will be required by clients who are seriously ill, have difficult in standing, or confused. Some clients may need assistance in bathroom, whereas others require bedpan or urinal on bed. Elderly clients in particular may have difficulty in maintaining balance and raising or lowering toilet seat.
- In uncircumcised males, fore skin must be retracted for effective cleansing of meatus and during voiding.
- Never store specimens in food refrigerator.
- Female clients need to be instructed to discard toilet or into waste bag rather than with urine because it makes analysis of urine invalid.
- If female is menstruating, notes it on specimen requisition in case red blood cells appear in urine.

Urinary Catheterization

Definition

Urinary catheterization is the insertion of a special catheter into the urinary bladder using aseptic technique, for the purpose of evacuating or instilling fluids.

Purposes

- To empty the contents of the bladder, e.g., before or after abdominal, pelvic, or rectal surgery and before certain investigations.
- To determine residual urine.
- To allow bladder irrigation.
- To bypass on obstruction.
- To relieve retention of urine and incontinence.
- To introduce cytotoxic drugs in the treatment of papillary bladder carcinoma.
- To perform bladder function tests.
- To measure urinary output accurately.

In the female, urinary catheterization may be carried out for the eight reasons listed above and for the one further reason:

- To empty the bladder before childbirth, if though that necessary.
- To avoid complications during intracavitary insertion of radioactive cesium.

Equipment

- Clean trolley
- Sterile catheterization pack containing forceps, receiver, gauze swabs
- Lubricant
- Disposable pad
- Sterile gloves
- Appropriate sterile urinary catheter
- Antiseptic solution or normal saline
- Sterile container for analysis is if required
- Sterile syringe and needle, sterile water
- Standing lamp, if available
- Draining bag
- Hypoallergenic tape
- Kidney tray

Procedure: Urinary Catheterization (Table 3.19)

Table 3.19: Procedure of urinary catheterization.

Nursing action	Rationale
1. Check the physician's order, progress notes, and nursing care plan.	To obtain specific instruction and/or information.
2. Identify the patient. Check identification against physician's order.	To perform the right procedure on the right patient.
3. Explain the procedure to the patient.	To allays fear and gain patient's confidence and cooperation. To reassure the patient and promote patient education.
4. Allow him to ask question. Ensure privacy.	To avoid unnecessary embarrassment to the patient during the procedure.
5. Assist the patient to get into supine position with knees bent. Do not expose the genital area at this stage.	
6. Direct the standing lamp (if available) for visualization of genital area.	
7. Wash and dry hands.	To prevent cross-infection.
8. Open sterile catheterization package and sterile catheter using aseptic technique. Prepare lubricant, aspirate sterile water into the syringe (refer to manufacturer's instructions).	Catheterization requires same aseptic technique precautions as in surgical procedure. To prevent fact infection.

Contd...

Contd...

Nursing action	Rationale
9. Place disposable pad across the patient's thighs and under buttocks.	To ensure urine does not leak onto bed clothes.
10. Wear sterile gloves.	To prevent cross-infection.
11. Apply lubricant to the nozzle of the catheter.	

Female

Nursing action	Rationale
12. Separate the labia minora, so that the urethral meatus is visualized. One hand is to maintain separation of the labia until catheterization is finished.	To prevent labia minora contamination of the catheter. To provide better access to the urethral orifice.
13. Cleanse around the urethral meatus with normal saline or antiseptic solution manipulate cleansing sponges with forceps, cleansing with downward strokes. Dispose of sponge after each use.	Bacteria that normally colonize the distal urethra may be introduced into the bladder during or immediately after catheter's insertion. Inadequate preparation of the urethral meatus is a major cause of infection.
14. Handle the tip of the catheter placing its end in the receiver between the patient's legs.	
15. Introduce the well-lubricated tip of the catheter into the urethral meatus using strict aseptic technique. Insert catheter in an upward and backward direction for 5–7 cm (2–3 inches). Avoid contaminating surface of catheter.	The direction of insertion and the length of catheter inserted should be areolation to the anatomy of the area.
16. Allow same bladder urine to flow through catheter before connecting the bag.	
17. Inflate the balloon according to the manufacturer's instruction, having ensured that the catheter is draining adequately.	Inadvertent inflation of the balloon in the urethra causes pain and urethral trauma.

Male

Nursing action	Rationale
18. Wash off penis around urinary meatus with normal saline or antiseptic solution. Cleanse urethral meatus from tip to foreskin with downward stroke. Dispose sponge after each use. Keep the foreskin retracted. Maintain sterility of dominant hand.	To prevent contamination and retraction of penis.

Contd...

Nursing action	Rationale
19. Grasp shaft of penis and elevate it. Insert catheter into the urethra applying gentle traction to penis while catheter is passed.	To straighten the penile urethra and facilitate catheterization.
20. Advance catheter 15–25 cm (6–10 inches)	Advancing catheter ensure sits position into the bladder.
21. Inflate the balloon according to the manufacturer's instructions.	
22. Withdraw the catheter slightly and connect to the drainage system.	This prevents traction and tension on the bladder and friction in the urethra.
23. Anchor the catheter by taping laterally.	
24. Dry area. Position the patient comfortably.	If the area is left wet and moist secondary infection and skin irritation may occur.
25. Measure the amount of urine.	
26. Dispose of equipment as appropriate.	
27. Wash and dry hands.	
28. Document the procedure appropriately. Record date and time type of catheter used and size, color and amount of urine, patient's tolerance and any other relevant observations.	

NUTRITIONAL NEEDS

Objectives

Mastery of content in this unit will enable the students to (Fig. 3.2):
- Diet in health and disease
- Factors affecting nutrition in illness

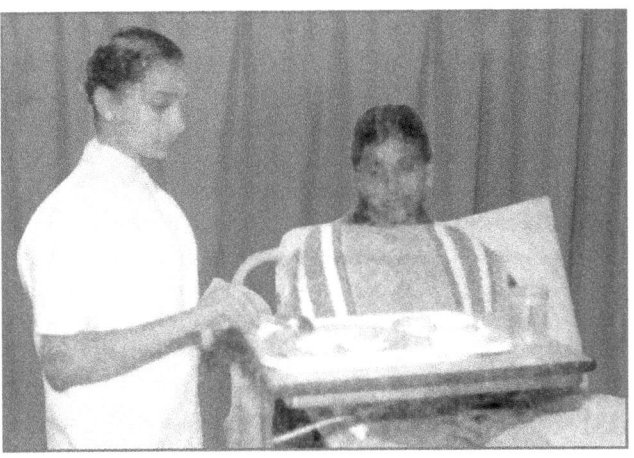

Fig. 3.2: Patient is taking meal.

- ❖ Nurses role in meeting patient nutritional need
- ❖ Modification of diet in illness
- ❖ Diet planning and serving
- ❖ Feeding helpless patients including artificial method of feeding

Adequate and appropriate nutrition is basic for the proper growth and development of an individual. Man and animals are born with the sensation of hunger. Primitive man learned to kill the animal by using different methods to satisfy his hunger. Later man started cultivating a variety of vegetables, fruits, grains, and started rearing animals and birds for use as food. Invention of fire made the man to cook and eat the tasty foods. But as the day passed scientists proved how important it is to take the right food in order to get proper energy and protection, which is necessary to promote health and prevent infection. Therefore, it is necessary for all the health professionals to understand the subject nutrition, to keep them fit as well as to teach their clients about healthy food habits as per the need.

Definition

Nutrition may be described as the sum of the processes by which the body utilizes food for energy, maintenance, and growth.

Importance of Diet in Health and Disease

Deficiency of protein and calories commonly occurs among weaned infants and preschool children usually it is seen in developing countries like India. Kwashiorkor and nutritional marasmus are common protein deficiency diseases. Protein energy malnutrition (PEM) is one of the largest nutritional problems in India and other developing countries. Mental retardation, stunted growth and development are also other problems seen in children with protein deficiency. Protein deficiency during pregnancy leads to stillbirth, low-birth weight, and anemia.

Carbohydrates

Carbohydrates, mostly plant products in origin, include sugars, starches, and cellulose are composed of the elements carbon, hydrogen, and oxygen. Carbohydrates are formed by all green plants by a complex process known as photosynthesis. Carbohydrates are either small single units (molecules) or larger units. Those which have special significance in nutrition are the simple sugars—glucose, fructose, and galactose; the double sugars—sucrose, lactose, and maltose; and the more complex forms—starch, glycogen, and cellulose. **Glucose** (grape, sugar, corn sugar, and dextrose) is found in fruits, certain roots, corn, and honey. It is less sweet than table sugar and is very inexpensive form of sugar. It is the form of sugar in the blood, as it is the end product of all carbohydrate digestion. It is also the form in which carbohydrates are absorbed, because it is the only fuel the central nervous system can use. Glucose is given for immediate energy (by mouth or intravenously), as it is ready for utilization by the body. It is stored as glycogen in the liver.

Fructose (fruit sugar) is found in honey and in many fruits and vegetables. It is combined with glucose in table sugar and gives honey its characteristic flavor.

Galactose is produced from lactase in milk, but does not occur free in nature.

Sorbitol, a sugar alcohol, is also simple sugar but without nutritive value. It is sometimes used as a "nonnutritive" sweetener in "dietetic" foods.

Sucrose (can sugar, sugar beets, and table sugar) is found in sugar cone, sugar beets, molasses, maple sugar and syrup, and many fruits and vegetables.

Lactose (milk sugar) is produced only by mammals. It is less soluble and less sweet than cane sugar, and is digested more slowly.

Maltose (malt sugar) is found in malt and malt products. It is made from the starch available in sprouting grain and is not found free in nature.

Starch is the form of the reserve store of carbohydrates in plants (grains, seeds, roots, potatoes, green bananas, and other plants) and is changed into glucose during digestion, through intermediate steps of dextrin and maltose.

Glycogen (animal starch) is the body's reserve form of carbohydrate, stored in the liver, and is quickly changed to and from glucose as necessary.

Cellulose (fiber) is found in the pulp and skins of fruit and vegetables, the structural parts of plants, and the covering of seeds and outer covering of nuts. It is indigestible, so it provides bulk and stimulation for the intestinal tract.

Dextrin is formed from starch breakdown by heat or by enzymes during digestion. For example, starch is converted to dextrin in the toasting of bread.

Sources

Plant sources

Cereal grains: Rice, wheat, corn, oats, rye, barley, buckwheat, and millets.

Fruits: Fruits contain a large proportion of water. Their carbohydrate content is mostly sugar, except in dried fruit it is low.

Sweets: Ordinary fable sugar, molasses, maple syrup and sugar, corn syrup, honey, and sorghum syrup are poor sources because they are concentrated with "empty" calories.

Animal sources

There is none of importance except possibly lactose in milk. Traces of glycogen are found in meat, poultry, fish, and eggs and small amounts are available in liver and scallops. If carbohydrate intake is limited, the body is capable of converting amino acids and the glycerol of fats into glucose. Therefore, there is no specific dietary requirement for carbohydrates.

Functions

The primary function of carbohydrate is to meet the body's specific need for energy. After these needs are met, carbohydrates are comparable to fats in protein-sparing action. Carbohydrates are readily converted to energy. One gram of carbohydrate yields 4 kilocalories.

1. To spare the burning of protein for energy (as protein has more important functions)
2. To aid in a more efficient and complete oxidation (burning) of fats for energy.
3. As sugar, to produce energy quickly.
4. As starch to provide an economical and abundant source of energy after change to glucose.
5. As lactose, carbohydrates has a certain laxative action (remains in the intestines longer and encourages desirable bacterial growth) and aids in the absorption of calcium.
6. As cellulose (insoluble and indigestible), it aids in the normal functioning of the intestines.

Requirements

Carbohydrates are a source of energy for the brain and other tissue cells and for the synthesis of lactose of milk. Carbohydrate is essential for the oxidation of fat, and for the synthesis of certain nonessential amino acids. At least 40–50% carbohydrates calories should be present in well-balanced diets. The list below shows the percentage of carbohydrate calories should be present into calories intake.

Adults (male and female)	50–70%
Expectant and nursing mothers	40–60%
Infants (1–12 months)	40–50%
Preschool children (1–5 years)	40–60%
Older children and adolescents	50–70%

Deficiencies

When carbohydrate (glucose) level goes beyond 40 mg% in the blood, person will go into the condition called hypoglycemia. But it is not common in healthy individuals. Diabetic patient usually gets this condition on poor compliance of medicine. Signs and symptoms are headache, giddiness, palpitation, tachycardia, confusion, slurred speech, staggering gait, lack-of coordination convulsion, and coma.

Fats

Fats constitute a second group of nutrients that provide energy in the diet. They and certain fat-like substances are classified as lipids. Fats are compounds of fatty acids—three molecules of fatty acids and one molecule of glycerol (triglycerides), which like carbohydrates, contain carbon, hydrogen, and oxygen but in different proportions. When oxidized, they give about two and half times more energy than carbohydrates. Most of the fats in food occur in triglycerides.

Fat-like substances having important roles in the body include phospholipids (fat plus the mineral phosphorus) and sterols (ergo sterol in plants, and cholesterol, either free or combined with fatty acids as cholesterol esters, in animal tissue).

Hydrogenated fats are made by treating liquid fats—vegetable oils such as cotton, corn, soybean, etc., with hydrogen to produce a plastic fat for cooking purposes or a table fat for a butter substitute.

Fatty acids, a variety of which are present in different food fats, are classified as "saturated" and "unsaturated" depending on the absence or presence of double bonds between the carbon atoms in the molecule.

Food fats contain a mixture of both kinds of fatty acids. If saturated acids predominate and the fat is solid, is called a poly saturated fat; if unsaturated acids predominate, the fat is called a poly unsaturated fat.

The relative amount of fatty acids ill foods and diets is referred to as a *PIS* ratio (P = polyunsaturated, S = saturated fatty acids). A ratio of polyunsaturated fat to saturated fat *(PIS),* less than 2: 1 is generally considered unsuitable.

Saturated fats are found in animal products such as whole milk, cream, butter, cheese mode from whole milk, egg yolk, meat and lord, and margarine, hydrogenated shortening, chocolate, and rich desserts.

Polyunsaturated fats are found in vegetable oils (including sunflower, corn, cotton seeds, soybean, and sesame oils), fish salad dressings, mayonnaise, and certain margarines.

Essential fatty acids (EFA) are necessary for nutritional well-being of all animals. The principal ones for the human are linoleic and arachidonic acids.

Cholesterol, one of the "fat-like" sterols, is found in various concentrations in all animal tissue and the blood and has important functions in the body, food intake synthesis within the body being responsible for its presence. A fatty deposit containing cholesterol (which interferes with the flow of blood) is characteristic of a cardiovascular disease known as atherosclerosis, the exact house of which is unknown. Cholesterol has an essential role in the structure of sex and adrenal hormones and is converted to vitamin D3 by the action of ultraviolet light on the skin. It is stored in the liver and also occurs in the form of lipoprotein in the blood, as less than 10% of the total body cholesterol.

Sources

Animal source

Whole milk, butter, lards, meat fats, bacon, cheese, cream, and egg yolk.

Plant source

Vegetable oils—corn, cotton, peanut, etc., margarines, chocolate, peanut butter, salad dressings, nuts, olives, avocados (butter fruit), are the main plant sources.

Functions

The primary function of fat is to serve as a concentrated source of heat and energy. One gram fat yields 9 calories, more than twice that of carbohydrate. About one-third to one-half of the kilocalories in the current American diet comes from fat. The body cells, except for the cells of the nervous system and erythrocytes, can use fatty acids directly as a source of energy. In addition, function of the fat is:
- Furnish essential fatty acids.
- Spare burning of protein for energy.
- Add flavor and palatability to the diet.
- Gives satiety value to the diet (fats slow the digestive process and retard the development to hunger).

Animal fats and fortified margarines not only contain some of the fat soluble vitamins (A, D, E, and K) but also aid in their absorption. They also play a role in the absorption of fatty acids. Excess fat, stored in the body as adipose tissue, insulates, and protects organs and nerves. Fats also lubricate the intestinal tract; and the phospholipids have an important role in metabolism.

Requirements

There are no specific requirements for fat other than meeting the body's need for essential fatty acids, usually found in a diet containing 15–25 g of appropriate food fats. The approximate percentage of fat calorie requirements of total calorie as per the different age group is as follows:

Adults (male and female)	10–20%
Expectant and nursing mothers	10–20%
Infants (birth–1 year)	25–30%
Children and adolescents (2–18 years)	15–20%

Deficiencies

Deficiency of essential fatty acids in infants leads to perianal irritation, and skin changes such as dryness. In adults, it may lead to phrynoderma.

Vitamins

- Vitamins are discovered during 20th century. They are organic food substances and essential in small amounts for growth, maintenance, and the functioning of body processes.
- Vitamins are found only in living things—plants and animals—and usually cannot be synthesized by the human body.
- Vitamins may be classified broadly into two, according to the substance in which they are soluble:
  a. Fat-soluble vitamins are those vitamins, which are soluble in fats and fat solvents and insoluble in water. They are vitamins A, D, E, and K.
  b. Water-soluble vitamins are those vitamins, which are soluble in water and insoluble in fat and fat solvents. They are vitamin B complex, vitamin C (ascorbic acid), and bio-flavonoids.
- Vitamins have no caloric value, but they are as necessary to the body as any other basic nutrients.
  (1) Currently, there are about 20 substances identified as vitamins. (2) Recent research is concerned with identifying even more of these substances since they are so essential to survival.

Factors Affecting Nutrition in Illness

There are many factors that affect illness, both the quality and quantity of vitamins in food. The following are the most important:
1. **Variety of food:** Some foods have more or less of a certain vitamin.
2. **Soil variation and climate:** The same food grown in one area may have more or less vitamin value than the same food grown elsewhere.
3. **Degree of maturity:** Some foods have more of a vitamin when under ripe; others when ripe.
4. Type of diet fed to the animal used as food.
5. **Storage after harvesting of production:** Improper storage may have a destructive effect on vitamins.
6. **Freezing:** Some vitamins are lost in preliminary blanching.
7. **Drying:** Certain vitamin losses occur during this process.
8. **Canning:** Although some vitamins will be lost in canning, there is less lost in acid food than in nonacid food.
9. Cooking of food affects vitamins in various ways.
10. **Antivitamin factors:** Certain substances may inactivate vitamins, be antagonistic to them, and interfere with their absorption and metabolism or synthesis in the body. Antibiotics and other drugs may kill intestinal bacteria which help in the synthesis. Oxidation may also be destructive.

Nurses Role in Meeting Patient's Nutritional Needs

Understanding Nutrition in Health

Balanced diet

An adequate and balanced diet is one that meets all the nutritional needs of an individual for maintenance, repair, the living processes, and growth or development. It includes all nutrients in proper amounts and proportion to each other.

Ideal nutrition

Evidence of optimal nutrition is a well-developed body, ideal weight for body composition (ratio of muscle mass to fat) and height, and good muscle development and tone. The skin is smooth and clear, the hair is glossy, and the eyes are clear and bright. Well-nourished persons are much more likely to be alert, mentally and physically. They are not only meeting their day-to-day needs but also are maintaining essential nutrient reserves for resisting infectious diseases and generally extending their years of normal functioning.

Clinical signs of good nutritional status

Features	Good signs
General appearance	Alert, responsive
Hair	Shiny, lustrous, healthy scalp
Neck glands	No enlargement
Skin, face, neck	Smooth, slightly moist, good color, reddish-pink mucus membrane
Eyes	Bright, clear, no fatigue circles
Lips	Pinkish and moist
Tongue	Good pink color, no swelling or bleeding, firm
Gums	Good pink color, surface papillae present, no lesion
Teeth	Straight, no crowding, well-shaped jaw, clean, no discoloration
Skin general	Smooth, slightly moist, good color
Abdomen	Flat
Legs, feet	No tenderness, weakness, swelling, discoloration
Skeleton	Normal formation
Weight	Normal for height, age, body builds
Posture	Erect, arms and legs straight, abdomen in, chest out
Muscles	Well-developed, firm
Nervous control	Good attention span for age, does not cry easily, not irritable or restless.
Gastrointestinal functions	Good appetite and digestion, normal, regular elimination

Basic food group guides

To interpret and apply sound nutrient standards, health workers need practical food guides to use in nutrition education and food planning with individuals and families. In 1985, Government agency in the United States issued a guide to food groups with different groups of foods and the recommended daily servings. The Basic Food Groups and the number of servings are intended to represent a total daily diet. They are:

1. Grains: Bread, cereal, rice, pasta: 6–11 servings.
2. Vegetables: 3–5 servings
3. Fruits: 2–4 servings
4. Milk, yoghurt, cheese: 2–3 servings
5. Meat, poultry, fish, drybeans, eggs, nuts: 2–3 servings
6. Fats, oils, sweets: Use sparingly

Dietary guidelines

Dietary guidelines are general statements to provide persons with direction toward a healthy diet. The guidelines are directed not only toward general health promotion, but also toward reducing risk of disease. Therefore, they reflect the current emphasis on prevention of the major diseases, such as heart disease and cancer. The dietary guidelines for the American public developed by Government agencies are a good example of guidelines that can be used in many countries. They are:

Eat a variety of foods

The greater the variety of foods ingested, the more likely the person receives the required nutrients. Good nutritional status exists when the necessary nutrients are consumed in sufficient amounts and are used appropriately by the body to meet needs. All persons need the same nutrients throughout life. The major effects of good nutrition include the following:

a. Growth and development of tissues/organs
b. Source of energy for metabolic processes and physical activity
c. Tissue healing and repair
d. Resistance to infection

One way to ensure a good variety of foods is to follow the guidelines of the Basic Food Groups Guide.

Maintain ideal weight

Weight control is a major concern of many people. The term overweight, obesity, and underweight must be differentiated and are defined as follows:

Overweight: Any weight between the high point and 20% above the ideal body weight as established by height and weight standards.

Obesity: Any weight more than 20% above the height and weight standards.

Underweight: Any weight, which is 20% below the height and weight standards. There is a condition called massive obesity, in which the person is much more than 20% above his/her weight. Such a condition predisposes the individual to numerous health problems. Similarly, unplanned weight loss may be an early sign of a medical disorder and medical evaluation should be sought. Some weight loss may be due to inadequate calorie intake or failure to increase caloric intake when physical activity is increased. People who are underweight may have nutritional deficits that affect growth and development, metabolism, and the body's protective mechanisms.

Thus, health promotion usually includes, helping persons to maintain their ideal body weight by restricting energy input (high calorie foods) while increasing energy output (physical activity).

Avoid too much fats and cholesterol

Excess fats that the body cannot use are deposited in the tissue, adding to body weight. In addition, research strongly supports a relationship between dietary fat and the incidence of cancer, especially cancer of the breast, colon, rectum, and prostate. The public is becoming better informed about the effects of high levels of serum cholesterol as a risk factor of coronary heart disease, but it remains the role of the nurse to continue this education at every opportunity.

Eat foods with adequate starch and fiber

Starch is the most important source of carbohydrate because it contains more nutrients than sugar. Dietary fiber contains cellulose and some noncellulose polysaccharides. Cellulose is not digestible, therefore, it remains in the gastrointestinal tract, providing bulk to help, stimulate peristalsis in the intestines. The noncellulose polysaccharides absorb water to odd to the bulk. Noncellulose substances also bind dietary cholesterol, preventing its absorption. The high intake of dietary fiber decreases the risk for colon cancer. Sources of dietary fiber include whole grains (wheat, rye, and oats) used in cereals and breads, bran, fruits, and vegetables.

Avoid too much sugar

Excess amounts of sugar odd to caloric intake without supplying nutrients, they also contribute to the formation of dental caries.

Avoid too much sodium

Sodium, a major body electrolyte, can affect blood pressure levels. A decreased sodium intake can help decrease blood pressure.

Therapeutic Nutrition

It is diet therapy or diet in disease. It involves the modification of adaptation of the normal or basic diet according to the needs of the individual.

Purposes of Therapeutic Nutrition

- ❖ To maintain or improve the nutritional status.
- ❖ To improve clinical or subclinical nutritional deficiencies.
- ❖ To maintain increase or decrease in body weight.
- ❖ To rest certain organs or the whole body.
- ❖ To eliminate particular food constituents to which the individual may be allergic.
- ❖ To adjust the composition of the normal diet to meet the ability of the body to adjust, metabolize and excrete certain nutrients and other substances.

Basic Hospital Diet

The basic routine diet referred to, from hospital to hospital as the house, general, regular, standard or full diet, is served to ambulatory patients and those patients who do not require a therapeutic diet. There are some differences from hospital to hospital in the foods allowed in each category, as well as the number of kinds of diets. When a patient is admitted to the hospital, the type of diet will be selected by the physician. This may be changed, if and when the patient's condition makes it desirable.

The method of feeding and the time of feeding may also vary. For example, sometimes hourly feeding or several small meals a day or preferred to three meals daily.

Modification of Hospital Diet for Therapeutic Purpose

The basic diet becomes therapeutic when it is modified in the following ways:

- ❖ The energy value (kilocalories) may be increased or decreased.
- ❖ Fiber (bulk, roughage) may be increased or decreased.
- ❖ Specific nutrients (one or more) may be increased or decreased.
- ❖ Specific foods or types of foods (such as allergens for persons with allergies, fried foods, or gas forming foods) may be increased or decreased.
- ❖ Any of these modified diets may be further altered to become a soft or liquid diet.
- ❖ Condiments and any specific foods that are not tolerated by the individual may be eliminated from the diet.

Prescription of Therapeutic Diet

Therapeutic diets are named in terms of the diet modification without reference to the disease (except in case of the diabetic diet). Adaptation are sometimes classified as qualitative, when the adaptations are in types of foods or consistency and quantitative, when the modifications consist of increases or decreases of certain nutrients or calories.

The diet prescription is written in terms at energy requirements, based on the individual's weight and activity requirements for protein, fat, carbohydrates, minerals, vitamins, and fiber with regard for the increased or decreased needs for each because of the patient's illness. This prescription is translated into foods and meals by the dietician, who in turn, instructs the patient regarding the diet, its importance as a single therapeutic measure or as a supplement to medication and how to prepare and serve it at home.

Modifications in Carbohydrate, Protein, and Fat

1. **Diabetic diet:** This diet is carefully calculated for each patient to minimize the occurrence of hyperglycemia and glycosuria and to attain or maintain ideal body weight and promote good health.
2. **Low kilocaloric diet:** This diet is used ·to achieve weight loss in individuals with cardiovascular and diseases, hypertension, gallbladder disease, gout or hypothyroidism, and for severely ill patients.
3. **High protein, high fat, low carbohydrate diet: This diet is used for patients with hyperglycemia.**
4. **Ketogenic diet:** In some cases, a ketogenic diet is used to control epilepsy. This diet is high in fat, and protein and carbohydrate are controlled.

Modification in Fat

1. **Restricted fat diet:** Fat is restricted for patients with disease of the liver, gallbladder, or pancreas in which

disturbance of digestion and absorption of fat may occur.
2. **Fat controlled, low cholesterol diet:** This diet is used in individuals with elevated blood cholesterol levels and for those with atherosclerosis.
3. **Dietary management of hyperlipoproteinemia:** This diet is important for lowering the risk for cardiovascular disease.

Modification in Protein

1. **Restricted protein diet:** This diet is used for patients in hepatic coma or with chronic uremia, renal disease, or liver disease.
2. **Gluten-free diet:** Individuals with celiac disease or nontropical have gluten intolerance and must be on a gluten-free diet.
3. **Restricted-phenylalanine diet:** This diet is used in confirmed cases of phenylketonuria (PKU), in which phenylalanine cannot be processed by the body.
4. **Restricted purine diet:** A decrease in purines is useful in lowering the blood uric acid leveling out.
5. **High protein diet:** A high-protein diet is used to correct a protein inadequacy from any source—pre and postoperative, high lever, burns, injuries, increased metabolism, nephrosis (in children), chronic nephritis (unless there is nitrogen retention), pernicious anemia, ulcerative colitis, hepatitis, celiac and cystic fiber cysts. Tuberculosis and other wasting diseases, wounds, or nutritional anemia.

Modification in Carbohydrate, Minerals, and Vitamins

1. **Lactose-free diet:** Patients who have a total or partial inability to metabolize this milk sugar must avoid lactose in their diet.
2. **Dumping syndrome diet:** Patients who have had a gastrostomy or gastric bypass surgery may require the special diet.
3. **Restricted sodium diets:** These diets are far more common and are prescribed for patients with congestive heart failure, hypertension, and renal disease with edema, cirrhosis of the liver with ascites, pre-eclampsia and eclampsia (toxemia) and adrenocorticotropic hormone (ACTH) therapy.
4. **Restricted copper diet:** Wilson's disease, oliguria, or anurias all calls for the restriction of copper intake.
5. **High-calcium and high-phosphorus diet:** An increase in calcium and phosphorus intake is desirable in rickets, osteomalacia, tetany, dental caries, and acute lead poisoning.
6. **High iron diet:** Nutritional or hemorrhagic anemia calls for a high intake of dietary iron.
7. **High vitamin diet:** If a specific vitamin deficiency is diagnosed, an increased intake of vitamins may be necessary. An increase in vitamin A is necessary to combat night blindness and xerophthalmia; increased intake of vitamin D is recommended for rickets and osteomalacia; increased vitamin K is needed in liver and gallbladder disease, in which the vitamin is not stored; increased thiamine is necessary to avoid beriberi and polyneuritis; increased niacin is needed to combat pellagra; and increased ascorbic acid (vitamin C) will improve wound healing and fight scurvy.

Important Consideration in Meal Service

Attractive food service plays an important role in stimulating the appetite and enjoyment of food. The patient's attitude toward food may reflect a more general attitude toward illness.

General Consideration in Meal Service

- The table or tray should be appropriately and properly set.
- Clean linen or good quality paper products, and clean light weight, attractive utensils should be used.
- Food portions should be of appropriate size, attractively arranged on dishes and garnished.
- Hot foods should be served hot and cold foods should be served cold.
- Meal time conversation should be pleasant, without discussion of disagreeable subjects.
- Trays or plates should be light weight and sufficiently large to hold all the necessary articles and foods.
- There should be no spilled foods or liquids.
- Patient should be placed in comfortable position and food should be placed within easy reach.
- Meals should be served according to scheduled times.
- Enough time should be given for eating.
- The patient's name and diet should be tallied before serving.
- Empty tray should be removed without hurry.

Suggestion for Assisting Patient

- It is important for the person assisting a patient to be seated and relaxed.
- Engage in pleasant conversation with the patient.
- Explain the reasons for the various foods offered, especially if the patient does not understand the diet well.
- Alternate one food with another if the patient must be fed.
- If the patient is blind, describe the foods before starting.
- Avoid criticism of the meal and of the patient.

Diet Planning and Serving

1. **Mechanical diet (edentulous):** This type of diet is used for the individual who has difficulty in chewing because of lack of dentures or teeth due to inflammation of the oral cavity.
2. **Tube feeding:** This type of feeding is used for patients with an esophageal obstruction or severe burns or those who have undergone gastric surgery or who have additional inability to chew or swallow. It is also sometimes necessary for patients with anorexia nervosa.
3. **Restricted residue diet:** This diet may be used for patients with gastritis, Crohn's disease, severe diarrhea, ulcerative colitis, diverticulitis, typhoid fever or partial intestinal obstruction, and after gastrointestinal surgery.

4. **High residue or high-fiber diet:** This type of diet may be prescribed for atonic constipation (intestinal stasis) or for diverticulitis. It is also being promoted for the prevention or therapy of gastric ulcers, cancer of the colon, hypercholesterolemia, diabetes, and obesity.

On the other hand, there are favorable foods handling practices that will enhance vitamin retention.

- Store vegetables properly to avoid wilting and drying out, which cause loss of vitamin A.
- Cook vegetables whole as often as possible. Cutting releases oxidative enzymes and increases cut surfaces where water-soluble vitamins leach out.
- Use cooking water and canned food juices to conserve soluble nutrients.
- Avoid use of baking soda in cooking vegetables, as it is destructive to thiamine and ascorbic acid. Also avoid long cooking for the same reason.
- Store fats properly to prevent rancidity, destructive factor for vitamin A.
- Keep milking glass containers away from light, which is destructive to riboflavin.
- Use drippings when cooking meat to conserve thiamine and niacin.
- Keep fruit juice covered and cold to prevent oxygen from destroying ascorbic acid.
- Do not stir while cooking foods containing ascorbic acid as oxygen destroys vitamin C.
- Cook vegetables covered and just until fork-tender. Store leftovers covered and cold. Reheating causes further loss of vitamins.

Assessing Nutritional Status

Nutritional assessment is a specific measurable means of identifying clients who are malnourished. Nutritional status is evaluated by patient's diet history, performing physical examination, taking anthropometric and biochemical measurements. The diet history identifies the patient's eating patterns and habits. The physical examination discloses objective data on the body's health or conditions that is directly related to nutrition. Biochemical measurements like albumin and hemoglobin level provide other clues to the patient's basic nutritional status.

Purposes

- To identify nutritional deficiencies that adversely affects health.
- To obtain information to plan and deliver nutritional care.
- Evaluate the effectiveness of nutritional care.

Equipment Required

- Balance scale
- Height measuring scale
- Clippers (to measure skin folds)
- Measuring tape (to measure skin folds)

Procedure: Assessing Nutritional Status (Table 3.20)

Table 3.20: Procedure to assess nutritional status.

Steps	Rationale
1. Assess patient's appetite, usual pattern of food intake and recent changes.	Changes in food intake may occur with illness
2. Determine the number of meals eaten daily and types of meals.	To determine eating patterns and habits.
3. Review results of relevant laboratory tests, albumins, hemoglobin.	To determine circulating proteins status.
4. Measure the patient's weight.	Weight is a very useful index of client's state of nutrition.
5. Measure patient's height.	To identify nutritional parameter.
6. Compare the height and weight with standards for the patient's age. If they are not within normal limits, determine what percentage of the weight is over or under for the age.	To avoid muscular contraction that may alter the measurement slightly. Normal mid arm circumference (MAC) Male: 29.3 cm. Female: 28.5 cm.
7. With thumb and forefinger, pinch a double flood of fat lengthwise about 1 cm. above midpoint of MAC. With other hand place teeth of calipers on either side of the fat fold. Calipers are placed below fingers so pressure is exerted from calipers and not fingers. Take three separate readings in mm and record.	Skin-fold measurements are used to estimate fat content of subcutaneous tissue (i.e., Biceps, scapula, abdominal muscles). Triceps skin fold (TSF) is most common and easiest to measure. Average the three readings of TSF: Normal TSF male; 12.5 mm Female 16.5 mm.
8. Assist the patient to comfortable positions.	To promote comfort.
9. Calculate midarm muscle circumference (MAMC) $$MAMC = \frac{MAC - TSF \times 3.14}{10}$$	MAMC is the estimation of skeletal muscle mass. Normal MAMC Male = 2.5 cm Female = 23.2 cm
10. Determine whether weight, height, midarm circumference and stain fold measurements are falling within normal range of accepted standards for the age and sex.	To assess normal nutritional status.
11. Document the assessment data and indicate if recommendations are made.	To report information to other healthcare providers.

Assisting Adult Patient with Oral Nutrition

Feeding Helpless Patients Including Artificial Method of Feeding

Assisting an adult patient with or malnutrition requires time, patience, knowledge, and understanding. Generally, people eat without assistance. With illness or trauma, the patient may be unable to eat without any assistance. Patients who need assistance in feeding are elderly, handicapped, immobilized, and children.

Purposes
1. To maintain adequate nutritional status.
2. To maintain good health.

Equipment/Requirements
1. Diet tray with food.
2. Napkins.
3. Towel.
4. Gloss with water.
5. Soap and water.

Procedure: Feeding Helpless Patients Including Artificial Method of Feeding (Table 3.21)

Table 3.21: Procedure of feeding helpless patients including artificial method of feeding.

Steps	Rationale
1. Wash hands	Reduces spread of microorganisms.
2. Determine to what extent the patient is able to self-feed. Assess level of consciousness, motor skills and vision.	Patients with any level of independence should not be to fully feed by hospital staff.
3. Check for food allergies.	Prevents allergic reaction to food items.
4. Remove all unpleasant objects from the client's bedside environment.	Remove noxious odors that decrease appetite. Prepare a pleasant atmosphere for eating.
5. Assist patient to urinate or defecate as necessary.	Enhances patient's comfort.
6. Assist the patient with washing hands face or doing mouth case as desired.	Removes potentially harmful microorganisms and refreshes the patient.
7. Check tray for completeness and correct diet.	To prevent mistakes.
8. Pull curtain around the bed (if needed). Assist patient to comfortable sitting position. If patient is unable to sit, turn patient onside.	Prevent mistakes. Proper positioning reduces risk of aspirations.

Contd...

Contd...

Steps	Rationale
9. Place a towel under the patients chin covering the chest, if he/she is likely to dribble food or fluid.	Allows more independence.
10. For the patient who cannot eat independently, assist in feeding by standing next to the client.	Standing close to the patient during feeding promotes psychologically comforting and caring environment, which may increase appetite.
11. Feed the patient in the order he would like to eat, allow ample time between the bites.	Allows sufficient time to chew and swallow.
12. Provides fluids as requested. Do not allow patients to drink all liquids at beginning of meal.	Prevents patient from filling up on liquids.
13. Talk to patient during meals.	Conversion promotes socialization.
14. Utilize the opportunity to educate patient during meal time, especially related to nutrition.	Educate whenever the nurse and patient are together.
15. Remove tray and assist patient to wash hands and mouth.	Allows patients to refresh himself/herself after eating and helps to prevent dental caries.
16. Assist patient to comfortable resting position.	Patient may feel tired after a full meal.
17. Return patients tray to appropriate place and wash hands.	Reduces spread of microorganisms.
18. Document in patient's chart, tolerance to food, amount eaten intake and output.	Documentation facilitates communication among healthcare professionals.

Nasogastric Intubation

Definition
Passing of tube through the nose to the stomach.

Purposes
- To remove fluid and gas from gastrointestinal (decompression) tract.
- Prevent or relieve nausea and vomiting after surgery.
- To treat patients with mechanical obstruction and bleeding of the upper gastrointestinal tract.
- To obtain a specimen of gastric contents for laboratory studies.
- Administer medications and feeding directly into gastrointestinal tract.

Equipment/Requirements
- Nasogastric intubation
- Lubricant

- ❖ Syringe
- ❖ Adhesive tape
- ❖ Lubricant jelly
- ❖ Blue litmus paper
- ❖ Stethoscope
- ❖ Specimen container
- ❖ Towel
- ❖ Glass with water
- ❖ Soap and water.

Procedure: Nasogastric Intubation (Table 3.22)

Table 3.22: Procedure of nasogastric intubation.

Nursing action	Rationale
1. Check the physician's order, progress notes, and nursing care plan.	To obtain specific instructions/information.
2. Identify the patient.	To perform the right procedure on the right patient.
3. Explain the procedure to the patient.	To allay fears and gain patient's consent and cooperation.
4. Predetermine a signal by which the patient can communicate if he/she requires the nurse to halt the procedure, e.g., raise his/her hand.	The patient is often less frightened if he/she feels able to have some control over the procedure.
5. Collect and prepare the equipment.	This may include placing the Nasogastric tube in freezer for up to 30 minutes. This assists in the easy passage of the tube that becomes slightly rigid when cold.
6. Ensure the patient's privacy	To avoid unnecessary embarrassment.
7. Help the patient into a comfortable position. Sitting upright either in a bed or on a chair. Support the patient head with pillows.	To allow easy passage of the tube. This position enables easy swallowing and ensures that the epiglottis is not obstructing the esophagus.
8. Observe the patient throughout this procedure.	
9. Remove the patient's dentures, if present place in labeled container.	
10. Wash and dry hands.	
11. Check the patient's nostrils and request patient to sniff each nostril in turn or clean the nostrils if necessary.	To identify/clear any obstruction.
12. Ask the patient of any nasal defect or tenderness in order to avoid attempting to pass the tube through a defective nasal passage.	
13. Establish the distance that the tube is to be passed by measuring the distance on the tube from the patient's ear lobe to the bridge of the nose to the bottom of the Xiphisternum	To indicate approximately the length of tube required entering into the stomach.
14. Using clean technique, assemble the equipment.	
15. Lubricate about 15–20 cm of the tube with water soluble jelly, which has been placed on a gauze swab.	To reduce friction between the mucus membrane and the tube.
16. Ask the patient to relax as much as possible while the tube is passed.	
17. Insert the tube and slide it gently but firmly inward and backward along the floor of the nose to the nasopharynx. If an obstruction is felt, withdraw the tube and try again or use another nostril.	To facilitate the passage of the tube by following the natural anatomy of the nose.
18. Encourage the patient to swallow and breathe through his mouth when the tube reaches the pharynx keeping the chin down and head forward to assist the passage of the tube.	To focus the patient's attention on something other than the tube. The swallowing action closes the glottis enabling the tube to pass into the esophagus.
19. Advance the tube until the length previously measured has been inserted and the mark has reached the external nares. If the patient shows any signs of distress, e.g., gasping or cyanosis, remove the tube immediately.	Distress may indicate that the tube is in the bronchus.
20. Ascertain whether the tube is in the stomach by: • Aspirating the contents of the stomach with a syringe. The aspirate should turn blue litmus papered. • Place the stethoscope over the epigastria and inject 2–3 mL of air to the tube.	The acidic nature of the stomach contents verifies the position of the tube. Air can be detected by a whooshing sound when entering the stomach.
21. Secure the tube to the patient's nose with tape. Secure the free-end of the tube in the suitable position avoiding visual obstruction.	To secure the tube and ensure the patients comfort.

Contd...

Nursing action	Rationale
22. Aspirate the stomach contents as per the order of the doctor (If required, dispatch specimen to laboratory).	
23. Ensure that the patient is left feeling as comfortable as possible.	
24. Clean and dispose off the equipment.	
25. Wash hands.	
26. Initiate and maintain intake and output chart.	
27. Document the nursing procedure appropriately, monitor after–effects and report any abnormal findings immediately.	

Nasogastric Tubefeeding

Enteral feeding via nasogastric tube is preferred over parenteral nutrition because it improves utilization of nutrients, for patients prevent dislocation of bacteria from the gut, and is less expensive. If the bowel can handle nutrients, this method should be used. Nasogastric feeding or gastric lavage is the instillation of specially prepared nutrients into the digestive tract through a tube that is inserted through one of the nostrils, down the nasopharynx and into the alimentary tract.

Purposes

- To supply the body with adequate nourishment, when the patient is unable to take food by mouth (e.g., unconscious, semiconscious, and delirious patients) or for patients who will not eat (e.g., psychosis patients, elderly, or confused).
- To supply with adequate nutrients when conditions of mouth or esophagus make the chewing or swallowing difficult or impossible, e.g., patients with fractured jaw, structure esophagus, surgery of mouth, and esophagus.

Requirements/Equipment

- A clean tray containing.
- Large volume syringe.
- Required feed, fluid.
- Kidney tray.
- Stethoscope.
- A glass with water for flushing the tubings.
- Continuous infusion set is continuous drip method is ordered.
- Towel.
- Disposable gloves (if needed).
- Measured glass to measure the fluid intake.

Procedure: Nasogastric Tubefeeding (Table 3.23)

Table 3.23: Procedure of nasogastric tubefeeding.

Steps	Rationale
1. Explain procedure to patient.	To prevent anxiety.
2. Ask patient for any history of allergies.	Early identification helps to prevent food allergies.
3. Auscultate for bowel sounds before feeding.	Bowel sounds indicate presence of peristalsis and ability of GI tract to digest nutrients.
4. Wash hands and put on clean gloves (optional).	Remove harmful microorganisms. Protect hands from contact with body sections.
5. Check placement of gastric tube by means of aspiration of gastric juice is by checking with stethoscope while introducing air into the stomach.	To confirm whether the tip of the tube is in the stomach.
6. Position patient to high Fowler's position or elevate head of bed to 30 degrees.	Elevated head helps to prevent aspiration.
7. Place a towel under the chin.	To protect the patients clothing's and bed linen.
8. Examine the appearance of aspirated contents.	To determine whether the previous feed has digested or not.
9. Pinch proximal end of the feeding tube and elevate to 18 inches above the patients head. Fill syringe with the required feed. Allow syringe to empty gradually, refill until prescribed amount has been given to the patient.	Prevents air from entering patient's stomach.
10. If continuous drip method is used, hang the feeding bag to the pole above 18 inches above patient's head and connect end of bag to the proximal end of the feeding tube and set rate.	Continuous feeding method is designed to deliver prescribed hourly rate of feeding. This method reduces risk of diarrhea.
11. Regulate the drip rate to permit the formula to infuse over 20–30 m by adjusting the height of the feeding bag or adjusting the rate of flow.	Prevents large amount of formula infusion in a short time.
12. When tube feedings are not being administered, clamp the proximal end of the tube.	Prevents air from entering stomach between feeding.

Contd...

Contd...

Steps	Rationale
13. Rinse the tube with plain water at the end of feeding.	Rinsing tubing with water cleans old tube feedings and prevents bacterial growth.
14. Reclamp the gastric tube.	To prevent return flow of feeds.
15. Remove gloves and wash hands.	To limit transfer of microorganisms.
16. Record amount of feeding, patient's response to tube feeding and untoward effects in nurses' notes and record intake in fluid balance chart.	To document amount of feeding administered to patient. Intake and output are indicators of fluid status. Documentation allows the other health team members to plan for next feeding.

PSYCHOLOGICAL AND SPIRITUAL NEEDS

* Psychological and spiritual needs
* Importance
* Nurses role-diversional and recreational therapy

CARE OF TERMINALLY ILL AND DYING PATIENT

* Dying patient's sign and symptoms need of dying patient and family,
* Nursing care of dying: special considerations, advance directives, euthanasia, will dying declaration, organ donation, etc.
* Medicolegal issues
* Care of the dead body
* Care of unit
* Autopsy
* Embalming

Provide Care for Terminally Ill

Terminal Illness

Much chronic illness, which is not responding to medication or medical therapies and changes in life style, keep progressing with complication of specific disease is called terminal illness. Example any malignancy, chronic renal failure not responding to dialysis and not able to arrange transplant, heart failure, etc., is termed as terminal illness.

Terminal illness lead to fear of death causes disturbances to physical, psychological, social well-being, create uncertainty about life. Individual experiencing terminal illness often find themselves reviewing and asking, why this happens to me? What I have done? Terminal illness always affects family members specially life partner and children.

It is very essential to consider the terminal illness patient's physical and psychological symptoms, experiencing at the end of life, regardless of whether the client receive care in a hospital, or at home. Providing complete care is important for patient, which includes physical, social, psychological, and spiritual support.

One of the examples in Indian context that, Mr. Murthy age 30 years suffering from both kidney failures underwent dialysis twice a week. His family consists of father, mother, two sisters, and two brothers all are younger to him. Father is a driver having his own taxi and whole family depends on his earning. For managing Murthy's dialysis, his father sold the taxi, started working as a driver due to this his income reduced to 50% and at the end he could not able to arrange kidney transplant to his son, which is required for his survival. After struggling 8 years Mr. Murthy expired. When we examine the incident, we can understand that how much struggle whole family has to undergo with this type of terminally ill clients.

Death—Definition, Meaning, Types (Brain and Circulation Death)

A person who has sustained either irreversible cessation of all functions of circulatory and respiratory functions or irreversible cessation of all function of the entire brain, including the brainstem is dead. A determination of death must be made in accordance with accepted medical standard.

Biological Death

This is the irreversible cellular damage, due to the lack of oxygen. The declaration of death is made through a physical examination that includes absence of breathing and heart sound, immediate cessation of vital functions, the body becomes bluish, cool, and passes urine and stool. After death declaration, family members are informed and involve in their grief and manage care of the body after death.

Clinical Death

This is the absence of vital signs; heart beats and breathing. This process is irreversible, difficulty for swallowing, urinary incontinence, loss of reflexes; body becomes cold and clammy, decrease in vital signs or restlessness at the end loss of consciousness.

Circulatory Death

Circulatory death occurs when the heart has irreversibly stopped beating and when circulation and oxygenation to the tissue irreversibly stops.

Brain Death

Brain death when a person on artificial life support machine no longer has any brain functions. This means they will not regain consciousness or be able to breathe without support. A person who's brain dead is legally confirmed as dead.

Sign of Impending Death

Sign of impending death include:
* Loss of movement, sensation, and reflexes
* Decreasing body temperature, pulse, blood pressure

- Cheyne-Stokes respiration
- Cold and clammy skin
- Decreased urinary/bowel secretion
- Cyanosis of extremities

Dying Patient Bill of Rights

- I have the right to be treated as a living human being until I die
- Respecting advance care directives and living wills
- Provide emotional, spiritual, and physical care
- Courtesy, respect, dignity, and timely responsive attention to his or her needs
- Competent terminal ill treatment
- Right to obtain medical record
- Right to make treatment choice
- Be free of pain
- Maintain sense of hopefulness
- Have their questions answered honestly

Care of Dying Patient

Death

Death may occur due to the result of acute illness, age, accident, or chronic illness. Death may result with irreversible cessation of all functions, including brain, respiration, and cardiovascular system and person not responding to deep painful stimuli and lack of all reflexes.

Many patient prefer to die at home in familiar setting, some individual prefer to die in hospital. Family members and healthcare providers try to support the client wishes.

- Provide daily basic care, offer help with hygienic needs and manage symptoms
- Maintain pain, daily pain management
- Discuss with family members and medical team regarding available treatment facility.

Care after Death

- Deceleration of death by qualified doctor and confirm death.
- Confirm any organ donation example eye donation inform concerned authority, assist for the procedure.
- Provide support for grieving family members while dealing with extreme stress of loosing loved one.
- Take consent for autopsy, the surgical dissection of a body after death to determine exact cause of death. According to country law, an autopsy is performed when suspecting unnatural death.
- Document death certificate as per institutional policy to provide an accurate and reliable medical record.
- Document time and date of death, name of the medical officer certifying. Nursing document becomes very important for legal purpose.

Physiological Changes Occurring After Death

Death is declared either when there is brain death or breathing and circulation cannot be restored.

After 1 hour

At the movement of death, all of the muscle in the body relax and allow urine feces to pass, a state called primary flaccidity, pupil dilate, the jaw might fall open, and body joints and limbs are flexible. At the same time, body begins to cool from its normal temperature or death chill, the expected decrease in body temperature during algor mortis can help forensic scientists to calculate approximate time of death. Beginning approximately in the third hour after death, chemical changes within the body cells cause begin stiffening known as rigor mortis

Death declaration certification

Death certificate will be given to relatives of person who expired and certificate will be given by last attending doctor (by qualified registered doctor) as per state regulation, form will be filled and signed forwarded to medical record section.

Autopsy

An autopsy (postmortem examination) is a surgical procedure that consists of a thorough examination of a corpse by dissection to determine the cause, mode, and manner of death or to evaluate any disease or injury that may be present for research or educational purpose.

Embalming

This is the art and science of preserving human remains by treating them to forestall decomposition. This is usually to make the deceased suitable for public or private viewing as part of the funeral ceremony or keep them preserved for medical purposes in an anatomical laboratory.

In the modern procedure of embalming, the blood is drained from one of the veins and replaced by a fluid, usually based on Formalin injected into one of the main arteries, cavity fluid is removed with a long-hallow needle called a trocar and replaced with preservative.

Last office/Death care

When patient dies at hospital nurses provides postmortem care, the care of a body after death. Nurses should respect dead body. Same respect as living person based on individual religion and cultural practice as follows:

- Clean and prepare the body ask family members in preparation of the body or support the preparation such as wearing special cloth artifacts
- Remove all connection such as tubes, catheter, Ryle's tube, artificial denture
- Dress the hair, cover the body with clean sheet, and close eyes gently. Dress any wound in the body. Respect religious beliefs and practices. Allow the family members to view the body
- Handover personal belonging, valuables to the family as per the institution policy
- Complete recording in death register, nursing notes, write time and date of death, person to be notified to hand over the body, time of body transfer and destination.

Equipment
- Bath towels
- Wash cloth
- Bed linen
- Basin
- Soap solution
- Cotton buds
- Gauze pads
- Documentation paper

Euthanasia while dying

Assisted death at the end of life. Providing assistance for suicide by another person or by healthcare providers by providing dangerous dose of medication or withholding of medication and food and fluids, for the purpose of ending someone life but not legally supported. Although assisted suicide is prohibited under common law.

Autopsy

The surgical opening to find out the causes of death. The medical officer incharge determine need for autopsy as per regional law or legal requirements such as unnatural death, road side accident, poison, drugs, suspicion on death, and all medicolegal cases. While doing autopsy inform the family members, if consent is required depends upon nature of death should be taken. Autopsy provides a legal record. After autopsy cause of death will be ruled out and report will be send to the concern authority.

Terminal illness

Much chronic illness, which is not responding to medication or medical therapies and changes in life style, keep progressing with complication of specific disease is called terminal illness. Example any malignancy, chronic renal failure not responding to dialysis and not able to arrange transplant, heart failure, etc., termed as terminal illness.

Terminal illness lead to fear of death causing disturbances to physical, psychological, social well-being, create uncertainty about life. Individual experiencing terminal illness often find themselves reviewing and asking, why this happens to me? What I have done? Terminal illness always affects family members especially life partner and children.

It is very essential to consider the terminal illness patient's physical and psychological symptoms, experiencing at the end of life, regardless of whether the client receive care in a hospital, or at home. Providing complete care is important for patient, which includes physical, social, psychological, and spiritual support.

One of the examples in Indian context that, Mr. Murthy age 30 years suffering from both kidney failures had undergone dialysis twice a week. His family consists of father, mother, two sisters, and two brothers all are younger to him. Father is a driver having his own taxi and whole family depends on his earning. For managing Murthy's dialysis, his father sold the taxi, started working as a driver due to this his income reduced to 50% and at the end he could not able to arrange kidney transplant to his son, which is required for his survival. After struggling 8 years Mr. Murthy expired. When we examine the incident we can understand that how much struggle whole family has to undergo with this type of terminally ill clients are there in the family.

Spiritual problems

Any individual suffering with terminal illness, major life changes occur, especially spiritual distress when there is a conflict between person beliefs about life. Person often becomes more spiritual, more aware of purpose and value of life, and adjusting his life according to situation. Their spiritual belief based on many factor such as religion, caste, education, culture, economic status, and life style. It is often based on a lifelong belief with religious practice, illness always threatens the spirituality. Spiritual distress causes person to feel alone, often ask their spiritual values, individual experience and accept with individual care giver and family members.

Counseling and supporting grieving relatives
- Allow freedom to express feeling and fear
- Use effective coping strategies
- Support appropriately
- Listening to their concern
- Being nonjudgmental listeners
- Be sure all family members able to participate in grieving process
- Remind family members about rest and food
- Preparing the family ahead of time
- Listening to the family expression of grief and loss
- Acknowledge their shock and listen to their grief

Placing the body in the mortuary

A mortuary is a room or area, often in a hospital, where a dead body is kept. A mortuary is a place where a body is kept until it is buried or cremated, if relatives not taking body directly or no medicolegal issues of dead person or cause of death body will be shifted to mortuary before postmortem, nurses responsibility to see, take care of dead body, and shifting the body to mortuary, while shifting keep an identity tag and following to be written in the tag:
- Name of the deceased
- Diagnosis or cause of death
- Address of relatives
- Identification of dead body
- Dr who certified the death
- Contact number of relatives

Caregiver role

Care provided by family members and healthcare providers either in hospital or at home, it will support individual to cope with the situation. Symptoms management is very important when dealing with terminally ill. Care givers confidence and therapeutic communication skill becomes an important aspect to build caring relationship with the client. Confidence building, trust development, meet and support client physical, psychological, emotional, spiritual needs, call for special skills, which enable the individual to understand the meaning of terminal illness.

Terminal Illness Health Model (Table 3.24)

Table 3.24: Terminal illness health model.

Available services	Client response
• Client experience available services offered by healthcare institution • Healthcare providers	• Exposure to treatment environment • Previous client exposure to treatment • Exposure to different choices of medical regimen
Terminally ill	
Support client • Helping client to adjust to loss or stressful life situation • Collaboration with different choices of medical intervention	**Building confidence** Client will improve personal harmony and connections with care givers

The client will improve personal harmony and connection with caregivers

Assessment

❖ Assess how illness affects his strength, faith, and belief.
❖ Identify activities that will help physically, emotionally, socially, and economically.
❖ Encourage to build relationship with his family members.
❖ Assess need for guidance and counseling, if necessary.

Nursing Implementation

❖ Careful evaluation of patient includes physical, psychological, and spiritual dimension, understanding how the patient and family are affected.
❖ Educating patient and their care givers.
❖ Supporting patient and family to adopt life with illness.
❖ Decide end of life goal.
❖ Encourage to discuss openly about illness.
❖ Discuss harmful effect of illness and its prognosis.
❖ Find out any difficulty which was not able to reveal.
❖ Discuss what message wants to communicate to family members or to community.
❖ Ask whom they wanted to communicate in their family.
❖ Coordinate with healthcare services with serious progressive illness.
❖ Careful management of symptoms.

Pain Management

❖ Pain assessment should be done during admission. Assess whenever patient condition changes to pain.
❖ Assess the area of pain, ask the patient to rate the severity of the pain.
❖ Ask the patient to describe nature of pain (description such as sharp, shooting, or burning, onset, and duration).
❖ The comprehensive pain assessment is the basis of pain management.
❖ Accept patient report while assessing pain.
❖ Administer analgesics as prescribed.
❖ Educate patient and family on appropriate pharmacological intervention.

Managing Dyspnea

Breathing difficulties is common in patient approaching the end of life in terminal illness.

❖ Observe the signs of dyspnea associated with tachypnea, cyanosis for the patient with COPD, advanced heart disease, etc.
❖ Administer medication as prescribed
❖ Manage anxiety, advice relaxation technique, administer anxiolytic medication as prescribed
❖ Treat underlying disease
❖ Administer oxygen, if required.

Nurses Role in Caring Terminal Illness

Nurses role involve educating and counseling the patient and their care giver, supporting to adapt to life with illness.

❖ Nurses approaches toward patients and family should be open.
❖ Understand cultural differences among patient in Indian context.
❖ As Indian tradition death is an untimely violent and unprepared. A good death is timely in the right place.
❖ Signs and symptoms in terminal illness may be caused by the disease itself or by medication adverse effect. Complication of disease should carefully and systematically assessed and managed.
❖ Observe how symptoms disturb the client physical functioning, mobility, nutritional status, and elimination activities.
❖ Discuss with patient and family about the nature of symptoms, i.e., particular time of the day, how frequent and intensity of symptoms appear and how the patient coping with the symptoms.
❖ Pharmacological and nonpharmacological methods of symptoms management may be used, specifically for pain, nausea, dyspnea, constipation and use of relaxation technique to achieve desired effect.
❖ Planning for intervention for symptoms management is given more importance.

Procedure: Care of Dead Body (Table 3.25)

Table 3.25: Procedure of care of dead body.

Sl. No.	Nursing action	Rationale
1.	No preparation of the body may be began until the physician has officially pronounced the patient is dead	To avoid legal implication To issue death certificate

Contd...

Contd...

Sl. No.	Nursing action	Rationale
2.	Provide privacy for relatives to express their grief in whatever manner they choose. Make certain that families have all the information	To be at ease To aid in official leg document
3.	Invite the relatives to call if they have lingering question or concerns that they wish to discuss	To avoid confusion
4.	Inform appropriate person	To inform relatives, if they are not in the hospital
5.	Wash and dry hands	To prevent cross-infection
6.	Involve relatives if they wish to participate in the procedure	To give them self-satisfaction
7.	Do disposable gloves	To prevent cross-infection
8.	Place the diseased in his/her back. Close his/her eyelids, remove pillows. Support the jaw by placing the pillow on the chest underneath the jaw. Remove any mechanical aids such as foam rings, heel pads, etc. Straighten the limb	If the procedure is delayed after rigor mortis (stiffening of body occur 2–4 hour after death) it is difficult to handle the body.
9.	Wash the deceased, clean the nostrils, ear, and mouth. Replace any denture, trim the nails	For esthetic reasons
10.	Drain the bladder by pressing on the lower abdomen. Pack all orifices. Remove dressing and drainage tubes are left in position (by medical instruction) cut them to just above skin level, cover with a dressing pad, and secure them with tape or loose bandage	The body continues to secrete fluids after death. Leaking orifices pose a health hazards to any staff coming into contact with the body Procedure prevents bad odor from the body

Contd...

Sl. No.	Nursing action	Rationale
11.	Redress any wound	Clean dressing are applied to prevent any further leakage from wounds site
12.	Label one wrist and one ankle with identification label (name, medical record numbers, age, sex, ward, date and time of death, hospital name and nurse initial)	To ensure correct identification of the body
13.	Wrap the body in a mortuary sheet ensuring that the face and feet are covered and that all limbs are held securely in position	To avoid possible damage to body
14.	Tape the second notification of death card to the outside of the sheet	For easy identification of the body in the mortuary
15.	Clean away the equipment used during the procedure	
16.	Remove gloves, wash hands	
17.	Hand over to the body to relatives, if present or remove to hospital mortuary	
18.	Document the procedures appropriately	

Contd...

UNIT 4

Assessment of Patient/Client

LEARNING OBJECTIVES

After completing this unit, learner will be able to:
- Discuss physical assessment
  - Importance, principles, and methods of assessment
  - Height, weight, and posture
  - Head to toe examination
- Explain physiological assessment
  - Vital signs, normal-abnormal characteristics, and factors influencing the variations
  - Observation and collection of specimen: urine, stool, vomitus, and sputum
- Describe psychological assessment

HEALTH ASSESSMENT

Interview Technique

Collecting patient data is a core step in the nursing process. Often referred to as a nursing health assessment interview, nurses must systematically collect patient information so patients can receive the care they need. Health assessment in nursing is so much more than asking questions, it is the gateway to building an effective nurse-patient relationship that will make patient feel at ease, supported, and empowered.

Essential elements of a nursing health assessment is expressing to the patient that you are committed or dedicated to his or her wellness.

The respect model, which is widely used to promote nurse's awareness of their own cultural bases and develop their rapport with patient from different cultural backgrounds.

Elements of interview technique:
- Establish rapport
- Respect patient privacy
- Empathy
- Support
- Partnership
- Explanations
- Cultural competence
- Do not use medical terminology

Communication skills are the fundamental link between the nurse and the patient. Although, communication with patients may seem like a simple task, it actually takes practice and knowledge.

Observation Techniques

Observation is the process of watching someone or something. Often, observation is an informal action, but it can also be formal and involve data collection. An observation can also be the collected information itself.

Observation techniques involve observing actual behaviors, which are subsequently scored. There are many types of observations, covert and overt observation and participant and nonparticipant, which all have their strengths and weaknesses.

Observational learning is a major component of Bandura's social learning theory. He also emphasized that four conditions were necessary for any form of observing and modeling behavior, attention, retention, reproduction, and motivation.

Observation is way of gathering data by watching behavior, events, or nothing but physical characteristics in their natural setting. Observations can be overt (everyone knows they are being observed) or covert (no one knows they are being observed and observer is concealed).

Importance of Observation Technique

Observation provides the most accurate information about people, their tasks, and their needs. Since healthcare providers need to know their client's behavior, observing is the most important because it provides the most accurate information about client's problems and needs.

Observations, often perceived as a basic routine, are a vital part of the information gained to ensure safer patient care and early recognition, of clinically deteriorating condition.

Importance of Health Assessment
- To obtain base line data about the client's functional activities.
- To supplement, confirm, or refuse data obtained in the nursing history.
- To identify disease in its early stage.
- Determine the cause and extent of the disease
- To obtain data that determines the nature of the treatment or nursing care needed for the patient.
- To find out whether the person is medically fit or not for a particular task.
- To screen for the presence of disease.

Process of Health Assessment

There are several types of nursing assessment; each one is conducted at different times and for different purposes.
- **Initial assessment:** This is aimed at providing a complete database for identifying problems and planning care. It also provides the baseline data for comparison when evaluating the effectiveness of care. It is, therefore, performed as close to the time of admission as possible. It includes taking a comprehensive nursing history and performing a physical examination.
- **Focused assessment:** This is aimed at providing data about a specific problem. It may be carried out at the time of the initial assessment, once a problem is identified or as part of the ongoing assessment after problems are confirmed.
- **Time lapse assessment:** This provides current data to compare with the baseline data collected previously. It is undertaken sometime after the initial assessment.
- **Emergency assessment:** This is used to identify life-threatening problems that may occur whenever a physiological or psychological crisis presents itself. These assessments are carried out as and when needed.

Basic Skills for Assessment

The basic skills needed for assessment are:
- Good communication skills.
- **Accurate observation skills:** These enable the nurse to secure objective and subjective data needed to identify nursing problems and to plan, provide, and evaluate care. They have been the focus for learning fundamentals of nursing.
- Examination skills are also needed to obtain objective physical data and these skills will be the focus of this unit.

PHYSICAL EXAMINATION AND ASSESSMENT

Physical examination or physical assessment is an integral part of the nursing assessment. It is performed following the health history. A complete health assessment is generally conducted from the head to the toe; however, the procedure can vary in many ways according to the age of the client/individual, severity of the illness, the preference of the nurse and the agency's priorities and procedures regardless of what procedure is used, and the patient's energy and time need to be considered. The health assessment is, therefore, conducted in a systematic and efficient manner that requires the fewest position change for the patient.

Definition

Physical examination or physical assessment is a thorough investigation of the entire body or some parts of the body to determine the general physical or mental condition of the body (client).

Techniques of Physical Examination

The nurse depends on his/her own senses and uses them in five examination techniques that enable her to collect a broad range of physical data about the patients. These are:
1. **Inspection (using sight)**
2. **Palpation (using touch)**
3. **Percussion (using hearing and touch)**
4. **Auscultation (using hearing)**
5. **Olfaction (using smell).**

Inspection

Inspection is a visual examination, i.e., assessing using the sense of sight. The nurse inspects with the naked eye and with a lighted instrument such as an otoscope (used to view the ear). Nurses frequently use this technique to assess color, rashes, scars, body shape, facial expressions that may reflect emotions, and body structures, e.g., the inner eye. Inspection is an active process, not a passive one. The nurse must know what to look for and where. Inspection should be systematic, so that nothing is missed. Lighting must be sufficient; either natural or artificial light can be used.

Palpation

Palpation is the examination of the body using the sense of touch. The pads of the fingers are used because their concentration of nerve endings makes them highly sensitive to tactile discrimination.
- Texture, e.g., of the hair
- Temperature, e.g., of a skin area
- Vibration, e.g., of a joint
- Position, size, consistency, and mobility of organs or masses
- Distention, e.g., of urinary bladder
- Presence and rate of peripheral pulses
- Tenderness or pain.

There are two types of palpation: (1) Light and (2) Deep. Light (superficial) palpation should always precede deep palpation, because heavy pressure on the fingertips can dull the sense of touch. Deep palpation is a technique used more commonly by nurse practitioners and clinical specialists than by nurses in general practice.

The effectiveness of palpation depends largely on the patient's relaxation. Nurses can assist a patient to relax by:

- Gowning and/or draping the patient appropriately.
- Positioning the patient comfortably.
- Ensuring that their own hands are warm before beginning, e.g., running them under warm water, if they are cold.
- Commencing palpation with areas that are not painful.
- During palpation, the nurse should be sensitive to the patient's verbal and facial expressions indicating discomfort.

Percussion

Percussion is an assessment method in which the body surface is struck to elicit sounds that can be heard or vibrations that can be felt.

Purposes

Percussion is used to determine the size and shape of internal organs by establishing their borders. It indicates whether tissue is fluid-filled, air-filled, or solid. Percussion elicits five types of sound; flatness, dullness, resonance, hyper resonance, and tympany.

- Flatness is an extremely dull sound produced by very dense tissue, such as muscle or bone.
- Dullness is a thud-like sound produced by those tissues, such as the liver, spleen, or heart.
- Resonance is a hollow sound such as those produced by lungs filled with air.
- Hyper resonance is not produced in the normal body. It is described as booming and can be heard over an emphysematous (pathological distention of lung tissues by air) lung.
- Tympany is a musical or drum-like sound produced from an air-filled abdomen.

Types of percussion

There are two types of percussion: (1) Direct percussion and (2) Indirect percussion. In direct percussion, the nurse strikes the areas to be percussed directly with the pads of two, three, or four fingers or with the pad of the middle finger. The strikes are rapid and the movement is from the wrist. This technique is not generally used to percuss the thorax but is useful in percussion an adult's sinuses.

The second type, indirect percussion, is the striking of an object (e.g., a finger) held against the body area to be examined. This technique is generally used to percuss the thorax.

Auscultation

Auscultation is the process of listening to sounds produced within the body. Auscultation may be direct or indirect.

- Direct auscultation is done by the use of the unaided ear, e.g., to listen to a respiration wheeze or the grating of a moving joint.
- Indirect auscultation is done by the use of stethoscope, which amplifies the sounds and conveys them to the nurse's ear. A stethoscope is used primarily to listen to sounds from within the body, e.g., heart, lungs, and bowel sounds.

Olfaction

Olfaction is the sense of smell. Certain alterations in the body function create characteristic body odors. The sense of smell can detect abnormalities that go unrecognized by any other means (**Table 4.1**).

Table 4.1: Example of odors.

Odor	Site or source	Potential causes
Alcohol	Oral cavity	Ingestion of alcohol
Ammonia	Urine	Urinary tract infection
Halitosis	Oral cavity	Poor dental and oral hygiene, gum disease
Sweet fruity, ketones	Oral cavity	Diabetes ketoacidosis

Preparation for examination patient and unit

Before beginning a physical assessment, the nurse should make necessary arrangements to properly prepare the examination room, equipment, and patient. Poor preparation may result in a haphazard examination that yields incomplete or inaccurate assessment findings.

Preparing the environment: To promote the patient's comfort and ensure an efficient examination, the examination room should have the following features:

- Privacy of the patient
- Curtains or dividers to enclose the patient's bed
- A warm comfortable temperature
- Proper examination clothing for the patient
- Adequate lighting
- Control of outside noises
- Precautions to prevent interruptions by visitors or other healthcare personnel
- A bed or table set at examiner's waist level.

Preparing the equipment: The nurse uses a variety of equipment throughout the assessment process. To facilitate the examination, the equipment should be readily accessible, in proper working order, and warmed. The following is a list of equipment and supplies for general physical examination. There may be a need for specific instruments in a special examination.

Equipment and supplies needed for performing a physical examination (**Table 4.2**).

Preparing the patient: To ensure an accurate assessment and physical examination, the patient must be properly prepared physically and psychologically. A tense, anxious patient will not go through any of the physical maneuvers required during examination or cooperate with the nurse's instructions. To prepare the patient properly, the nurse will:

Table 4.2: List of equipment and supplies for general physical examination.

Equipment	Functions
Incontinent sheet	Protects bed linen from getting soiled
Drapes	Ensures privacy for the client
Forms	Documents pertinent information
Gloves	Prevents cross-infection
Gown for patient	For easy access of different body parts of the client
Paper towel	Dry hands and arms, and to wipe equipment
Percussion hammer	Test various reflexes of the body
Height-weight scale	Measures body weight and height of the client
Specimen containers	Collect specific sample for laboratory evaluation
Sphygmomanometer and cuff	Measures blood pressure
Stethoscope	Auscultate different body sound, e.g., heart sound
Measuring tape	Measures body parts, e.g., abdominal girth
Thermometer	Measures body temperature
Tongue depressor	Facilitates visualizing pharynx or to test gag reflex
Wristwatch with second hand	Records time of examination and used when checking vital signs
Cotton applicators	Examine superficial sensations of the skin including corneal reflex
Eye chart (e.g., Snellen's chart)	Test visual acuity
Flashlight	Facilitates visualization of ear, nose and throat and to check pupil reaction
Lubricant	Lubricant instrument is used in rectal and vaginal examination
Ophthalmoscope	Examines fundus of the eye
Otoscope	Examines outer ear and the tympanic membrane
Sterile safety pin	Examines deep sensation of the skin
Tuning fork	Test hearing acuity
Vaginal speculum	Facilitates vaginal examination
Proctoscope	Facilitates rectal examination

❖ Provide for patient's physical comfort by allowing the opportunity to empty the bowel or bladder (a good time to collect the needed specimens).
❖ Provide privacy while the patient changes into a gown and gives the patient time to undress, assisting, if necessary.
❖ Drape body parts that need not be exposed.
❖ Help the patient assume proper positions during examination so that body parts are accessible and the patient stays comfortable. The nurse adjusts drapes accordingly.
❖ Thoroughly explain what will be done, what the patient should expect to feel, and how the patient can cooperate.
❖ Use simple terms when describing steps of the examination.
❖ Encourage the patient to ask questions and mention discomfort felt during the examination.
❖ Have a witness or third person present in the examination room during examination of genitalia when patient and nurse are of opposite genders. The witness is a third person to the examiner's proper conduct.
❖ Pace or time of the examination process according to the patient's physical and emotional tolerance.

It is difficult to examine patients on beds or stretchers. Special examination tables make patients easily accessible and help them assume special positions. The tables are high and narrow, so the nurse must carefully assist patients so that they do not fall while getting on and off the tables. Confused or noncooperative patients should not be left on an examination table without supervision. A patient can be made comfortable by raising the head of the table to a position of 30 degree and by offering a small pillow.

General survey

The general survey is a study of the whole person, covering the general health state, and any obvious physical characteristics. It is an introduction to the physical examination that will follow. It should give an overall impression of the person. Objective parameters are used in the general survey, but these apply to the whole person, not just to one body system.

Start a general survey at the moment you first encounter the person. Does the person respond promptly when his or her name is used? Does he or she walk easily to meet you? Or does the person look sick, rising slowly, or with effort, with shoulders slumped? Is the hospitalized person conversing with visitors, involved in reading or television, or lying perfectly? Even as you introduce yourself and shake hands, you collect data. Does the person fully extend the arm, shake your hand firmly, make eye contact or smile? Are the palms dry or wet and clammy? As you proceed through the health history, the measurements, and the vital signs, note the following points that will add up to the general survey. Consider these four areas:

1. **Physical appearance:**
   * **Age**—Is the appearance congruent with stated age?
   * **Sex**—Is development appropriate for age?
   * **Level of consciousness**—Is he/she alert, oriented responding appropriately to questions?
   * **Skin color**—What is the color tone, is there any pigmentation or lesions?
   * **Facial features**—Is there symmetry with movement?

2. **Body structure:**
   - **Stature**—Is height within normal limits for age?
   - **Nutrition**—Does weight appear to be within normal range?
   - **Symmetry**—Do the body parts look equal bilaterally and in proportion?
   - **Posture**—How does the person stand?
   - **Position**—Are there any signs of discomfort, is the person relaxed?
   - **Build and contor**—Do proportions appear normal, are there any deformities?
3. **Behavior:**
   - **Facial expression**—Is there eye contact, what expressions are evident?
   - **Mood and affect**—Is the person comfortable, cooperative?
   - **Speech**—Is speech clear and understandable?
   - **Dress**—Is it appropriate according to the climate and culture, clean, well fitting?
   - **Personal hygiene**—Is the person clean and well groomed?

   All data should be judged against expected normal findings and any deviation from normal should be noted. The **Table 4.3** gives examples of some of the general survey observations and their comparison to normal findings.
4. **Vital signs:**

   Establishing baseline data for the patient's temperature, pulse, respiration and blood pressure, are part of the general physical survey.

Detailed Physical Examination

This is often referred to as a "head-to-toe" examination but may be carried out system-by-system. Whichever way it is approached it should be systematic, comprehensive, and appropriate to the nurse's competence. A detailed physical examination will require the nurse to use all the skills already covered to collect objective physical data, which is then weighed against his/her knowledge base. Abnormalities are detected and from them health problems are identified.

Students in this course will be required to complete physical examinations with an emphasis or inspection and observation of the client's health indicators. This will include examination of:

- **Sensory perception:** Sight, hearing, taste, smell, and touch
- Skin and other body surfaces and features such as mucous membranes, hair, nails
- Respiration
- Circulation
- Nutrition
- Elimination
- Neurological responses
- Immune system responses
- Sexual health

SPECIFIC AREAS OF EXAMINATION

Frequently, nurses assess a specific body area instead of the entire body. These specific assessments are made in relation to patient's complaints, the nurse's own observation

Table 4.3: General survey observations.

Assessment	Normal findings	Deviation from normal
Observe body build, height and weight	Varies with lifestyle	Excessively thin or obese
Listen to relevance and organization of thoughts	Logical sequence. Makes sense or has sense of reality	Illogical sequence. Flight of ideas, confusion
Observe the client's posture and gait	Relaxed, erect posture, coordinated movement	Tense, bent posture, uncoordinated movement, tremors
Observe the client's overall hygiene and grooming	Clean, neat	Dirty, unkempt
Note body and breath odor in relation to activity level	No body odor or minor body of odor related to work	Foul body odor, ammonia odor, acetone breath odor, foul breath
Observe for signs of distress in posture	Relaxed, erect posture	Tense, slouched, bent posture
Note obvious signs of health or illness	Healthy appearance	Pallor, weakness, obvious illness
Mental status		
Assess the client's attitude	Cooperative	Negative, hostile, withdrawn
Note the client's mood	Relaxed and happy	Tensed and sad
Assess orientation to self, place, and time	Oriented	Disoriented
Listen to relevance and organization of thoughts	Logical sequence. Makes sense has sense of reality	Illogical sequence. Flight of ideas, confusion

Table 4.4: Examples of specific situations and assessments.

Situation	Physical assessment
Patient complains of abdominal pain	Inspect, palpate, and auscultate the abdomen; assess vital signs
The nurse administers a cardio tonic drug to a patient	Assess apical pulse and compare with baseline data
The nurse administers postural drainage	Auscultate lungs before and after the procedure
The patient has just had a cast applied to the lower leg	Assess peripheral perfusion of toes, capillary blanch test, pedal pulse if able and vital signs
The patient's fluid intake is minimal	Assess tissue turgor, fluid intake and output, and vital signs

of problems, the patient's presenting of problems, nursing intervention provided, and medical therapies.

Table 4.4 shows some examples of these situations and assessments.

Assessment

1. Note if the client has had any acute distress: Difficulty in breathing, pain, anxiety, if such signs are present.
   Rationale: Signs establish priorities regarding what part of the examination has to be conducted first.

> **Critical Decision Point**
> Findings may change the direction of the examination. Any client in acute distress will require an immediate assessment of the body system(s) affected.

2. Review graphic sheet for temperature, pulse, respirations, and blood pressure and consider factors or conditions that may alter reading of vital signs.
   Rationale: Provides baseline and historical data regarding client's signs.
3. Reconfirm (after reviewing history) the primary reason why the client has sought health care or take the health history, if not already completed.
   Rationale: Keeps assessment focused on client to ensure that client's expectations are addressed.
4. Identify client's normal height and weight. If a sudden gain or loss in weight has occurred, determine the amount of weight change and period of time in which it has occurred.
5. Assess if client has recently been dieting or following exercise program.
   Rationale: Generally, weight of 15–20% above standard indicates excess body fat; however, fluid retention is one factor that must be ruled out. A person's weight can fluctuate, cause of fluid loss or retention.
6. Review client's past fluid intake and output (I and O) records.
   Rationale: Fluid and electrolyte balance maintains health and functions of all body systems. Intake includes all liquids taken orally by feeding tube, and parenteral. Liquid output includes urine, diarrhea stool, fistulas, vomitus, drainage from gastric suction, and drainage from postsurgical tubes, such chest tubes or drains.
7. Identify client's general perceptions about personal health.
   Rationale: Assessment of client's general appearance coupled with client's own perceptions may reveal specific problems.

Implementation

1. **Prepare the client:** Tell the client that you will be doing a routine process to check for areas of concern. Ask client to tell you, if any area you examine hurts when touched.
   Rationale: Behaviors may reflect specific physical or psychological abnormalities. Dementia and level of consciousness influences ability to cooperate. Timing of recent medications, especially pain medication and sedatives, may alter assessment data.
   a. If a client's responses are inappropriate, ask short, answer to-the-point questions regarding the information the client should know, e.g., "Tell me your name". "What is the name of this place?" "Tell me, where you live?" "What day is this?" "What month is this?" or "What season of the year is this?"
   Rationale: Measure client's orientation to person, place, and time. This may be noted in documentation as "Oriented × 3". If disoriented in any way, include subjective or objective data rather than just documenting disorientation.
   b. If client is unable to respond to questions or orientation, offer simple commands, e.g., "squeeze my fingers" or "move your toes".
   Rationale: Levels of consciousness exist along the continuous including full responsiveness, inability to consciously initiate meaningful behaviors, and unresponsiveness to stimuli.
2. **Observe the appearance of the client:** Gender, race, and age. Note the client's physical features.
   Rationale: Gender influences the type of examination performed and manner in which assessments are made. Different physical characteristics and predisposition to illnesses are related to gender and race.
3. **Assess posture, movement, and position**, noting alignment of shoulders and hips while client stands and sits. Observe whether the client has a slumped, erect, or bent posture.
   Rationale: May reveal musculoskeletal problem, mood, or presence of pain.
   a. Body movements: Are they purposeful? Are there tremors of the extremities? Are any body parts immobile?

b. Note if movements are coordinated or uncoordinated.
Rationale: May indicate neurological or muscular problem or emotional stress.

Psychological Preparation

Clients are easily embarrassed when forced to answer sensitive questions about bodily functions or when body parts are exposed and examined. The possibility that the examiner will find something abnormal also creates anxiety. The nurse should convey an open, receptive professional approach; nurse should first explain the examination in general terms. For example, nurse can tell the client—I am going to do a complete physical examination so that I can have a good idea of whether you have any health problems as we go along.

Mental Status and Speech

The assessment regarding mental status and speech can begin during the client's health history. An observation can be made regarding grooming, dress, and hygiene, you may ask yourself—is the person clean and well kept? Is the person's hair, skin, and nails clean and well groomed? Is the clothing appropriate for the present weather condition?

Nutritional Status

The person's nutritional status can reflect the level of general health.

Judgment

A person's judgment can be affected by the level of intelligence, education level, socioeconomic level, and cultural orientation.

Orientation

An assessment is made of a person's orientation to time, place, and person.

Memory

When assessing memory, you need to test the person's immediate, recent, and remote memories. Immediate memory is tested by asking, telephone number, or digits such as code number. Recent memory is tested by asking about events of the day, like breakfast, weather condition of the day. Remote memory is tested by asking about past events, like birthdays, anniversaries.

Affect

Affect is on emotional state such as fear, anger, depression, elation, and frustration.

Consciousness

Assess consciousness with noting whether the client is awake and alert. Note whether the person is able to answer your questions.

Speech

Need to note the characteristics of the person's speech, speech is assessed for quantity (talkative or silent) rate (fast or slow), loudness.

Integumentary System (Skin)

Assessment of the skin reveals a variety of conditions including changes in oxygenation, circulation, nutrition, local tissue damage, and hydration (**Fig. 4.1**).

Cyanosis (bluish discoloration) is best observed on the lips and nail beds. The best site to inspect for jaundice (yellow or orange discoloration) is the client sclera. Erythema (red discoloration) may indicate circulatory changes, e.g., an area of erythema may be due to sun burn or fever.

Color

Inspect the skin color hues seen in the palm, soles of the feet, lips, tongue, and nail beds. Increased color (hyperpigmentation) and decreased color (hypopigmentation) are common.

Moisture

The hydration of skin and mucous membranes helps to reveal body fluids imbalance. Skin surface is lightly rubbed; scaling involves fish-like scales that are easily rubbed off the skin surface. Dry skin includes lack of humidity exposure to skin, smoking, stress, excessive perspiration, and dehydration.

Temperature

Temperature is more accurately assessed by palpating the skin with the dorsum or back of the hand.

Texture

Localized changes may result from trauma, surgical wounds, or lesions. The nurse should ask if the client has had a recent injury to the skin.

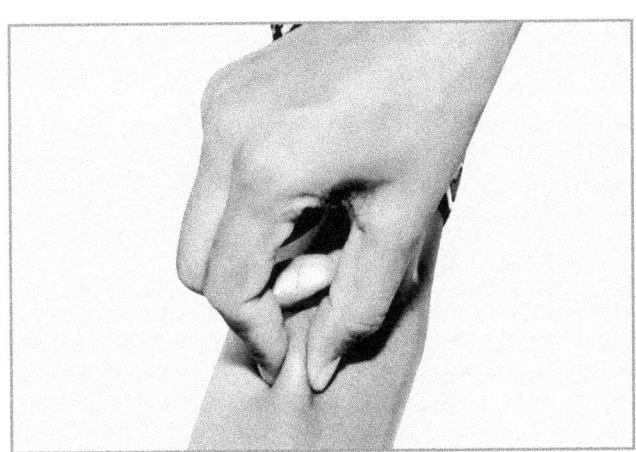

Fig. 4.1: Nurse assesses skin.

Turgor

Turgor is the skin's elasticity, which can be diminished by edema or dehydration. To assess the skin's turgor, fold of skin on the back of forearm or sternal area is grasped with the fingertips and released.

Edema

Areas of skin became swollen or edematous from a build up of fluids in the tissue.

Hair and Scalp

The nurse begins the inspection by noting the color distribution, quality, thickness, and lubrication of the body hair. Note hair loss (alopecia) or thinning of the hair, pediculus humans' capitis (body lice), pediculus corporis (body lice), and pediculus pubis (crab lice). The discovery of lice requires immediate treatment.

Nails

The condition of the nails can reflect general health, state of nutrition and a person's occupation. Before assessing the nails, the nurse asks if the client has had any recent trauma, or asks the client to describe his or her nail care practice.

Head and Neck

An examination of the head and neck includes assessment of the head, eyes, nose, ears, mouth, pharynx, and neck (lymph nodes, carotid arteries, thyroid glands, and trachea).

Head

History of intracranial injury and local or congenital deformities. The examination continues with nurse noting the size, shape of the skull, hydrocephalus, and acromegaly (disorder caused by excessive secretion of growth hormone).

Eyes

Examination of the eyes includes assessment of visual acuity, visual field, extraocular movement, and external and internal structure of the eye.

Visual Acuity

The assessment of visual acuity includes the ability to see small details. Assessment of distant vision requires use of Snellen chart. The client sits or stands 20 feet (6.1 m) away from the chart and tries to read it.

Extraocular Movement

Small skin muscles guide the movement of each eye. The client keeps the head in a fixed position facing the nurse and follows the movement of the fingers (six movements), i.e., lateral rectus, medial rectus, inferior rectus, superior rectus, inferior oblique, and superior oblique.

External Eye Structure

Inspect external eye structure

Position and alignment

The nurse assesses the position of the eyes in relation to one another.

Eyebrow

Inspect for size, extension texture of hair alignment, and movement.

Eyelids

The nurse inspects the eyelids for position, color, condition of the surface, condition and direction of the eye lashes, papillary reaction. Test for eye reaction to light, dilatation, or construction.

Ears

Inspection and palpation are the techniques used to examine the ears. Ear area to be assessed is the external (auricle) and ear canal, internal ear canal, and tympanic membrane (by performing an otoscopic examination).

Auricle

Inspect the auricle for color, size configuration, location, and angle of attachment to the head. The color of the ear should be same as that of the person's skin. Palpate the external ear for nodules and tenderness.

Otoscopic examination

An otoscope must be used to inspect the internal ear canal and tympanic membrane. Inspect the internal canal for impacted cerumen, foreign bodies, discharges, masses, redness, and swelling. Normally, you will view some cerumen, which varies in color (yellow, brown). Inspect the tympanic membrane, which is usually a shiny pearly gray or light pink.

Acoustic Nerve

The acoustic nerve is assessed by auditory acuity. Webber lateralization test, Rinne air, and bone conduction test. The watch assesses test auditory acuity. And in the whisper test, if abnormalities are detected, further testing using an audiometer is needed.

Webber lateralization: To perform the Webber lateralization, place the stem of a vibrating tuning fork in the center of the forehead (**Fig. 4.2**). Ask the person where the sound is heard well. Normally, sound is heard equally well in both ears as it is conducted through the bones. Note any lateralization of sound (sound heard better in one ear than the other). A person with a unilateral conductive hearing loss will hear the sound best in the impaired ear.

Rinne air condition and bone conduction test: The Rinne air and bone conduction test compares bone-conducted sound with air-conducted sound in one ear at a time.

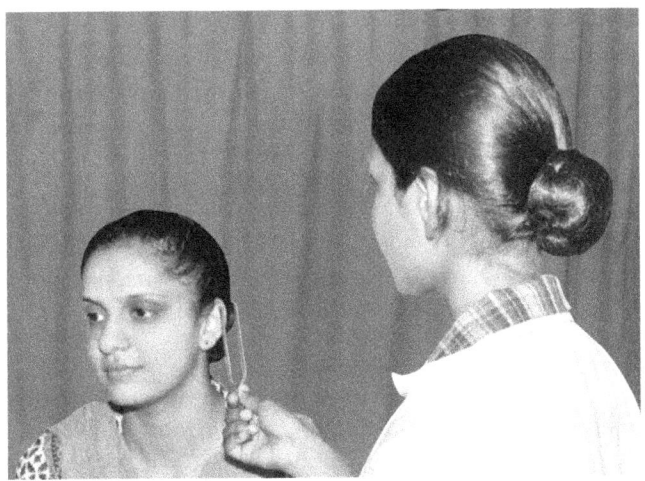

Fig. 4.2: Rinne test: Placing vibrating tuning fork 1–2 cm from ear canal.

Nose and Sinuses

Nose is assessed by inspection and palpitation. Inspect the external surface of the nose for symmetry in color, shape, and size. Palpate the external nares for tenderness to assess the patency. Ask the patient to occlude one ala nasi (one nostril) while breathing through the other.

Frontal and Maxillary Sinuses

Frontal and maxillary sinuses are palpated for tenderness, swelling, and thickening of secretions. Palpate the frontal sinuses by pressing up on the skull on either side of the nose under the eyebrows. Do not press on the eyes. Palpate the maxillary sinuses by pressing up over the lower part of the cheek bones on either side of the nose (**Fig. 4.3**).

Olfactory Nerve

To assess the sensory function of the olfactory nerve, instruct the person to close the eyes and occlude one ala nasi. Provide a familiar scent such as coffee or cinnamon for the person to smell. Test both nares. An absence of the sense of smell may result from excessive smoking, cocaine use, or sinus condition.

Mouth and Pharynx

The mouth and pharynx are assessed through inspection and palpation. Areas to be assessed include the lips, buccal mucosa, gums and teeth, tongue, soft and hard palate, and pharynx. Penlight tongue blade, gauze, and a pair of gloves will be needed.

Lips

Inspect the lips for symmetry, color, edema, and any surface abnormalities. Note that the lips are more pigmented than the facial skin. Common lesions associated with the lips are fissures, commonly seen with chapped lips and herpes simplex (cold sores). Using a gloved hand, palpate the lips for moistness, induration, intactness, and lesions (**Fig. 4.4**).

Gums and Teeth

Inspect the gums by placing your gloved hands in the lower lip and gently pulling it down to expose the gums. Normally, the gums are pink in color and free of lesions, inflammation, and bleeding.

The teeth should be clean, white, straight, firm, evenly spaced, and free of decay. Normally, there are 32 teeth, and inspect for caries, plaque, missing, or loose teeth. Inspection of the teeth can also provide information regarding the person's attitude toward general hygiene.

Tongue

Inspect and palpate the tongue using gloved hands and a piece of gauze. Note the symmetry movement, and color of the tongue. Normally, it should be pink, moist, and smooth. Ask the person to extend the tongue, so that you may palpate it from front to back. Wrap a piece of gauze around the tongue

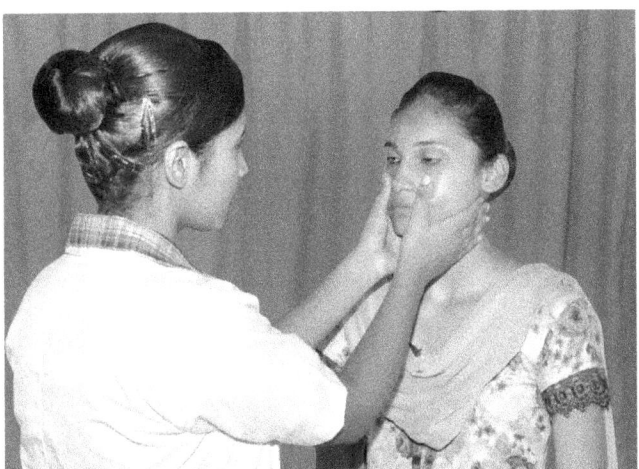

Fig. 4.3: Palpation of maxillary sinuses.

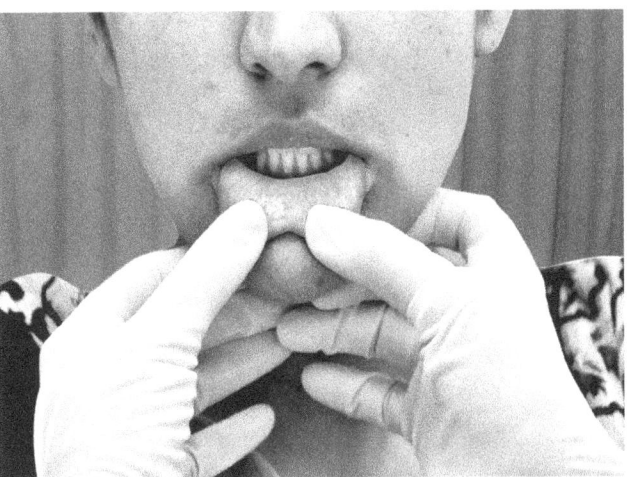

Fig. 4.4: Inspection of inner oral mucosa of lower lip.

during palpation. The floor of the mouth is a common site for oral cancer.

Neck

Assessment is performed using the techniques of inspection and palpation. Upon examination, the person should be in an upright position to facilitate the rotation of the neck. Inspect the neck for color, symmetry, masses, enlargement of the thyroid, or lymph nodes, abnormal pulsation, impaired range of motion, lesions and scars.

Lymph nodes (one of the many small oval structure that filters the lymph and fights infection and in which there are formed lymphocytes, monocytes and plasma cells). Palpate the lymph nodes using the pads of your index finger and middle fingers. Move the skin over the node, gently palpate in sequence, bilaterally, the posterior auricular occipital tonsillar, submaxillary, and submental.

Thyroid

Inspect and palpate the thyroid gland for sizes, shape, and any masses by instructing person to swallow water while extending the neck normally. The thyroid gland and the cricoids cartilage will rise as the person is swallowing. The enlarged thyroid gland is called Goiter; you may palpate the thyroid gland by standing in front or behind the person. Ask the person to swallow. You will be able to feel the thyroid isthmus rise beneath your finger.

Trachea

Inspect and palpate the trachea for any deviation from the midline by placing two fingers. The trachea is present at the suprasternal notch (**Fig. 4.5**).

Carotid Arteries

Inspect and palpate the carotid arteries to assess symmetry, amplitude, rate, and rhythm of pulsation. Palpate only one carotid artery at a time, remembering that these arteries supply essential blood to the brain.

Spinal Accessory Nerve (CN XI)

Innervates the major neck muscles (trapezes and sternocleidomastoid). Assess this nerve and muscle strength by asking the person to shrug the shoulder against the resistance of your hands and to turn the head from one side to the other as you try to resist these movements.

External Jugular Veins

Inspect the jugular veins for abnormal or unusual distention. The jugular veins are not normally distended.

Chest

Examination of chest involves assessment of respiratory system (lungs) and cardiovascular system (chest).

A thorough examination of the chest requires you to use the techniques of inspection, palpation, percussion, and auscultation. The posterior chest is examined first with the person in a sitting or supine position. During the assessment of the thorax, bear in mind the thoracic reference lines and familiar landmark, e.g., ribs, sternal documentation of the location of findings.

The posterior chest is inspected for any skeletal deformities that could affect the status of the respiratory system. Some common abnormalities are kyphosis (an exaggerated curvature of the thoracic vertebra), scoliosis (a lateral curvature of the spine), and lordosis (an exaggerated curvature of the lumbar vertebra) (**Fig. 4.6**).

- ❖ **Anterior thoracic reference line:**
    - Midstream line
    - Midclavicular line
    - Anterior axillary line
    - Midaxillary line
    - Posterior axillary line
- ❖ **Posterior thoracic reference line:**
    - Midspinal line
    - Midscapular line
    - Posterior axillary line

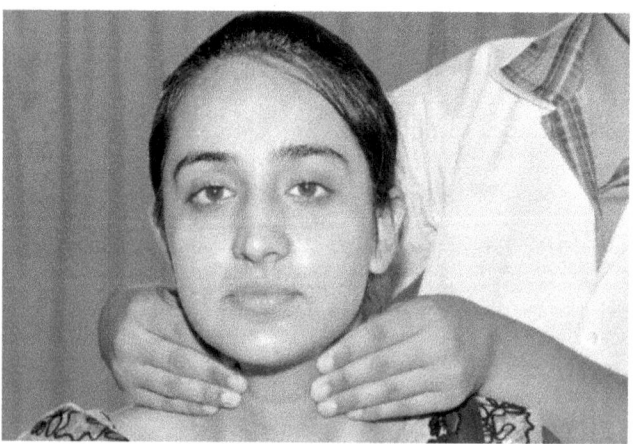

Fig. 4.5: Placement of the fingertips over the trachea to begin palpation of the thyroid gland.

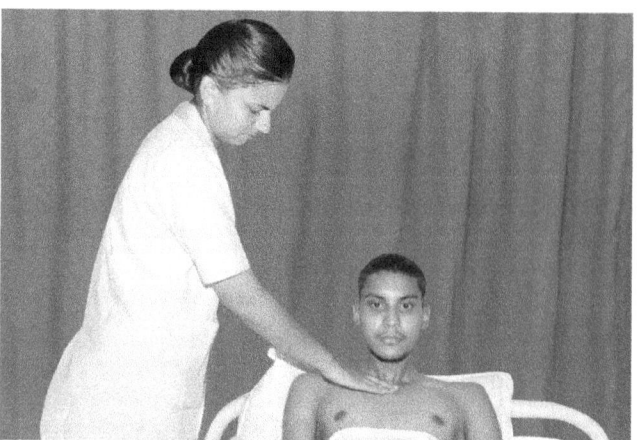

Fig. 4.6: Nurse locating the angle of Louis.

- Midaxillary line
- Anterior axillary line

Lung Assessment

Assess history of tobacco, cough (productive, nonproductive), chest pain, shortness of breath, history of pneumonia, or bronchitis, HIV infection, persistent cough, hemoptysis, unexplained weight loss. Review family history of cancer, tuberculosis, and allergies.

Inspect lungs: Color, intercostals space, chest symmetry, rib space, respiratory rate, shape and position of sternum, position of trachea, and chest expansion.

Palpation

The posterior chest is palpated for costal space, intercostal space, and any tenderness. Masses palpate with the palmar surface of the hand. Assessing the chest and comparing the right side to the left side make the client take deep breath and observe their movement.

Vocal fremitus: During speech, the sound created by the vocal cords is transmitted through the lungs to the chest wall. The sound waves create vibration that can be palpated externally, these vibration are called tactile or vocal fremitus. The building of mucus secretions, the collapse of lung tissue, or the presence of lung lesions can block the vibrations from reaching the chest wall.

Palpate the vibrations with the palmar surface or ulnar side of the hand. Ask the person to repeat the words "ninety nine" or "one, one, one". Use only one hand to palpate fremitus to avoid any discrepancies, differing sensitivity between the hands. You will cover the entire chest by moving back and forth from one side to the other. Also note an increase in fremitus during an inflammatory process.

Percussion

The posterior chest is percussed to determine whether the underlying tissue is air-filled, fluid-filled, or solid. The normal lung should be air-filled producing resonance (loud low pitched).

Auscultation

Auscultation is useful in assessing airflow, the presence of fluid mucus, or obstruction in the surrounding lung and pleural space. Whole auscultation, instruct the person to take deep breaths through the mouth. Listen to at least one full breath in each location following the percussion sequence.

Normal breath sounds: Normal breath sounds are vesicular, bronchial, and bronchovesicular. Breath sounds are soft and low-pitched fine resulting sounds.

Adventitious breath sounds: These are superimposed over normal sounds. The four types of adventitious sounds include crackles, also called rales; ranchi also called gurgles; wheeze; and floral friction rub. Each sound is caused by a specific entity and is characterized by a typical auditory feature.

Anterior Chest

Inspection

The anterior chest is inspected for any skeletal deformities. Some common abnormalities are barrel chest, pigeon chest, and funnel chest.

Palpation

The anterior chest is palpated for areas of tenderness, respiratory excursion, and fremitus.

Percussion

Percuss the anterior and lateral chest.

Auscultation

Auscultation for vesicular, bronchial, and bronchovesicular breath sounds.

Heart

Assessment of heart function is closely compared with findings from the vascular examination. In adults, the heart is located at the center of chest behind and to left of the sternum.

Health history should focus on risk factors for heart disease. The nurse assesses the history of smoking, alcohol intake, caffeine intake, use of recreational drugs, exercise habits and dietary patterns, stressful lifestyle, medication for hypertension, chest pain, and discomfort, anginal pain radiating to one or both the arms history of heart disease.

Inspection, percussion, palpation, and auscultation are the techniques used in the examination of the heart to identify the precordial points. You must be familiar with the landmarks and the angle of Louis is palpated as a prominence on the upper third of the sternum. Palpate this area and move the fingers laterally to identify the second intercostal space. The aortic area is located from the second intercostal space to the right sternal border. The pulmonic area is located at the second intercostal space to the left sternal border. Erbs point is located at the third intercostal space to the left sternal border. The tricuspid area is located at the fourth or fifth intercostal space to the left sternal border the mitral (apical) area is located at the fifth intercostal space medial to the midclavicular line. The epigastric area is the area overlying the xiphoid process.

Inspection

Position the person in a supine position or lying with the head of the bed at a 30°–45° angle inspect the precordial points of the chest for any abnormal pulsation and the apical impulse. The apical impulse is a pulsation located over the apex of the heart at the fifth intercostals space medial to the midclavicular line.

Palpation

The precordial points of the chest are palpated for any abnormal pulsation, thrills, apical impulse and aortic pulsation. A thrill is a palpable cardiac murmur. To palpate the apical impulse, place the heel of the hand on the sternum with your fingers stretched across the chest just under the breast area. Palpate it with your fingertips.

Percussion
Cardiac dullness is located in the third to fifth intercostal space. The auscultation technique assess the normal heart sounds (s1–s4) and murmur. Auscultate over the precordial area with both the stethoscope diaphragm and bell; listen to each area through several breathe through the nose to decrease the interference of breath sounds.

First heart sounds
The first heart sounds (s1) is produced by the closure of the mitral and tricuspid heart valves. It is best heard at the apex of the heart.

Second heart sounds
The second heart sounds (s2) is produced by the closure of the aortic and pulmonic heart valve. It is best heard at the base of the heart (aortic area). Remember that heart is upside down with its apex located at the fifth intercostal space. Along the sternal border, sl and s2 are both high-pitched sounds.

Third heart sound
Third heart sound (s3) is a low-pitched sound heard in the cardiac cycle immediately after s2.

Fourth heart sounds
The fourth heart sounds (s4) is low-pitched sound heard in just before s1.

Heart murmur
This is a harsh rumbling, blowing sounds caused by blood flow across a defective valve.

Examination of Breasts
It is important to examine the breasts of female clients. A small amount of glandular tissue, a potential site for the growth of cancer cells is located in the middle breast. In contrast, the majority of the female breast is glandular.

Female breast
Breast cancer is secondary to lung cancer, the leading cause of death in women with cancer. Early detection is the key to cure. A major responsibility for nurses is to teach client health behavior such as breast self examination (BSE).

History: Factors that affects and increase the risk of developing breast cancer are:
- Null parity
- Late childbearing
- Early menarche
- Family history, especially first-degree relative
- Obesity in postmenopausal women
- Premenopausal exposure to ionizing radiation
- History of benign breast disease
- Previous breast cancer.

Factors still under evaluation
- Alcohol
- High fat diet
- Oral contraception and hormone replacement therapy.

About 80% of symptomatic breast carcinomas appear as a palpable mass. A mobile lump appears, most frequently, in the upper outer quadrant of the breast. There may or may not be pain. If no lump is present, attention may be drawn to a problem by localized discomfort such as burning, stinging, or aching. Less common presentations such as nipple discharge and retraction, Paget disease, dimpling, or orange-peel appearance of the skin may be observed.

BSE should be performed monthly by women aged 20 years and older. An examination by a physician should be performed over 3 years, from the ages of 20–40. Over 40 women a year with a family history of breast cancer should have a yearly physician examination.

Inspection: Inspect the breast and nipple of the patient in sitting position.

Palpation: When pressing deeply on the breast you may mistake a normal rib for hard breast mass. Nodules in the tail of the breast are sometimes mistaken for enlarged axillary lymph.

Breast and axillae examination
Put the client in a standing or sitting position, disrobed to the waist, with her arm at her side.

Inspect the breast:
- Size symmetry
- Contour, masses, dimpling (retraction sign), or flattening
- Appearance of the skin color, (orange peel) thickening, edema, or venous prominence.

Patient education, breast self-examination (BSE)
- **Step 1:**
  - Stand before mirror.
  - Check both breasts from the nipple, dimpling in the contour of the breasts. As you do them you should be able to feel your muscles tighten.
- **Step 2:**
  - Watch closely in the mirror as you clasp your hands behind your head and press your hands forward.
  - Note any change in the contour of your breasts.
- **Step 3:**

Next, press your hands firmly on your hips and bow slightly toward the mirror as you pull your shoulders and elbows forward.

Note any change in the contour of your breasts.

Note: Women should do the next part of the examination in the shower. Your fingers will glide over soapy skin, so you can concentrate on feeling for change inside the breast.

- ❖ **Step 4:**
  - ◆ Raise your left arms
  - ◆ Use 3-4 fingers of your right hand to feel your left breast firmly, carefully, and thoroughly
  - ◆ Beginning at the outer edge, press the flat part of your fingers in small circles
  - ◆ Gradually work toward the nipple
  - ◆ Be sure to cover the whole breast
  - ◆ Pay special attention to the area between the breast and the underarm
  - ◆ Feel for any unusual lumps or masses under the skin.
- ❖ **Step 5:**
  - ◆ Gently squeeze the nipple and look for a discharge
  - ◆ If you have any discharge during the month—whether or not it is during your BSE—see your doctor
- ❖ **Step 6:**
  - ◆ Step 4-5 should be repeated while lying down.
  - ◆ Lie flat on your back with your left arm over your head and pillow or folded towel under your left shoulder.
  - ◆ Repeat on your right breast.

Male breast

The assessment of the male breast is relatively easy, the nipple and areola are inspected for nodules, edema, and ulceration. An enlarged breast may result from obesity or glandular enlargement. Cancer in men is relatively rare. Routine self-examinations are unnecessary (enlarged male breast is called gynecomastia).

Abdominal examination: Assess for nutritional history, appetite, weight gain or loss, gastrointestinal (GI) symptoms, dysphagia, nausea, vomiting, indigestion, belching, flatulence, hematemesis, black or tarry stools (Melina, heart burns, diarrhea, or constipation). Assess for family history of cancer, renal problems, alcoholism, hypertension, or heart disease.

Previous abdominal surgery or trauma

- ❖ Assess client's normal bowel habits, frequency, characteristics of stools. Measures used to promote elimination such as laxatives, enemas, dietary intake, eating, and drinking habits.
- ❖ Assess for abdominal or low back pain location onset, frequency, intensity, duration, relationship to infestation of foods, use of medication, aspirin, anti-inflammatory drugs, steroids, and GI diagnostic test.
- ❖ Determine if female client is pregnant.

The technique used to assess the abdomen involves inspection, auscultation, percussion, and palpation. It will also include the assessment of abdominal reflexes. Remember that the order of techniques is different from the examination of other body parts.

Auscultation is performed after inspection to ensure that the motility of the bowel and bowel sounds are altered.

Before you can begin the abdominal assessment, you need to be familiar with the four quadrants of the abdomen. The abdomen is divided into four quadrants, right upper, right lower, left upper, and left lower. The abdomen may also be divided into nine regions.

PHYSIOLOGICAL ASSESSMENT

Vital signs, normal abnormal, characteristics, and factors influencing the variations.

Assessing Vital Signs

The vital or cardinal signs are body temperature, pulse, respiration, and blood pressure. These signs should be looked at in total, to monitor the vital functions of the body. The signs reflect changes in functions that otherwise might not be observed. Monitoring a patient's vital signs should not be an automatic or a routine procedure; it should be thoughtful and scientific assessment.

Guidelines for Taking Vital Signs

Times to assess vital signs

When and how often to assess a specific patient's health status. Some hospitals have policies about taking patient's vital signs and physicians may specifically order assessment of a vital sign, e.g., "Blood pressure q2h".

Examples of times to assess vital signs are listed below:

- ❖ On patient's admission to a healthcare facility.
- ❖ In hospital, on routine schedule according to physician's order or hospital policy.
- ❖ During patient's visit to clinic or physicians office.
- ❖ Before and after any surgical procedure.
- ❖ Before and after any invasive diagnostic procedure.
- ❖ Before and after administration of medication that affect cardiovascular, respiratory, and temperature control function.
- ❖ When the patient's general physical condition changes, e.g., loss of consciousness or increase in intensity of pain.
- ❖ Before and after nursing interventions influencing any one of the vital signs, e.g., before ambulating a patient previously on bed rest or before patient performs range of motion exercises.
- ❖ Whenever patient reports to nurse any nonspecific symptoms of physical distress, e.g., "feeling funny or different".

Body Temperature—Definition, Physiology, Regulation, Factors Affecting Body Temperature

Definition

Body temperature is the balance between the heat produced by the body and the heat lost from the body. Temperature is a measure of the average kinetic energy of the particles in a object.

Physiology, regulation, factors affecting body temperature:
The physiologic control of the body's core temperature takes place primarily through the hypothalamus, which assumes the role as the body's thermostat. This organ possesses control mechanisms as well as key temperature sensors, which are connected to nerve cells called thermoreceptors.

There are two kinds of body temperature:
1. **Core temperature:** It is the temperature of the deep tissues of the body, e.g., cranium thorax and abdominal cavity. It remains relatively constant (37°C or 98.6°F).
2. **Surface temperature:** It is the temperature of the skin, the subcutaneous tissue, and fat. By contrast, rises and falls in response to the environment.

When measured orally, the average body temperature of an adult is between 36.7°C (98°C) and 37°C (98.6°F).

When the amount of heat produced by the body exactly equals the amount of heat lost, the persons is in heat balance.

Factors affecting body heat production and heat loss
A number of factors affect the body's heat production. The most important factors are:
- **Basal metabolic rate (BMR):** The BMR is the rate of energy utilization in the body to maintain essential activities such as breathing. BMRs vary with sex and age.
- **Muscle activity:** Muscle activity, including shivering can greatly increase metabolic rate.
- **Thyroxin output:** Increased thyroxin output increases the rate of cellular metabolism throughout the body.
- **Epinephrine, norepinephrine (hormones), and sympathetic stimulation:** These immediately increase the rate of cellular metabolism in many body tissues.
- **Increased temperature of body cells (fever):** The presence of fever acts to increase the body's temperature by increasing cellular metabolic rate.

Heat Loss
Heat is lost from the body through radiation, conduction, convection, and vaporization (evaporation).

Radiation
It is the transfer of heat from the surface of one object to the surface of another without contact between the two objects. Most heat loss or lost through radiation is in the form of infrared rays. Radiation accounts for 60% of the heat lost by a nude person standing in a room at normal temperature.

Conduction
It is the transfer of heat from one molecule to another. The heat transfer to the molecule of lower temperature, conductive transfer cannot take place without contact between the molecules. The amount of heat transfer depends on the temperature difference, the amount, and duration of contact.

Convection
It is the dispersion of the heated air current. There is usually a small amount of warm air adjacent to the body. This warm air rises and is replaced by cooler air, so people always lose a small amount of heat through convection.

Vaporization
It is continuous evaporation of moisture from the respiratory tract and from the mucosa of the mouth and from the skin. This continuous and unnoticed water loss is called insensible water loss.

Factors Affecting Body Temperature
Nurse should be aware of the factors that can affect a client's body temperature, so that they can recognize the normal temperature variations and understand the significance of body temperature measurements that deviate from normal.
- **Age:** The infant is greatly influenced by the temperature of the environment and must be protected against extreme changes. Elderly people are also particularly sensitive to extremes in the environmental temperature due to decreased thermoregulatory controls.
- **Diurnal variations:** Body temperatures normally change throughout the day, varying as much as 2.0°C (1.8°C between the early morning and the late afternoon).
- **Exercise:** Hard work or strenuous exercise can increase body temperature to as high as 38.3-40°C (101-104°F) measured orally.
- **Hormones:** In women, progesterone secretion at the time of ovulation raises body temperature. Thyroxin, norepinephrine, and epinephrine also affect body temperature.
- **Stress:** Stimulation of the sympathetic nervous system can increase the production of epinephrine and norepinephrine, thereby increasing the metabolic activity and heat production.
- **Environment:** Extremes in environmental temperatures can affect a person's temperatures regulatory systems.

Alterations is Body Temperature
Pyrexia: A body temperature above the usual range is called pyrexia, hyperthermia, or fever. A very high temperature, e.g., 41°C (105°F) is called hyperpyrexia.

Common Types of Fevers
- **Intermittent fever:** During intermittent fever, the body temperature alternates at regular intervals between periods of fever and periods of normal temperatures.
- **Remittent fever:** During a remittent fever, a wide range of temperature fluctuations occurs over the 24-hour period, all of which are above normal.
- **Relapsing fever:** In a relapsing fever, short febrile periods of a few days are interspersed with periods of 1-2 days of normal temperature.

❖ **Constant fever:** During a constant fever, the body temperature fluctuates minimally but always remains elevated.

Clinical Signs of Fever

The clinical signs of fever vary with the onset, course, and abatement stages of the fever.

Onset (cold or chill stage)
- Increased heart rate and respiratory rate and depth
- Shivering due to increased skeletal muscle tension and contraction
- Cold skin due to vasoconstriction
- Complaints of feeling cold
- Cessation of sweating
- Rise in body temperature

Course
- Skin feels warm
- Increased pulse and respiratory rate
- Increased thirst
- Mild to severe dehydration
- Drowsiness, restlessness, or delirium and convulsions due to the irritation of the nerve cells
- Loss of appetite with prolonged fever
- Malaise, weakness, and aching muscles due to protein break down.

Abatement stage
- Skin that appears flushed and feels warm
- Sweating
- Decreased shivering
- Possible dehydration

Nursing Interventions for Patients with Fever

Nursing interventions for a patient who has a fever are designed to support the bodies, normal physiologic processes, provide comfort, and prevent complications.

Following are the examples of nursing interventions for patients with fever:
- Monitor vital signs
- Assess skin color and temperature
- Monitor white blood cell count and other pertinent laboratory records
- Remove excess blankets when the patient feels warm, but provide extra warmth when the patient feels chilled
- Provide adequate food and fluids to meet increased metabolic demands and prevent dehydration.
- Measure intake and output.
- Maintain prescribed intravenous fluids.
- Reduce physical activity to limit heat production.
- Administer antipyretics (drugs that reduce the level of fever) as ordered.
- Provide a tepid sponge bath to increase heart loss through conduction.
- Provide cool circulating air by using a fan to increase heart loss through convection.

Assessment of Body Temperature

There are a number of methods of measuring body temperature. The three most common are oral, rectal, and axillary, each of the sites has advantages and disadvantages which are mentioned in **Table 4.5.**

Hypothermia

Hypothermia is a core of the body temperatures below the lower limit of normal. The ability of the hypothalamus to regulate temperature is greatly impaired when the body temperature falls below 34.5°C (94°F), and death usually occurs when the temperature falls below 34°C (93.2°F).

The three physiologic process of hypothermia are:
1. Excessive heat loss.
2. Inadequate heat production to counteract the heat loss.
3. Impaired hypothalamic thermoregulation.

Table 4.5: Advantages and disadvantages of three sites for body temperature measurement.

Site	Advantages	Disadvantages
Oral	Most accessible	• Mercury in glass thermometers can be broken, if bitten thereby injuring the client. Children under 6 years and clients who are confused or who have convulsive disorders, inaccurate, if client has just eaten very hot or cold food. • Inaccurate, if client breathes through the mouth, therefore contraindicated for clients who have nasal surgery, may inure the mouth following oral surgery.
Rectal	Most reliable measurement	Inconvenient and more unpleasant for clients; difficult for client who cannot turn to the side. May injure the rectum following rectal surgery. Placement of thermometer at different sites within the rectum yields different temperatures, yet placement at the same site each time is difficult. A rectal thermometer does not respond to changes in arterial temperatures as quickly as an oral thermometer, a fact that may be potentially dangerous for febrile clients, since misleading information may be acquired. Presence of stool is soft the thermometer may be embedded in stool rather than against the wall of the rectum. If the stool is impacted, the depth of thermometer insertion may be insufficient.
Axillary	Safest and most noninvasive	The thermometer must be left in place a long time to obtain an accurate measurement. More chance for eternal contact with air and in cause inaccurate measurement.

People at risk for hypothermia:
- Infant and children whose thermoregulatory systems are immature.
- Elderly people who have insufficient food, clothing, or fuel.
- People who have neurological deficits and are unable to identify or respond to cold.
- Alcoholics who have extreme heat losses con develop to vasodilatation.
- Hypothermia.

The major clinical signs of hypothermia include the following:
- Decreased body temperature
- Severe shivering (initially)
- Feelings of cold and chills
- Pale, cool, waxy skin
- Hypotension
- Decreased urinary output
- Lack of muscle coordination
- Disorientation
- Drowsiness progressing to coma

Management includes: Removing the patient from the cold environment to the rewarming of the patient's body, include the application of blankets for mild hypothermia and the application of hyperthermia blankets (electronically controlled).

Wet clothing should be replaced by dry clothing. Because rapid rewarming can cause vasodilatation and subsequent additional heat loss, the patient should be monitored closely.

Equipment and technique

Types of thermometers

Body temperature, measured with a variety of devices:
- Electronic and digital thermometer,
- Tympanic membrane thermometer,
- Temporal artery thermometers,
- Disposable single-use thermometer,
- Automated monitoring device.

No matter, which type of thermometer is used, it is very important to follow the manufacturer's instructions.

Note: Traditionally, body temperatures have been measured by using mercury-in-glass thermometers. However, patients may still have mercury thermometer at home and in some hospitals may be continuing to use them.
- **Oral thermometer** may have long-slender tips, short-round tips, or pear-shaped tips. The round thermometer can be used at the rectal as well as other sites. Disposable thermometers are also manufactured; these are used only once.
- **Digital thermometer:** A thermometer is a device that measures temperature. A thermometer has two important elements, a temperature sensor in which some change occurs with a change in temperature and some means of converting this change into a numerical value.
- **Electronic thermometers** offer another method of assessing body temperatures. They can provide a reading in only 2–60 seconds, depending on the model. The equipment consists of a battery operated portable electronic unit, a probe that the nurse attached to the unit, and a probe cover, which is usually disposable. Chemical disposable thermometers are also used to measure body temperatures. They come in an individual case and are discarded after use. One type has small chemical dots at one end that respond to body hearty changing color, thereby providing a reading of the body temperature.

Other types of thermometer

Temperature scales: The body temperature is measured in degrees on two scales: Celsius and Fahrenheit. The Celsius scale normally extends from 34 to 42°C. The Fahrenheit scale usually extends from 94 to 108°F. Body temperatures rarely extend beyond these scales.

Sometimes a nurse needs to convert a Celsius reading to Fahrenheit, or vice versa.

To convert from Fahrenheit to Celsius, deduct 32 from the Fahrenheit reading and multiply by the fraction 5/9, i.e.,

$$C = (\text{Fahrenheit temperature} - 32) \times 5/9$$

For example, when the Fahrenheit reading is 100:
$$C = (100 - 32) \times 5/9$$
$$= (68) \times 5/9$$
$$= 37.7$$

To convert from Celsius to Fahrenheit, multiply the Celsius reading by the fraction 9/5 and then add 32, that is:

$$F = (\text{Celsius temperature} \times 9/5) + 32$$

For example, when the Celsius reading is 40:
$$F = (40 \times 9/5) + 32$$
$$= (72) + 32$$
$$= 104$$

Guidelines for Taking Vital Signs
- The primary nurse caring for the client is the best one to take vital signs, interpret their significance, and make decisions about care.
- Equipment used to measure vital signs must be appropriate and work properly to ensure accurate finding.
- Knowing the normal range for all vital signs helps the nurse detect abnormalities.
- A client's normal range may differ from the standard range for that age or physical state. Normal values for a client serve as a baseline for comparing in condition overtime.
- Know the client's medical history and therapies or medication, for vital sign changes.
- Control or minimize environmental factors that may affect vital signs. Measuring a pulse after client experiences an emotional upset, many yield values that are not clear indicators of the client's current status.

❖ An organized, systematic (step-by-step) approach when taking vital signs ensures accuracy of findings.

Taking the Oral Temperature

Definition

Body temperature: Temperature is the "hotness" or 'coldness'. The body temperature is the difference between the amount of heat produced and the amount of the heat lost to the external environment.

Purpose
❖ To determine the body temperature of the patient.
❖ To aid in making diagnosis.

Equipment
1. Oral clinical thermometer disinfected in a container **(using mercury in glass thermometer)**
2. Swab in a container.
3. Kidney basin or thermometer container.
4. Blue pen.
5. Watch with second hand.
6. Graphic TPR chart.
7. Paper bag.

Procedure
Taking the oral temperature using (mercury thermometer) **(Table 4.6)**

Using Digital Thermometer
Follow above step except thermometer, and follow as:
❖ Clean the thermometer with cold water and soap, then thoroughly rinse it
❖ Turn the thermometer on
❖ Put the tip under tongue, towards the back of the patient mouth
❖ Close the lips around the thermometer

Table 4.6: Procedure of taking oral temperature.

Steps	Rationale
Determine the need to measure client's body temperature.	Certain conditions place clients at risk for temperature.
Assemble equipment.	To save time and energy.
Identify the patient, greet the patient, and explain the procedure.	To prevent error. To relieve anxiety and gain cooperation.
Place the client in comfortable position, assess site most appropriate for temperature measurement.	To carry out the procedure.
Wait 20–30 minutes before measuring oral temperature, if client has smoked or ingested hot or cold liquid or foods.	Smoking and hot or cold substances can cause false temperature reading in oral cavity.

Contd...

Contd...

Steps	Rationale
Hold color-coded end or system glass thermometer with fingertips.	Reduces contamination of thermometers bulb.
If thermometer stored in disinfectant solution, rinse in cold water before using.	Removes solution irritating to oral mucosa. Hot water can cause mercury to expand break bulb.
Take swab and wipe thermometer bulb end toward fingers in rotating fashion. Dispose off tissue.	Reduce contamination of thermometer bulb.
Read mercury level while holding thermometer horizontally and gently rotating at eye level. If mercury is above desired level, grasp the tip of thermometer securely and sharply flick wrist downward. Continue shaking until reading is below 35.5°C.	Mercury level should be below 35.5°C (96°F). Thermometer reading must be below body temperature before use.
Ask client to open mouth and gently place thermometer under tongue in posterior sublingual, lateral to center of lower jaw (**Fig. 4.7**).	Heat from superficial blood vessels in sublingual pocket produces temperature reading.
Ask client to hold thermometer with lips closed. Caution against biting down on thermometer.	Maintains proper position of thermometer during recording. Breakage of thermometer may injure the mucosa and cause mercury poisoning.
Leave thermometer in place for 2 minutes or according to agency policy.	Studies vary as to proper length of time for recording.
Carefully remove thermometer and read at eye level while holding thermometer horizontally.	Ensure accurate reading.
Wipe secretions from thermometer with soft issue. Wipe in rotating fashion from fingers towards bulb. Dispose of tissue.	Avoids contact of microorganisms with nurse's hands. Wipe from area of least contamination to area of most contamination
Wash thermometer in lukewarm water, rinse in cool water, dry and replace in container.	Mechanically removes organic material that can harbor microorganisms and hinder action of disinfectant. Storage container prevents breakage.
Record the temperature on the chart	To document nursing procedure. To avoid chances or forgetting the exact reading
Wash hands.	To prevent cross-infection.
Report any unusual variation to the charge nurse.	To take necessary action.

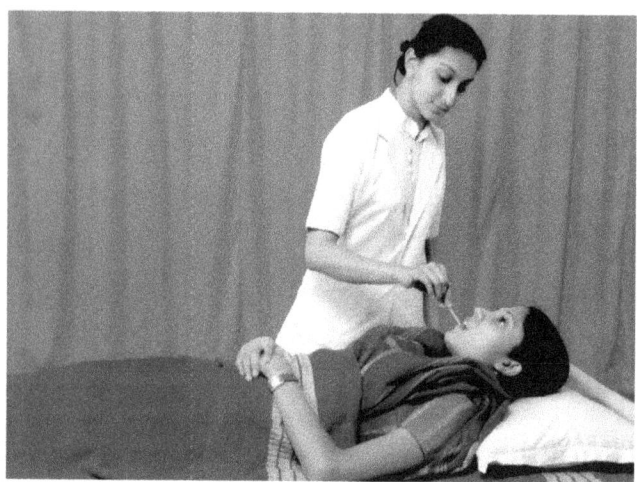

Fig. 4.7: Ask client to open mouth and gently place thermometer.

- Wait until it beeps or flashes
- Check the temperature on the display.
- Digital thermometers accurate reading in about 1 minute or less

Taking the rectal temperature purposes

1. To determine body temperature mainly for infants, young children, adult unconscious patient, and postoperative patient.
2. To aid making diagnosis.

Equipment

- Rectal clinical thermometer
- Swab in a container
- Tissue paper
- Lubricant (Jelly)
- Disposable gloves
- Kidney basin or thermometer container
- A blue pen
- Watch with secondhand
- Graphic TPR Chart
- Paper bag.

Procedure:

Taking the Rectal Temperature **(Table 4.7)**

Taking Axillary Temperature

Purposes

- To determine the body temperature of the patient when oral and rectal methods are contraindicated.
- To aid in making diagnosis.

Equipment

- Oral clinical thermometer (disinfected) in a container
- Swab in container
- Kidney basin or thermometer container

Table 4.7: Procedure of taking rectal temperature.

Steps	Rationale
Complete preparation steps 1-9.	
1. Draw curtain around clients' bed or close room door. Assist client to Sims position with upper leg flexed. Move aside bed linen to expose only anal area.	Maintains client privacy and minimizes embarrassment. Exposes anal for correct thermometer placement.
2. Squeeze liberal portion of lubricant on tissue. Dip thermometer's bulb end into lubricant, covering 2.5–3.5 cm (1–1.5 inches) for adult or 1.2–2.5 cm (0.5–1.5 inch) for infant.	Lubrication minimizes trauma to rectal mucosa during insertion. Use of tissue avoids continuation of all lubricant in container.
3. With nondominant hand, separate client's buttocks to expose anus. Ask client to breathe slowly and relax.	Fully exposes anus for thermometer insertion. Relaxes anal sphincter for easier thermometer insertion.
4. Gently insert thermometer into anus in direction of umbilicus Insert 1.2 cm (0.5 inch) for infant and 3.5 cm (1.5 inches) for adult do not force thermometer.	Ensures adequate exposure against blood vessels in rectal wall.
5. If resistance is felt during insertion withdraw thermometer immediately	Prevents trauma to mucosa. Glass thermometers can break.
6. Hold thermometer in place for 2 minutes or according to agency policy.	Hold thermometer to prevent injury to client recommended times vary among institutions.
7. Carefully remove thermometer and wipe-off secretions with tissue. Wipe in rotating fashion from fingers toward bulb. Dispose of tissue.	Avoids nurse's contact with microorganisms. Wipe from area of least contamination to area of most contamination.
8. Read thermometer at eye level rotate until scale appears.	Ensures accurate reading.
9. Wipe client's anal area to remove lubricant or feces and discard tissue help client return to comfortable position.	Provides for client's comfort.
10. Wash thermometer in lukewarm water, rinse in cool water, dry, and replace in storage container.	Mechanically removes organic material that can harbor microorganisms and hinder action of disinfectant. Storage container prevents breakage.
11. Record the temperature on the chart.	To document nursing produced. To avoid chances of forgetting the exact reading.
12. Wash hands.	Prevents cross-infection
13. Report any unusual variations to the charge nurse.	Take correct action.

- Blue pen
- Watch with secondhand
- Graphic TPR chart
- Paper bag

Procedure:

Taking Axillary Temperature **(Table 4.8)**

Follow-up Activities

For temperature above normal expected range, initiate the following nursing measures:
- Increase fluid intake to at least 3L daily (unless contraindicated by client's condition).
- Control environmental temperature at 21-27°C (70-80°F).
- Remove excess blankets or bed coverings.
- Reduce frequency of exhaustive care activities.
- Keep clothing and bed linen dry.
- Implement measures to prevent or control spread of infection, e.g., wound care, and adequate urinary elimination.
- If fever persists or reaches unacceptable level as defined by physician, implement sponging with tepid water, administer antipyretics as ordered.

For temperature below normal expected ranges initiate the following nursing measures:
- Cover client with warm blankets.
- Close room doors or window initiate the following measures.
- Turn client every 1-2 hours and perform passive ROM exercise of extremities.
- Monitor apical pulse rate rhythm since hypothermia causes bradycardia and cardiac dysrhythmias.

Special Consideration
- Temperature should be taken approximately 30 minutes after administering antipyretics, and every 4 hour until temperature stabilizes.
- Caution while clients using oral thermometer against moving mouth or repositioning thermometer.

PULSE

Physiological Basis of Pulse

The pulse is a wave of blood created by contraction of the left ventricle of the heart. The heart is a pulsatile; the blood enters the arteries with each heart beat, causing pressure pulses or pulse waves. Generally, the pulse wave represents the stroke volume output and compliance of the arteries. Stroke volume output is the amount of blood that enters the arteries with each ventricular contraction. Normally, the heart empties about 70% of its volume with each contraction, i.e., about 70 mL of blood in healthy adult. Compliance of the arteries is the dispensability of the arteries, i.e., when a person's arteries lose their ability or contract and expand their distensibility as

Table 4.8: Procedure of taking axillary temperature.

Steps	Rationale
Complete preparation steps 1-9.	
1. Dry the axilla.	To prevent moisture altering the skin temperature.
2. Insert thermometer into center of axilla, low arm over thermometer, and place arm across client's chest.	Maintain proper position of thermometer against blood vessels in axilla.
3. Leave the thermometer in place for 3 minutes or placement of thermometer in the center of the axilla for checking body temperature (**Fig. 4.8**)	To get accurate reading.
4. Remove the thermometer from the axilla.	To get the reading.
5. Wipe the thermometer using a spirit swab from stem to bulb use a firm twisting motion.	To clean the thermometer. To prevent contamination of the finger.
6. Discard the used swab into the paper bag.	For proper disposal of work.
7. Read the thermometer holding it horizontally at the eye level, rotate it unit the mercury column is seen.	To get accurate reading of the mercury column.
8. Place thermometer in the kidney basin (thermometer container)	To keep the used thermometer separately.
9. Record the temperature on the chart using blue pen and mention axillary.	To document nursing procedure. To avoid chances of forgetting the exact reading.
10. Wash hands.	To prevent cross-infection.
11. Report any unusual variations to the charge nurse.	To take necessary action.
12. Recording and reporting. Record temperature on vital sign flow sheet's or nurse's notes. Also record any signs or symptoms of temperature alterations.	Vital sign measurements should be recorded promptly on flow sheets to avoid omissions from client's record.

can happening old age, greater pressure is required to pump the blood into the arteries.

When an adult is resting, the heart pumps 4-6 L of blood each minute. This volume is called the cardiac output. The cardiac output (CO) is the result of the stoke volume (SV) times the heart rate (HR) per minute.

$$CO = SV \times HR$$

In a healthy person, the pulse reflects the heartbeat, i.e., the pulse rate is the same as the rate of the ventricular

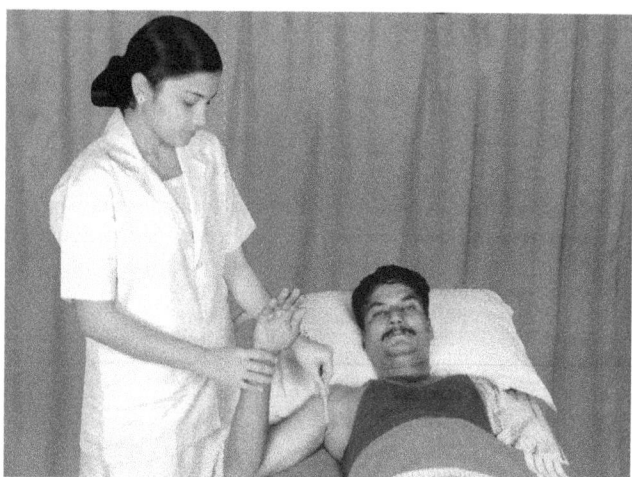

Fig. 4.8: Placement of thermometer.

contractions of the heart. However, in some types of cardiovascular disease the heartbeat and pulse rates can differ. For example, a client's heart may produce very weak or small pulse waves that are not detectable in a peripheral pulse. In these instances, the nurse should assess the heartbeat and the peripheral pulse. A peripheral pulse is a pulse located in the periphery of the body, e.g., in the foot, hand or neck. The apical pulse, in contrast, is a central pulse, i.e., it is located at the apex of the heart.

The pulse rate is regulated by the autonomic nervous system (ANS). When impulses pass through the parasympathetic branches to the sinoatrial node (SA node), which is the pacemaker of the heart. These impulses decrease the heart rate. When body demands indicate a need for an increased heart rate, the impulses of the parasympathetic system are inhibited and the impulses of the sympathetic system increase.

Factors Affecting Pulse Rate

A pulse rate varies according to a number of factors. The nurse should consider each of the following when assessing a client's pulse:
- **Age:** As age increases, the pulse rate gradually decreases.
- **Sex:** After puberty, the average male's pulse rate is slightly lower than the female's pulse rate.
- **Exercise:** The pulse rate normally increases with activity.
- **Fever:** The pulse rate increases (1) in response to the lowered blood pressure that results from peripheral vasodilatation associated with elevated body temperature and (2) because of the increased metabolic rate.
- **Medications:** As medications decrease the pulse rate, and others increases it. For example, cardiotonics decrease the heart rate, whereas epinephrine increases it.
- **Hemorrhage:** Loss of blood from the vascular system (hemorrhage) normally increase pulse rate. An adult has about 5 L of blood in the system and can usually lose up to 10% without adverse effects.
- **Stress:** Stress increases the rate as well as the force of the heartbeat. Emotions such as fear and anxiety stimulate the sympathetic system.
- **Position changes:** The rate changes with the position because of changes in blood flow volume and sympathetic stimulation.

Pulse Sites

Nine sites where a pulse is commonly taken are the following:
1. Temporal, where the temporal artery passes over the temporal bone of the head. The site is superior (above) and lateral to (away from the mid line of) the eye.
2. Carotid, at the side of the neck below the lobe of the ear, where the carotid artery runs between the trachea and the sternocleidomastoid muscle.
3. Apical, at the apex of the heart. In an adult this is located on the left side of the chest, not more than 8 cm (3 inches) to the left of the sternum (breast bone) and under the fourth, fifth, or sixth intercostal space.
4. Brachial, at the inner aspect of the biceps muscle of the arm (especially in infants) or medially in the antecubital space (elbow crease).
5. Radial, where the radial artery runs along the radial bone, on the thumbs side of the inner aspect of the wrist.
6. Femoral, where the femoral artery passes along the inguinal ligament.
7. Popliteal where the popliteal artery passes behind the knee. This point is difficult to find, but it can palpate, if the client flexes the knee slightly.
8. Posterior tibia, on the medial surface of the ankle where the posterior tibia artery passes behind the medial malleolus.
9. Pedal (dorsalis pedis). Where the dorsalis pedis artery passes over the bones of the foot. This artery can be palpated by feeling the dorsum (upper surface) of the foot on an imaginary line drawn from the middle of the ankle to the space between the big and second toes (**Fig. 4.9**).

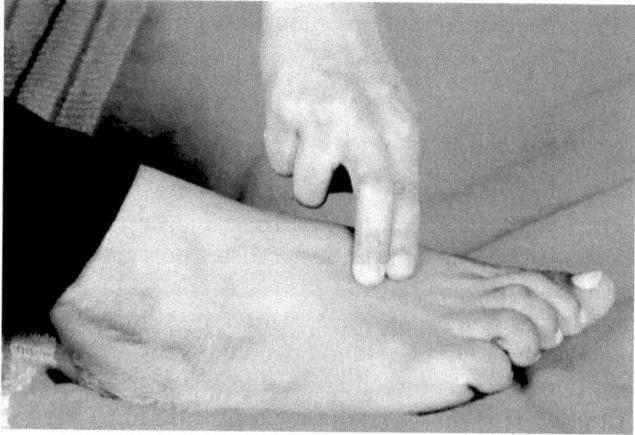

Fig. 4.9: Dorsalis pedis pulse can be palpated by feeling the dorsum (upper surface) of the foot.

A pulse is normally palpated by applying moderate pressure with the three middle fingers of the hand. The pads on the most distal aspects of the fingers are the most sensitive areas of detecting a pulse. With excessive pressure, one can obliterate a pulse, whereas with too little pressure, one may not be able to defect it. Before the nurse assesses the resting pulse, the client should assume a comfortable position, whether the client has been physically active, if so, wait 10-15 minutes until the client has rested and the pulse has slowed to usual rate.

Any baseline date about normal heart rate for client, e.g., a physically fit athlete may have a heart rate below 60.

Characteristics of the Pulse

When assessing the pulse, the nurse collects the following data: the rate, rhythm, volume, arterial wall elasticity, and presence or absence of bilateral equality.

The pulse rate is expressed in beats per minute. An excessively fast heart rate, e.g., over 100 beats per minutes in an adult, is referred to as tachycardia. The heart rate in an adult of 60 beats per minute or less is called bradycardia. If a client has either tachycardia or bradycardia, the apical pulse should be assessed.

The pulse rhythm is the pattern of the beats and the intervals between the beats. Equal time elapses between beats of a normal pulse. A pulse with an irregular rhythm is referred to as a dysrhythmias or arrhythmia. It may consist of random, irregular beats, or a predictable pattern of irregular beats. When a dysrhythmias detected, apical pulse should be assessed. An electrocardiogram (ECG or EKG) is necessary to define the dysrhythmia further.

Pulse volume, also called the pulse strength or amplitude, refers to the force of blood with each beat. Usually, pulse volume is the same with each beat. It can range from absent to bounding. A normal pulse can be felt with moderate pressure of the fingers and can be obliterated with greater pressure. A forceful of full blood volume that is obliterated only with difficulty is called a full or bounding pulse.

A pulse that is readily obliterated with pressure from the fingers is referred to a weak, feeble, or thread. The elasticity of the arterial wall reflects its expansibility or its deformities. A health, normal artery feels straight, smooth, soft, and pliable. Elderly people often have inelastic arteries that feel twisted (tortuous) and irregular upon palpation.

Pulse Technique

Peripheral Pulse Assessment

A peripheral pulse, usually the radial pulse, is assessed by palpation for all individual sex except.

- Newborns and children up to 3 years. Apical are assessed in these clients.
- Very obese or elderly clients, whose radial pulse may be difficult to palpate. Doppler equipment may be used for this client's or the apical pulse is assessed.
- Individuals with a heart disease, they require apical pulse assessment.
- Individuals in whom the circulation to a specific body parts must be assessed. For example, following leg surgery the pedal (dorsalis pedis) pulse is assessed.

The cardiac monitoring machine is another device for assessing the apical pulse. It indicates the rate on a screen or read out graph.

Apical Pulse Assessment

Assessment of the apical pulse is indicated for clients whose peripheral pulse is irregular as well as for clients with known cardiovascular, pulmonary, and renal diseases. It is commonly assessed prior to administering medications that affect heart rate. The apical side is also used to assess the pulse for newborns, infants, and children up to 2-3 years old.

Procedure

Radial pulse assessment **(Table 4.9)**.

Special Considerations

1. If redial pulses are inaccessible because of dressings, bandages, carts, or IV placement, use apical pulse when radial pulse reveals irregularities.
2. Do not palpate radial pulse with thumb because the nurse's own pulse may be felt.

RESPIRATION

Physiological Basis for Respiration

Respiration is the act of breathing; it includes the intake of oxygen and the output of carbon dioxide. Reference is often made to external respiration and internal respiration. The former or the external respiration refers to the interchange of oxygen and carbon dioxide between the alveoli of the lungs and the pulmonary blood. Internal respiration in contrast, takes through the body. It is the interchange of these gases between the circulating blood and the cells of the body tissues.

Respiration is controlled by the respiratory center in the medulla oblongata and the Pons of the brain and by the chemoreceptor's located centrally in the medulla and peripherally in the carotid and aortic bodies. These centers and receptors respond to changes in the concentration of oxygen (O_2), carbon dioxide (CO_2), and hydrogen (H^+) in the arterial blood.

Definition

Respiration is the act of breathing. It includes the intake of oxygen and the output of carbon dioxide, i.e., respiration consists of inspiration and expiration.

Table 4.9: Procedure of radial pulse assessment.

Steps	Rationale
1. Wash hands.	Reduces transmission of microorganisms.
2. If supine, place client's forearm across lower chest with wrist extended straight. If sitting, bend client's elbow 90 degree and support lower arm on chairs or on nurse's arm. Slightly extend wrist with palm down.	Relaxed position of lower arm and extension of wrist permits full exposure of artery to palpation.
3. Place tips of first two or middle three fingers of dominant hand over groove along radial or thumb side of clients (**Fig. 4.10**).	Fingertips are the most sensitive parts of hand to palpate arterial pulsation. Nurse's thumb has palpation that may interfere with accuracy.
4. Lightly compress against radius obliterates pulse initially, and then releases pressure so pulse becomes easily palpable.	Pulse is more accurately assessed with moderate pressure. Too much pressure occludes pulse and impairs blood flow.
5. When pulse is easily palpable, look at watch's second hand and begin to count rate: when sweep hand hits number on dial, start counting with zero, then one, two, and so on.	Rate is determined accurately only after nurse is assured pulse can be palpated. Timing begins with zero. Count of one is first beat palpated after timing begins.
6. If pulse is regular count rate for 30 seconds and multiply total by 2.	Research indicates that 30-second pulse check is most accurate for rapid pulse rates, and that 15-second check is often inaccurate for resting and rapid heart rates.
7. If pulse is irregular count for full minute.	Longer time period ensures accurate count.
8. Assess regularity and frequency of any dysrhythmias.	Inefficient contraction of heart fails to transmit pulse wave and can interfere with cardiac output. Determines and to assess for pulse deficit.
9. Determine strength of pulse. Note whether thrust of vessel against fingertips is bounding, strong, weak.	Strength reflects volume of blood ejected against arterial wall with each heart construction.
10. Assist client in returning to comfortable position.	Promotes sense of well-being.
11. Wash hands.	Reduce transmission of infection.
12. If pulse is assessed for first time establish as baseline.	Used to compare future pulse assessment.

Contd...

Contd...

Steps	Rationale
13. Assess pulse again by having another nurse conduct measurement, if pulse character is abnormal or irregular.	Original measurement may result from error by assessor
14. Record characteristic of pulse in nursing progress sheet or vital signs flow sheet. Also, record any accompanying signs and symptoms of pulse alterations.	Vital sign should be recorded immediately for accuracy and inclusion in medical record.
15. Report abnormal findings to the nurse are charge or physician.	Abnormalities may necessitate immediate medical therapy.

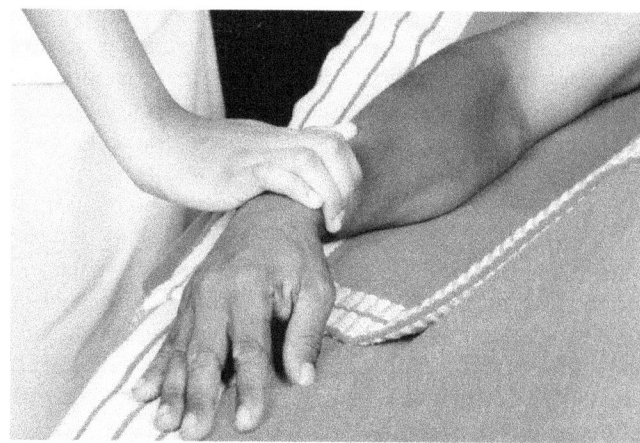

Fig. 4.10: Placing hand over groove.

Assessing Respiration

Resting respiration should be assessed when the client is at rest because exercise affects respiration, increasing their rate and depth (**Fig. 4.11**). Anxiety is likely to affect respiratory rate and depth as well. Respiration may also need to be assessed after exercise to identify the client's tolerance to activity. Before assessing a client's respiration, nurse should be aware of:

❖ The client's normal breathing pattern.
❖ The influence of client's health problems on respiration.
❖ Any medications or therapies that might affect respiration.
❖ The relationship of the client's respiration to cardiovascular function.

The characteristics of respiration should be assessed:

❖ The respiratory rate is normally described in breaths per minute. A healthy adult normally takes between 15 and 20

UNIT 4: Assessment of Patient/Client

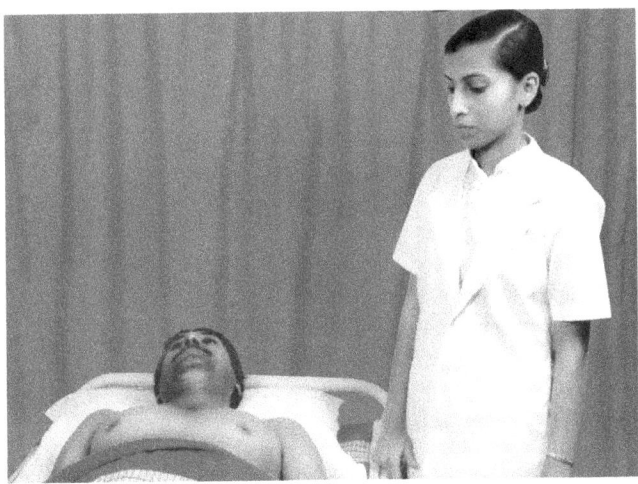

Fig. 4.11: Resting respiration should be assessed when the client is at rest.

breaths per minute. There is different respiratory rate for different age groups.
- The depth of a person's respiration can be established by watching the movement of the chest. Respiratory depth is generally described as normal, deep, or shallow.
- The rhythm and respiration can be assessed by intervals between the two respirations. During a normal inspiration and expiration, an adult takes in about 500 mL of air. This volume is called the tidal volume.
- Vital capacity is the total of the tidal volume plus the inspiratory reserve volume and the expiratory reserve volume. The capacity of the lungs varies with sex, age, stature, and physical development.
- Body position also affects the amount of air that can be inhaled and respiration.

Equipment
- Wrist watch with second-hand or digital display.
- Pen and flow sheet or record form.

Procedure: Assessing Respiration (Table 4.10)

Table 4.10: Procedure of assessing respiration.

Steps	Rationale
1. Determine the need to assess client's respiration.	
2. If client is active, wait 5 or 10 minutes before assessing respiration.	Exercise increases respiratory rate and depth. Respirations should be assessed at rest to allow for objective comparison of values.
3. Assess respiration as first vital sign in infant or child.	Avoid startling or arousing infant or child, which can falsely increase respiratory rates.
4. Assess respiration after pulse measurement in adult.	Inconspicuous assessment of respiration immediately after pulse assessment prevents client from conscious attempt to control breathing.
5. Be sure client is in a comfortable position, preferably sitting.	Position of discomfort may cause client to breath more rapidly sitting erect promotes full ventilator movement.
6. Be sure client's chest movement is visible. If necessary remove bed lines or gown.	Ensure clear view of chest wall and abdominal movements.
7. Place client's arm in a relaxed position across the abdomen or lower chest.	Position used during assessment of pulse allows client's to be inconspicuous.
8. Observe complete respiratory cycle (one inspiration and one expiration)	
9. After cycle is observed, look at watch's second-hand and begin to count rate, when sweep hand hits number on dial, begin time frame, counting one with first full respiratory cycle.	Timing begins with count of one. Respirations occur more slowly than pulse: thus timing does not begin with zero.
10. If rhythm is regular in adult, count number of respirations in 30 seconds and multiply by 2. In infant or young child count respirations for full minute. If adult has irregular rhythm or abnormally slow or fast rate, count one full minute.	Respiratory rate is equivalent to number of respirations per minute, young infants and children normally breathe irregularly. Accurate interpretation with irregularities requires assessment for at least 1 minute.
11. Note down depth of respirations. This can be assessed subjectively by observing degree of chest wall movement while counting rate.	Reveals volume of air moving to and from lungs. Character of ventilator movement may reveal specific alterations or disease status.
12. Note rhythm of ventilator cycle. Normal breathing is regular and interrupted. Infants breathe less regularly. Young child may breathe slowly for a few seconds and then suddenly breath fastens.	Characters of ventilation can reveal specific types of alterations.
13. Replace client's gown and covers with bed lines.	Restores client's comfort.
14. Wash hands	Reduce transmission of microorganisms.

Contd...

Contd...

Steps	Rationale
15. Compare client's respirations with previous baseline and normal respiratory rate for age group.	Allow nurses to assess for change in client's condition and for presence of respiratory alterations.
16. Record any accompanying signs and symptoms of respiratory alterations in nurse's notes or flow sheet.	Abnormalities may necessitate immediate medical therapy.

BLOOD PRESSURE

Blood pressure is the lateral force on the wall of an artery by the pushing blood under pressure from the heart.

The heart contraction forces blood under high pressure into the aorta. The peak of maximum pressure when ejection occurs in the systolic blood pressure, when the ventricles relax: the blood remaining in the arteries exert a minimum or diastolic pressure. The diastolic pressure is the minimal pressure exerted against the arterial walls at all the times.

Definition

Blood pressure may be defined as the force exerted by blood against the walls of the vessels in which it is contained. Differences in blood pressure between different areas of the circulation provide the driving force that keeps the blood moving through the body.

The standard unit for measuring blood pressure is millimeter of mercury (mm Hg) the measurement indicates, the height to which the blood pressure can raise a column of mercury. Blood pressure is recorded with the systolic reading before the diastolic (e.g., 120/80 mm Hg).

The difference between systolic and diastolic pressure is the pulse pressure for blood pressure of 120/80 mm Hg the pulse pressure is 40 mm Hg.

Physiology of Arterial Blood Pressure

Blood pressure reflects the interrelations of cardiac output, peripheral vascular resistance, blood volume, blood viscosity, and arterial elasticity.

Cardiac Output

Cardiac output is the volume of blood pumped by the heart (stroke volume) during 1 minute (heart rate).

Peripheral Resistance

Blood circulates through a network of arteries, arterioles, venules, and veins. Arteries and arterioles are surrounded by smooth muscles that contract or relax to change the size of the lumen, the size of the arteries and arterioles changes to adjust blood flow to the need of local tissues example, when more blood is needed by a major organ, the peripheral arteries constrict decreasing their supply of blood, more blood becomes available to the major organ because of the resistance change in the periphery.

Blood Volume

The volume of blood circulating within the vascular system affects blood pressure. However, if volume increases, more pressure is exerted against arterial walls.

Velocity

The thickness or viscosity of blood affects the blood flows through small vessels. The hematocrit or percentage of red blood cells in the blood determines blood viscosity. The heart must contract more forcefully to move the viscous blood through the circulatory system.

Elasticity

Normally, the walls of an artery are elastic and easily distensible as pressure within the arteries increases. The diameter of vessels walls increases to accommodate the pressure changes.

Factors Affecting Blood Pressure

Among the factors influencing blood pressure are age, exercise, stress, race, obesity, sex, medications, and diurnal variation.

1. **Age:** In older adults, the diastolic pressure often increases as a result of the reduced compliance of the arteries.
2. **Exercise:** Physical activity increases both the cardiac output and blood pressure thus, a rest of 20-30 minutes following exercise is indicated before the blood pressure can be reliably assessed.
3. **Stress:** Stimulation of the sympathetic nervous system increases cardiac output and vasoconstriction of the arterioles, thus increasing the blood pressure reading; however, severe pain can decrease blood pressure greatly and cause shock by inhibiting the vasomotor center and producing vasodilatation.
4. **Race:** Black males over 35 years have higher in some overweight and obese people than in normal weight.
5. **Sex:** After puberty, females usually have lower blood pressure than males of the same age; this difference is thought to be hormonal variations. After menopause, women generally have higher blood pressure than before.
6. **Medications:** In many cases medications, may increase or decrease the blood pressure, nurses should be aware of the specific medication that the client is receiving.
7. **Disease process:** Any condition affecting the cardiac output, blood viscosity, and or compliance of the arteries has a direct effect on the blood pressure.

Assessing Blood Pressure

Blood pressure is measured with a blood pressure cuff, a sphygmomanometer, and a stethoscope.

Sphygmomanometer

The sphygmomanometer consists of a compression bag enclosed in an unyielding cuff, and inflating bulb, pump, or other device by which the pressure increases, a manometer from which the applied pressure is read, and a control valve to deflate the system.

Manometer

Mercury in sphygmomanometers is reliable on the whole, it is easily maintained. Care should be taken to avoid loss of mercury. Substantial errors may occur if the manometer be kept patent. Aneroid sphygmomanometers are generally less accurate than mercury ones.

Cuff

The cuff is an inelastic cloth that encircles the arm and encloses the inflatable rubber bladder: it is secured around the arm of leg by wrapping its tapering end to the encircling material, Velcro surfaces, or by hooks. Croft and Cruikshank (1909) in studying adults found that in terms of precision there is no basis for using two different cuff sizes. Readings from large cuffs came close to intra-arterial pressure in large arms and were also accurate for small arms. They recommend the use of large cuffs only.

Inflatable Bladder

A bladder that is too short and/or too narrow will give false high pressure. The British Hypertension Society in 1986 that recommended the bladder length should be 80% of the arm circumference and the width at least 40%.

Control Valve, Pump, and Rubber Tubing

The control valve is a common source of error. It should allow the passage of air without excessive pressure need to be applied on the pump. When the valve is closed it should allow holding the mercury at a constant level and when released, it should allow a controlled fall in the level of mercury. The rubber tube should belong (approximates) and with airtight connection that can easily be separated.

Using the stethoscope, it is possible to identify a series of five phases as blood pressure falls from the systolic to the diastolic. These phases are known as Korotkoff's sounds. When the cuff pressure has fallen to just below the systolic pressure, a clear but often faint tapping sound is produced by the transient and turbulent blood flowing through the brachial artery during the peak of each systole.

As the pressure in the cuff is reduced further, the sound becomes louder, but when the artery is no longer constricted and the blood flows freely, the sounds becomes muffled and can no longer be heard. Diastolic pressure is usually defined as the cuff pressure at which "muffling" and not disappearance occurs. However, if there is an obvious difference between these both valves are reported. The stethoscope's bell should be placed lightly over the brachial artery; the bell is designed to amplify low frequency sounds such as Korotkoff's sound. Excessive pressures on the stethoscopes bell may partially occlude brachial artery and delay the occurrence of Korotkoff's sound. Korotkoff's sounds form five phases:

1. The appearance of faint, clear tapping sounds, which gradually increase in intensity.
2. The softening of sounds, which may becomes wishing.
3. The return of sharper sounds that become crisper but never fully regain the intensity of the phase 1 sounds.
4. The distinct muffling sound which becomes of and blowing.
5. The point at which all sounds cease.

Systolic Pressure

The systolic pressure is the maximum pressure of the blood against the wall of the vessels following ventricular contraction and is taken as an indication of the integrity of the heart, arteries and arterioles.

Diastolic Pressure

The diastolic pressure is the minimum pressure of the blood against the walls of the vessels following closure of the aortic valve and is taken as a direct indication of blood vessel resistance.

Common Errors in Assessing Blood Pressure

The importance of the accuracy of blood pressure assessment cannot be overemphasized. Many adjustments about a client's health are made on the basis of nursing intervention. Two possible reasons for the blood pressure errors are (1) hasten the part of the nurse and (2) subconscious bias. For example, a nurse may be influenced by the client previous blood pressure measurements or diagnosis and the practitioner's expectations. Some reasons for erroneous blood pressure reading are given in **Table 4.11**.

Table 4.11: Sources of error in blood pressure assessment.

Error	Effect
Bladder cuff too wide	Erroneously high
Bladder cuff too wide	Erroneously low
Arm unsupported	Erroneously high
Insufficient rest before the assessment	Erroneously high
Repeating assessment too quickly	Erroneously high-systolic and high-diastolic reading
Cuff wrapped too loosely or unevenly	Erroneously high
Deflation of cuff too quickly	Erroneously low-systolic and high-diastolic reading
Failure to use the same arm consistently	Inconsistent measurement
Arm above level of the heart	Erroneously low
Assessing immediately after a meal or while client smokes or has pain.	Erroneously high
Failure to identify auscultator gap	Erroneously low

Indication of Blood Pressure Measurement

1. To determine baseline blood pressure recording and monitor fluctuation.
2. To aid in the diagnostic disease.
3. To aid in the assessment of cardiovascular system.

Equipment

- Sphygmomanometer
- Bladder and cuff (appropriate size)
- Pen and vital signs flow sheet or record form.
- Alcohol swab.

Procedure: Measuring Blood Pressure (Table 4.12)

Table 4.12: Procedure of measuring blood pressure.

Assessment	Rationale
1. Determine the need to assess client's blood pressure. NOTE: Risk factors: History of cardiovascular disease, history of renal disease, history of diabetes mellitus, circulatory shock, acute or chronic pain, rapid IV infusion, or fluid or blood products, increased intracranial pressure, postoperative patient, taking blood pressure medicine, with toxemia pregnancy.	Certain condition place clients at risk for BP alterations.
2. Determine the best site for blood pressure assessment. Avoid applying cuff to arm with IV fluid infusing, in the pressure of arteriovenous shunt, when arm or hand has been traumatized in lower arm cast or bulky bandage.	Inappropriate site selection may result in poor amplification of sounds, causing inaccurate readings. Application of pressure from inflated bladder can temporarily impair blood flow and compromises circulation in extremity that already has been impaired circulation.
3. Determine previous baseline BP (if available) from clients record.	Will allow nurse to identify if change has occurred in clients status.
4. Encourage client to avoid exercise and smoking for 30 minutes before assessment.	These factors can cause false elevations in BP.
5. Have client assume sitting or lying position. Be sure room is warm and quite	Maintains clients comfort during measurements
6. Explain procedure to client and client have rest at least 5 minutes before measurement.	Reduces anxiety that can falsely elevate reading BP reading taken at different times can be objectively compared when all are assessed with client at rest.
Auscultation Method	
7. Wash hands	Reduces transmission of microorganisms.
8. Support clients forearm (while client is sitting or lying) with palm turned up.	It arm dangles, client may perform isometric exercise that can increase diastolic pressure 10%.
9. Expose upper arm fully by removing clothing.	Ensures proper cuff application.
10. Palpate brachial artery. Position cuffs 2.5 (1 cm) above site of brachial pulsation (antecubital space). Center bladder cuff above artery. With fully deflated, wrap cuff evenly, and snugly around upper arm.	Inflating bladder directly over brachial artery ensures proper pressure is applied during inflation. Loose fitting cuff causes false high readings.
11. Be sure manometer is positioned vertically at eye level. Observer should not be further than 1 yard away.	Eye level placement ensures accurate reading of mercury level.
12. Palpate brachial or radial artery with fingertips of an hand while inflating cuffs rapidly above point at which pulse disappears. Slowly deflate cuff and note point when pulse reappears.	Identifiers approximate systolic pressure and determine maximal inflation point for accurate reading to pressure 30 mm Hg. Prevents auscultator gap.
13. Deflate cuff fully and wait 30 seconds.	Prevent venous congestion and false high reading.
14. Place stethoscope ear pieces in ears and be sure sounds are clear, not muffled.	Each ear peace should following angle of ear canal to facilitate hearing.
15. Relocate brachial artery and place bell or diaphragm chest piece over it. Do not allow chest piece to touch cuff or clothing.	Proper stethoscope placement ensures optimal sound reception. Stethoscope improperly positioned causes muffled sounds that often result in false low systolic and false high-diastolic readings.
16. Close valve of pressure bulb clockwise until tight.	Tightening of valve prevents air leak during inflation.
17. Inflate cuff to 30 mm Hg above palpated systolic pressure.	Ensures accurate measurement of systolic pressure.
18. Slowly release valve and allow mercury to fall at rate of 2–3 mm Hg/Sec.	Too rapid or slow decline in mercury level can cause inaccurate readings.
19. Note point on manometer when first clear sound is heard.	First Korotkoff's sound indicates systolic pressure.
20. Continue to deflate cuff gradually, noting point at which muffled or dampened sound appears in on manometer at which sound disappears. Note down pressure to nearest 2 mm Hg.	Fourth Korotkoff's sound involves distinct muffing of sounds and is recommended by American Heart Association as indication of diastolic pressure in children. American Heart Association recommends recording fifth Korotkoff's sound as diastolic pressure in adult.

Contd...

Contd...

Assessment	Rationale
21. Deflate cuff rapidly and completely. Remove clients from arm unless measurement must be repeated.	Continues cuff inflation causes arterial occlusion, resulting in numbers and tingling of clients arm.
22. Assist client in returning to comfortable position.	Promotes participation in care and understanding of health status.
23. Inform client of BP reading.	Reduces transmission of microorganisms.
24. Wash hands.	Reduces transmission of microorganisms.

Palpation Method (Table 4.13)

Table 4.13: Palpation method.

Assessment	Rationale
1. Follow steps 1–5 of auscultation method.	
2. Palpate brachial or radial artery with fingertips of on hand. Inflate cuff to a pressure of 30 mm Hg above point at which pulse disappears.	Ensures accurate detection of true systolic pressure once pressure valve is released.
3. Slowly deflate cuff, allowing mercury to fall 2 mm Hg per sec.	Too rapid or slow a decline can result in inaccurate readings.
4. As soon as pulse is again palpable, note manometer reading.	Reading is the systolic pressure by palpation.
5. Deflate cuff rapidly and completely. Remove from clients arm unless reassessment is necessary.	Continuous cuff inflation causes arterial occlusion, resulting in numbness and tingling of clients arm
6. Assist client in returning to comfortable position and cover upper arm if previously clothed.	Restores clients comfort.
7. Wash hands.	Reduces transmission of microorganisms/germs.
8. If BP is mandible or difficult to obtain, try alternative method, are other arm.	Prevent venous congestion and false high readings. Alternate membrane of article pressure.
9. Record BP in medical record or flow sheet.	Record immediately of ensured accuracy.

Measuring Blood Pressure Using Digital Monitor

The digital monitor has a rubber pump on it for inflating the cuff and button for letting the air out. To measure blood pressure, the cuff is placed around the bare and stretched out upper arm, and inflated until no blood can flow through the brachial artery. No stethoscope is used.

- Turn the power on to start the unit
- On the automatic models, the cuff will inflate by itself with a push of a button
- After the cuff inflates, the automatic device will slowly let air out
- Look at the display screen to get blood pressure reading Upper arm monitors are the only type recommended by the American heart association because they are the most accurate.
- Observation and collection of specimens—urine, stool, vomitus, and sputum.

COLLECTION OF SPECIMEN

Phases of diagnostic testing (pretest, intratest, and post test) in common investigations and clinical implications.

Phases of Diagnostic Testing

Pretest Phase

Explain the procedure and purpose of test to the patient or parents to obtain informed consent. A warm moist compress may be applied to the puncture site, prior to the procedures to dilate the blood vessels. Assess for interfering factors, inadequate blood supply due to cold cyanosis, swelling, or edema will be ineffective in the process of collection. Reduces morphology caused by residual alcohol used for site cleansing or inadequate drying prior to puncture.

Intratest Phase

Observe universal precautions. Assess puncture site for interfering factors. Disinfect skin using 70% alcohol or betadine and wipe it dry with sterile gauze. Allow povidone iodine (betadine) to dry thoroughly for effectiveness. Create stasis by pressing on distal joint of finger to produce redness at the tip. Puncture the skin sharply, quickly, and deep enough to get a free flow of blood. After collection briefly apply pressure and a small sterile dressing to the puncture site. Label the specimen properly and document pertinent information.

Post-test Phase

Check patient on the puncture site, instruct patient to lie down and rest. Watch for signs of anxiety or other complications such as hematoma infection (septic phlebitis) or vasovagal syncope. If venous bleeding is excessive persists longer than 5 min, the physician should be notified. The dressing may be removed after a few hours when bleeding has stopped. Occasionally, a small bruise or minimal discomfort may occur.

Specific Guidelines for the Nursing Role
Assess for Interfering Factors

An action that may interfere with accurate test result includes:
- Incorrect specimen collection on handling, labeling wrong preservative or lock of preservative, delayed or improper storage of specimen, incorrect or incomplete patient

preparation, hemolysis of blood, incomplete specimen collection and old specimen.

❖ Factors that can alter test results include pretest diet, pregnancy, time of the day, age and sex, drug history, plasma volume, past and present illness history/health status, deficient patient knowledge/understanding, position or activity at time specimen was obtained. Stress, physical and emotional. Noncompliance postprandial status (the last time patient took food) and undisclosed drug or alcohol usage.

Prepare the Patient Properly

This process is crucial for obtaining accurate test result.

Fasting, special diet activity, restrictions with-holding of selected medications, or other preparations are some components of the pretest phase. When at doubt about holding medication, confer with laboratory staff, patient, and physician. Isolation precaution should be observed whenever necessary. Universal precautions are mandatory. In certain instances, sterile procedures may be necessary, e.g., contamination of a clean catch or sterile urine specimen with genital. Organisms could alter test results.

Be Aware of Legal Implication

These include the patient's right to information including risks and outcome properly signed with held consent forms.

Consider Ethical Implications

Maintaining confidentiality of information given, it becomes especially relevant when obtaining specimen from infectious disease like HIV.

Use Safety Measures

Patient safety and well-being should be optimized by detecting and/or by preventing complications after testing. The patients behavior, appearance, response should be observed and documented. For example, a patient with bleeding or immune system disorders needs to be protected from injury and infection.

Observe Infection Control and Universal Precautions

In spite of using universal precautions, caregivers hove the right to know the diagnosis of the patients they care for, so that they can obtain and handle diagnostic specimen properly in order to minimize risks to themselves. Proper protective clothing and device must be worn. The procurement and the disposal of specimen according to occupational safety and health act (OSHA) standards must be adhered to standard for universal precautions, isolation precautions.

Store and Transport Specimens

After the specimen is collected it should be stored properly or transported to the laboratory immediately. Failure to do so may result in specimen deterioration. For example, urine pH becomes alkaline due to bacterial growth, if the specimen stands for more than 30 minutes. Failure to follow protocol leads to repeat testing.

Nursing Protocol for Blood Specimen

Blood collection may be obtained through skin puncture, vein puncture, arterial puncture, or bone morrow aspiration. The type of blood sample whole blood plasma or serum varies with the specific test. Equipment type of blood sample collection, site technique, and patient age and condition determines methods of data collection.

Blood collection tubes have color-coded stoppers that indicate the type of additives in the tube.

Nursing Role

The nurse's role in blood collection will vary according to the type of specimen collected and patient's condition. Universal precautions must be observed with all blood collection procedures, including proper disposal of medical waste.

Skin Puncture (Capillary Blood)

Capillary blood samples require a skin puncture on the fingertip or earlobe of an adult. For children, the tip of the finger is often used, infant under 1 year of age and neonate yield the best. The toe may need to be used in adults when veins are sclerosed.

VENIPUNCTURE (VENOUS BLOOD)

Most blood studies requires venous blood sample. Core must be taken to avoid hemolysis or concentration of the sample and to prevent hematoma. Damage to the veins may result in infection and discomfort. The most common veinpuncture site is the antecubital fossa. However, the wrist area, forearm, or the dorsum of the hand or foot may be used.

Clinical Alert

Do not draw blood above as intravenous catheter of infusion site; choose a site distal to the IV site, if no other alternative site is available. Hemoconcentration may be caused by leaving the tourniquet on for more than 1 minute.

Nursing Standards and Protocols for Specimen Collection for Laboratory Investigation

The nurse follows agency protocols for specimen collections and handling. Uses universal precautions and sterile techniques, explaining the procedures to the patients/family in appropriate terminology, so as to educate, elicit cooperation, and obtain the desired expected outcomes.

Nursing Responsibilities

The nurse's role varies according to the type of specimen, purpose of test, the age, and the sex of the patient. The most common specimens collected are blood, urine and stool. It is important that the nurse, patient, and family understand collection requirements for these specimens and performs the procedure properly, including ordering of tests and timely coordination of activities. A thorough understanding of the principles, protocols, and standards related to specimen collection will prevent wrong results and injury.

Complete Blood Count (CBC)

It indicates oxygen carrying capacity of blood and presence of infection. Client is not fasting or nil by mouth.
- White Blood Cells (WBC): 5.000–19.000 mm^3
- Red Blood Cells (RBC):
  - Female: 4.2–5A/million/mm^3
  - Male: 4.7–6.1 million/mm^3

Hemoglobin (Hgb)

Measures the oxygen carrying capacity:
- Males: 13.5–17.5 g/dL
- Females: 12–16 g/dL

Culture and Sensitivity (C&S)

Determines presence of microorganisms, and antibiotics that will kill or inhibit growth of microorganisms. Normal values are negative for microorganism's growth.

Blood sample is done before administration of antibiotics.

Serum Electrolytes

Test determines blood electrolytes levels:

- Sodium (Na)   136–145 mEq/L
- Potassium (K)   3.5–5 mEq/L
- Chloride (Cl)   98–106 mEq/L
- Cells
- Phosphorus   1.8–2.6 mEq/L
- Carbon dioxide (CO_2) 22–30 mEq/L
- Magnesium (Mg)   1.5–2.5 mEq/L
- Client is not fasting
- Acid base imbalance can cause cardiac dysrhythmias
- Decreases level can cause dysrhythmias, decreased in CHF

Liver Function Test

Liver function test to examine the levels of certain enzyme found in the liver that helps to convert proteins into energy for the liver, test includes:

1. **Aspirate transaminase (AST):** AST is an enzyme that helps metabolize amino acids like ALT. AST is normally present in blood at low levels. An increase in AST levels may indicate liver damage. Normal value **8–48 U/L**
2. **Alanine transaminase (ALT)** is an enzyme found in the liver that helps convert proteins into energy for the liver cells. **Normal value 7–55 U/L**
3. **Alkaline phosphates (ALP):** ALP is an enzyme found in the liver and bone. Higher than normal levels of ALP may indicate liver damage. **Normal value 40–129 U/L**
4. **Albumin and total protein:** Albumin is one of several proteins to fight infections. Lower than normal levels may indicate liver damage. **Normal value—albumin 3.5–5.0 g/dL, total protein 6.3–7.9 g/dL**
5. **Bilirubin:** Bilirubin is a substance produced during the normal breakdown of red blood cells. Elevated levels indicate liver damage, **normal value 0.1–1.2 mg/dL**

Lipid/Lipoprotein Profile

The lipid and lipoproteins parameters, which are predominantly measured and effectively comprise of the traditional lipoprotein profile including total cholesterol, high-density lipoproteins (HDL) and low-density lipoproteins (LDL), cholesterol, and triglyceride.

Blood Lipids and Lipoproteins

Cholesterol and triglyceride level are important to evaluate a person's risk of developing atherosclerotic disease, cholesterol level is 150–250 mg/dL or 3.9–6.5 mmol/L. Decrease level of HDL and elevated levels of LDL increase the risk of development of atherosclerotic coronary artery disease. Normal value of HDL in 40–49 years of age is (80–90 mg/dL) over 50 years of age is (80–210 mg/dL).

Erythrocyte Sedimentation Rate (ESR)

Nonspecific test indicating presence of inflammation in:
Male: Upto 1–15 mm/hour
Female: Up 20 mm/hour (Westergren Method).

An examination that measures RBC has settled to the bottom of a test tube in 1-hour time frame. Level are increased, if the client has on inflammation, malignancy, etc.

Enzyme-linked Immunosorbent Assay (ELISA)

This is the basic screening test for the presence of antibodies to HIV normal—negative

Pretest counseling obtain informed consent—post-test counseling.

Western Blot

Confirmatory test for the presence of antibodies to HIV normal—negative

Pretest counseling obtains informed consent, and post-test counseling.

Polymerase Chain Reaction (PCR)

Detects HIV specific DNA (Virus) normal—negative

CD4 Cell Count

Predictor of HIV progression baseline taken after positive HIV test normal—500–1000/mm^3

Critical value + < 200 mm^3

Partial thromboplastin (PTT) also called activated partial thromboplastin time

Measures blood clotting time in seconds
Normal—PTT—60–70 seconds
Critical value—PTT > 100 Seconds

Activated Partial Thromboplastin Time (APTT)

Normal—30-40 seconds

When on anticoagulant therapy, the client's normal value is 1.5-2.5 times the control value, a blood specimen is drawn 30 minutes to 1 hour before the next heparin dose, if the client is on intermittent heparin therapy, but may be drawn at any time, if the client is on continuous heparin therapy.

* Assess any bodily discharge for the presence of blood.
* The antidote for heparin is protamine sulfate.
* Antihistamines, Vitamin C, and salicylates prolong the PTT time.

Bleeding Times

Measures the length of time for a platelet plug to occlude a small puncture wound
Normal—1-9 minutes
Critical value > 12 min (LVY method)

Coomb's Test (Direct Antiglobulin Test)

Detects if immunoglobins are attached to RBCs. Normal—Negative.

There are several drugs that causes false positive, e.g., ampicillin, captopril (capoten), indomethacin (indocin), and insulin.

Folic Acid (Folate Level)

Measures folic acid levels in the blood. Normal—5-20 ug/mL or 14-34 mmol/L

The client is not allowed to drink any alcoholic beverages before the test. The test is drawn before folic acid medication.

Hematocrit

Measures the percentage of blood cells in a volume of blood.
Normal—
Male: 42-52%
Female: 37-47%
Critical value: <15%
Client living in high altitude may have increased level

Schilling Test

Determines Vitamin B_{12} absorption by the intestine, differentiates between pernicious anemia and GI malabsorption problem.
Normal—8-40% of the radioactive Vitamin B_{12} is excreted in the urine within 24 hours.

Collect the urine for a 24-48 hours period. Laxatives are not given during the test as they decrease the absorption of B_{12}.

Sickle Cell Test

A screening test to determine the presence of Hgbs. Normal—No Hgbs.

If the exam results are positive a hemoglobin electrophoresis test is done, there are no food or fluid restrictions. Note on the laboratory slip, if the client has had a blood transfusion in the past 3-4 months.

White Blood Cells (WBCs)

Measures the number of WBCs in a sample of blood.
Normal—5.000-10.000/mm^3.

Aspirin, heparin, and steroids may increase WBC levels.

Differential Count

Determines the percentage of each type of WBC in a sample of blood:
Basophils: 0.5-1.0%
Eosinophils: 1-4%
Europhiles: 55-70%
Lymphocytes: 20-40%
Monocytes: 2-8%

Blood Urea Nitrogen Test (BUN)

Measures urea, end product of protein metabolism 5-25 mg/dL
Client nil by mouth for 8 hours preferred.
Note client hydration status.

Serum Creatinine

Specific indicator of renal disease.
Male: 0.6-1.5 mg/dL
Female: 0.6-1.1 mg/dL

Rheumatoid Factor (RF)

Abnormal protein in serum of about 80% of client and rheumatoid arthritis is formed as a result of the reaction of IgM and abnormal IgG. Also elevated in clients with other autoimmune disease, such as systemic lupus erythematous.
Normal: <1-20 L, elderly
Elderly: Slightly increased.

Uric Aid

Serum: Males 2.1-8.5 mg/dL
       Females 2.0-6.6 mg/dL
Urine: 250-750 mg/24 hours
       Elevated in gout.

Blood Glucose, Fasting Blood, Sugar

Measure of blood level of glucose (serum values), depends on the method used by the laboratory.
Normal: 70-115 mg/dL
Diabetic: >140 mg/dL
Critical value: > 400 mg
       < 50 mg/dL

Client must fast (except for water) for 6-8 hours withhold insulin or oral antidiabetics medication until blood drawn be certain that the client receive medications and meals after fasting specimen is drawn, as cortisone thiazide and loop diuretics cause increase.

2 hours Post Prandial Glucose (2h PPG) or 2 hours Post Prandial Blood Sugar (2h PPBS) Measure of blood glucose 2 hours after a meal

- Normal—70–140 mg/dL
- Diabetic: > 140 mg/dL
- Instruct the client to eat entire meal, and then not to eat anything until blood is drawn. Notify laboratory at the time meal is completed.

Glucose Tolerance Test (GTT)

- Evaluates blood and urine glucose 30 minutes before, and 1, 2, 3, and 4 hours after a standard glucose load.
- Normal—Blood glucose < 140 mg/dL
- Within 2 hours, urine tested negative.
- For more than 2 hours, Diabetic > 140 may never return to normal urine positive for glucose. Client must fast (except for water) 6–8 hours.
- With hold drugs that interfere with the results. After administration of glucose load, client may not eat anything else until test is completed. Should drink water and collect urine specimen at hourly periods. Administer medication after test is completed.

VDRL

- Blood test for the presence of syphilis.
- Normal—Negative or nonreactive.
- Explain the test to client including amount of blood to be drawn.

Thyroid Stimulating Hormone (TSH), Thyrotrophin

- This blood test determines thyroid function as well as monitors exogenous thyroid replacement.
- Normal—2–10 U/mL or 2–10 m U/I.
- Recent radiographic administration may affect test results.
- Severe illness may increase TSH levels include antithyroid.
- Drugs that may decrease TSH levels include aspirin, dopamine, heparin, steroids, and T3.
- Explain procedure to client, the client should be relaxed and recumbent for 30 minute before the test.

Thyroid Stimulating Hormone Stimulating Test (TSH, Stimulating Test)

- This blood test differentiates between primary and secondary hypothyroidism.
- Normal— nonreactive
- Explain procedure to client.
- Obtain baseline levels of radioactive iodine intake or serum T4 administer 5–10 unit of TSH intramuscularly for 3 days.
- Repeat radioactive iodine intake or T4 as indicated for comparison studies.

Serum Free Triiodothyronine (T3)

- This blood test measures the amount of free T3 that actually enters the cell and is active in metabolism.
- It is a true indicator of thyroid activity and can be used to diagnose thyroid status in pregnant females.
- Normal—0.2–0.6 ng/dL

Calcitonin, HCT, Thyrocalcitonin

This blood test determines thyroid and parathyroid activity.

It is also used as a tumor marker to detect thyroid cancer and several other cancers.

Normal = basal
Females = <14 pg/mL or <14 ng/L
Males = <19 pg/mL or <9 ng/L

Radioactive Iodine Uptake (RAIU) > Iodine Uptake Test

This nuclear scan uses oral radioactive iodine to determine. Normality to trap and retain iodine.

2 hours = 4–12% absorbed
6 hours = 6–15% absorbed
24 hours = 8–30% absorbed

The client who is allergic to iodine or shellfish or pregnant should not have the test done.

Parathyroid Hormone (PTH), Parathormone

This blood test measures the quantity of PTH to determine hyperparathyroidism or to distinguish if hypercalcemia is caused by parathyroid glands.

- Normal < 2000 pg/mL
- Recent radioisotope injection can interfere with test results.

Adrenocorticotropic Hormone Stimulation Test

Adrenocorticotropic hormone (ACTH) stimulation test, cortisol stimulation test, cosyntropin test.

This blood test monitors plasma cortisol levels to indicate adrenal gland response to ACTH. Normal
Rapid = – 7 µg/dL above baseline
24 hours = >40 µg/dL
3 days = >40 µg/dL for all tests, obtain baseline serum cortisol level.

Drugs that may increase plasma cortisol level include cortisol estrogen, gluco cortisol. For all tests obtain base line serum cortisol level. For rapid test, administer IV injection of cosyntropin over 2 minutes. Draw blood specimen at 30 and 60 minutes after injection, for 24 hours test. Start an IV infusion of cosyntropin 1 L normal saline and run 2 units/hour for 24 hours. Draw plasma cortisol level after 24 hours.

Arterial Puncture (Arterial Blood)

Arterial blood sample is necessary for arterial blood gases (ABGs) and are usually performed by a physician or a specially trained nurse or technician because of potential risks inherent in this procedure. They are normally collected directly from the radial brachial or femoral arteries. If patient has an arterial line in place (most frequently) in the radial artery sample can be drawn from this line.

Common Investigation Arterial Blood Gas

Direct measurement of pH, PO_2, PCO_2, and calculated measurement of HCO_3 and SaO_2 from samples of arterial blood.
pH = Expresses the acidic or alkaline content in the blood.
PaO_2 = Partial pressure of oxygen in the blood.
$PaCO_2$ = Partial pressure of carbon dioxide in the blood.
SaO_2: = Arterial oxygen saturation. The oxygen content of the blood expressed as a percent of the oxygen carrying capacity of the blood.

These explain why an arterial sample of blood is required. Arterial punctures cause more discomfort than venous. The client is instructed not to move. Assess the adequacy of collateral circulation. Apply firm pressure on the site for minimum of 5 minutes or until all bleeding stops.

Normal values
pH = 7.3–7.45
PCO_2 = 80–105 mm Hg
PO_2 = 35–45 mm Hg
HCO_3 = 22–26 mEq/L
O_2 saturation = 95–100%

Pulse Oximetry

- Noninvasive means of measuring oxygen saturation utilizing a light beam.
- SaO_2 > 95% (at sea level).
- Explain the procedure to the client.
- Assess peripheral circulation as this may alter results.
- Place the sensor on the earlobe, finger tip, or pinna of the ear.
- Keep sensor intact until a consistent reading is obtained.
- Observe and record readings.
- Report measurement below 95% to the physician.

Urine Tests	Urine Analysis
Color	Clear amber
Odor	Pleasantly aromatic until left standing, offensive, and unpleasant in kidney infection.
Albumin	(Protein)–negative
Acetone	(Ketones)–negative
RBCs	2–3/HPF
WBCs	4–5/HPF
Bilirubin	Negative
Glucose	Negative
Specific gravity	1.005–1.030
Bacteria	Negative
Costs	Rare
pH	4.6–8.0

Explain procedure purpose, assist with specimen collection. If needed ensure specimen is taken to the laboratory in a timely manner.

Creatinine clearance
Males = 95–135 mL/min
Females = 85–125 mL/min
Minimum = 10 mL/min to maintain life

Instruct client about 24-hours urine test, encourage water intake hourly. Keep urine on ice or in special refrigerator. Drugs affecting results, phenacetin, antibiotic steroids, thiazide, ascorbic acid, levodopa, and methyldopa (aldomet).

Stool for Occult Blood

- Fecal occult screening studies may be utilized as an indicator for possible colorectal cancer. Explain the method of stool collection to the client.
- Instruct not to mix toilet paper or urine with specimen.
- Wear gloves when obtaining and handling specimen.

Measuring Chemical Properties of Urine

Glucose, Ketones, Protein, Blood, and pH

These tests, which are a part of the routine urinalysis done by the laboratory, can be performed by the nurse easily, quickly, and more cheaply in the hospital patient-care divisions. Normally, glucose and ketones are not present in the urine and the appearance of other elements generally indicates that glucose is not effectively reaching the body's cells. When this screening test for the presence of glucose in the urine is positive, other tests are used to determine the diagnosis of diabetes mellitus. In the past, persons with diabetes mellitus routinely used urine testing of glucose to monitor the effectiveness of their medication, diet and exercise on their blood glucose levels. Today, the determination of blood glucose levels is done by finger sticks. Nevertheless, this traditional method of testing of urine for glucose will be described.

Assessing the chemical properties of urine can be accomplished by immersing a special chemically prepared strip of paper into a clean urine specimen or by combining drops of urine with chemically prepared tablets. The change in color of the strip or tablet will indicate the presence of any of these substances.

Equipment

- Specimen container, bedpan, urinal, or potty chair.
- Watch with second-hand or digital counter.
- Clean, disposable gloves (if person other than client test urine).

Reagent Tablet Testing

- 10 mL test tube
- Test tube holder
- Medicine dropper
- Clean container with 10 mL water
- Acetest tablets
- Tablet color chart
- Facial tissue

Reagent Strip Testing

- Reagent test strip
- Test strip color chart

Measuring Chemical Properties of Urine (Table 4.14)

Table 4.14: Measuring chemical properties of urine.

Steps	Rationale
Assessment	
1. Determine why physician has requested this particular urine test.	Allows nurse to consider other significant assessment to make.
2. Assess if the client or a family member performs urine testing at home or if there is need for the client to learn skill.	Client accustomed to testing own urine may prefer continuing to do so.
3. Determine if the physician has recommended specific type of reagent test for client to use.	Variety of reagent strips and tablets permit fast, accurate monitoring of urine glucose and ketones.
4. Assess whether the client, if diabetic, is familiar with double-voided specimens and uses the technique regularly.	Double-voided specimen is essential for accuracy of glucose test. Clients often do no perceive the importance of the procedure.
5. Assess type of medications the client receives; check drug literature for effects on reagent strips and tablets.	Certain drug components create false-positive glucose readings. Some drugs that can alter reagents include cephalothin sodium (Kelfin), ascorbic acid, chloral hydrate sulfonamides, tetracyclines, and levodopa.
6. Assess client for signs and symptoms of diabetes mellitus: increased thirst, polyuria, polyphagia, recent loss of weight, Pruritus of skin, fatigue.	Presence of these symptoms is often accompanied by glucose in the urine (Glycosuria).
7. If diabetic, assess client's ability to perform urine test.	Determine the level of instruction or assistance required from nurse. Diabetics may suffer from visual alterations or peripheral nerve damage that prevents them from performing a test.
Implementation	
1. Obtain double-voided specimen when testing of urine for glucose: a. Ask client to collect random urine specimen and discard. b. Have the client drink at least 500–1000 mL water or preferred liquid. c. 30–45 minutes later, have client collect another random specimen.	Stagnant urine stored in bladder overnight or for long periods does not reveal amount of glucose and ketones excreted by kidney at time of testing. Facilitates ability to void again within a short time period. Fresh specimen will provide accurate test measurements. If client is catheterized, single, fresh specimen from catheter is adequate.

Contd...

Steps	Rationale
2. Wear gloves.	Universal precautions advocated by CDC.
3. Perform glucose reagent tablet test 5-drop test: a. Use medicine draper to transfer 5 drops of well-mixed urine from container to the test tube. Use 2-drop or 1-drop test with young children: 2-drop test = 2 drops urine and 10 drops water;1-drop test = 1 drop urine and 11 drops water. b. Rinse dropper. c. Add 10 drops of water to the test-tube. d. Add reagent tablet to the test tube without touching to the bare skin. e. Place tube in holder or hold tube near top. f. Observe color change occurring as tablet boils. g. Fifteen seconds after boiling stops, shake tube gently and compare color of solution with color chart. h. Rinse test tube and drain.	Proper volume of urine is needed to ensure proper reaction of urine to agents in tablet. Prevents excess urine from being added to the tube. Reagent tablet contains sodium hydroxide, which boils in water. Combination of tablet and solution results in boiling effect. If fingers are moist, tablets will be caustic. Chemical reaction produces heat that can cause burn. Heat of reaction causes reduction of chemicals in tablet, if glucose is present. Concentration of glucose determines the color of urine solution. Comparison of color in test tube with standardized color chart indicates glucose concentration in urine. Delay in reading causes inaccuracy that can cause serious problems, if treatments are initiated because of results. Tube should be dry and free of chemicals for next test.
4. Perform glucose/ketones reagent test strip test: a. Immerse end of strip impregnated with chemical reagent into urine specimen. b. Remove strip immediately from the container and tap it gently against the container's side. c. Hold strip in horizontal position d. Time for number of seconds specified on container and compare color of strip with the color chart. e. Dispose of reagent strip in trash.	Strip test is often preferred over tablet test (3 above). Immersion exposes reagent to urine constituents. Although Test ape all measure quantity of glucose in urine, measurement scales are not interchangeable. Excess urine can dilute reagents. Prevents possible mixing of chemical reagents. Accurate interpretation of results depends on precise timing. Ketostix, 15 seconds; Test ape, 60 seconds. Compare darker part of tope with color chart. If results exceed 0.5%, wait another 60 sec and compare with second color chart. Maintains neat environment, which reduces spread of infection.

Contd...

Contd...

Steps	Rationale
5. Perform ketones (Acetest) tablet test: a. Place Acetest tablet on white tissue. b. Add one drop of urine to the tablet. c. Time for 30 seconds and compare tablet's color with Acetest color chart. d. Discard tablet and tissue in trash.	Unnecessary it Ketostix, Multistix, or Diastix reagent test strips are used. Color of tablet changes to shades of tan or gray that can be seen more easily on a white background. Begins chemical reaction. Time required for reagent to indicate ketones bodies. Reduces transmission of microorganisms.
6. Use Multistix reagent test strip to assess for chemical properties of pH, protein, glucose, ketones and/or blood simultaneously. a. Immerse end of chemically impregnated test strip into urine. b. Remove strip immediately from container and top it gently against the container's side. c. Hold strip in horizontal position. d. Time for number of seconds specified on container and compare color of strip with color chart (table).	Eliminates need for all previous testing discussed. Presence of these elements may indicate renal or other systemic diseases. Exposes reagent to urine. Excess urine can dilute reagents. Prevents possible mixing of chemical reagents. Accurate interpretation of results depends on precise timing.
7. Wash hands after removing and discarding gloves.	Reduces transmission of microorganisms.
8. Discuss test results with the client.	Client should participate with care to improve understanding and compliance.

Evaluation

1. Note presence of blood, protein, glucose, or ketones in the urine.	None of these substances should be in the urine; the pH should be slightly acidic (average = 6; normal = 4.5–8) Indicates need for further teaching.
2. Unexpected outcomes that may occur include: ➢ Client or family member is unable to perform urine test correctly. ➢ Test results are positive for: Glucose	When the blood glucose level exceeds 180 mg/dL (renal threshold), glucose spills into the urine. This most commonly occurs in poorly controlled diabetes mellitus, but also occurs with IV administration of fluids containing dextrose and with hyper alimentation.

Contd...

Contd...

Steps	Rationale
➢ Ketones	Ketones are the end products of fatty acid breakdown and are excreted in the urine when fat is burned for energy as occurs in low-carbohydrate diets, starvation, diabetes mellitus, and alcoholism.
➢ Protein	Protein in the urine is indicative of renal dysfunction and occurs only when the glomerular membrane fails to prevent its escape. A transient proteinuria may occur with excess exercise, cold baths, and severe stress.
➢ Blood	Blood in the urine may be indicative of renal damage, tumors, stones, infection or trauma in the urinary tract.
➢ Alterations in pH	Urine becomes excessively alkaline with alkalemia, infection of urinary tract, due to a diet high in vegetables or citrus fruits. Acidic urine is associated with academia, diarrhea, starvation, and a diet high in meat products or cranberries.

Recording and reporting

1. Record results immediately in nurses' notes or glucose testing flow sheet.	Timely documentation ensures accurate Therapeutic intervention.
2. Have the client in a home setting, record results of test on flow sheet.	Allow the client to see variations in testing over several days. Provides record of testing between visits to physician.

Follow-up Activity while Measuring Chemical Properties of Urine

❖ Consult with physician when results are unexpected.
❖ If client is a diabetic, nurse should determine if insulin should be given.

Note:
❖ Carefully read directions on bottles of test tablets and strips.
❖ Clarify with other health team members, if Clinitest is to be done with one drop, two drops, or five drops of urine.
❖ If client has difficulty in complying with double-void specimen, check first-voided specimen for sugar and acetone; however, this is not an accurate assessment of current blood glucose level.
❖ In the study done to evaluate diabetic client's home urine glucose, testing techniques, and ability to interpret result,

❖ Urine testing for glucose and acetone has been used for many years to monitor glucose control by diet and insulin. Test is acceptable to clients because it is easily performed and causes no pain; however, it is being replaced by testing capillary blood, which is obtained by skin puncture of fingertip. This change is being made because capillary blood monitoring directly reflects current serum glucose levels and is not affected by renal threshold for glucose or fluid volume. Hypoglycemia, which cannot be detected by urine testing, may be identified by sampling of serum glucose.

SPECIMEN COLLECTION

Definition

Specimen collection is the collection of a required amount of tissue or fluid for laboratory examination.

Indications

Specimen collection is required when microbiological; biochemical or other laboratory investigations are indicated. Specimen collection offers the first crucial step in investigations that define the nature of the disease and determine diagnosis and the mode of treatment.

CERVICAL SCRAPE

Definition

Obtaining a specimen from the cervix.

Purpose

For laboratory investigation as indicated.

Equipment

- Fixing agent
- Slides
- Cervical spatula
- Specimen
- Appropriate laboratory forms
- Good source of light
- Sterile gloves.

Procedure (Table 4.15)

Table 4.15: Procedure of cervical scrape.

Nursing action	Rationale
1. Check the physicians order, progress, notes, and nursing care plan.	To obtain specific instructions/information.
2. Identify the patient. Check identification against the physicians order.	To ensure that the right procedure is performed on the right patient.
3. Explain the procedure to the patient.	To obtain the patient's consent and cooperation.
4. Collect and prepare equipment.	
5. Ensure patient's privacy.	To avoid unnecessary embarrassment to the patient during the procedure.
6. Position the patient in a lithotomy position. Ensure that there is a good source of light.	To facilitate good visibility.
7. Wash and dry hands.	To prevent cross-infection.
8. Lubricate the speculum with warm tap water.	To ensure smooth insertion of the speculum.
9. Using the bilobed end of the cervical spatula, scrape firmly but gently around the squamocolumnar junction of the cervix. If the Os is sprayed open or scarred, a wider sweep with the brood end of the spatula may be necessary.	To obtain a usable amount of specimen.
10. Smear both sides of the spatula evenly on the slide with one stroke from each side of the spatula.	To ensure complete specimens.
11. Fix immediately and allow fixing agents to dry for 20 minutes.	Dry specimens are less likely to be damaged.
12. Place the slides in a transport container.	To safeguard delicate gloss slides.
13. Dispose off equipment appropriately.	
14. Wash and dry hands.	
15. Send specimen to the laboratory with appropriate laboratory forms filled and signed by the doctor.	

EAR SWAB

Definition

Collection of ear swab for laboratory investigation.

Purpose

Required for microbiological or other laboratory investigation.

Equipment

- Clinically clean tray.
- Sterile swab in a sterile container.
- Appropriate laboratory forms.

Procedure: Collection of Ear Swab (Table 4.16)

Table 4.16: Procedure of collecting ear swab.

Nursing action	Rationale
1. Check the physician's order, progress, notes, and nursing care plan.	To obtain specific instructions/information.
2. Identify the patient. Check identification against the physicians order.	To ensure that the right procedure is performed on the right patient.
3. Explain the procedure to the patient.	To obtain the patient consent and cooperation.
4. Ask the patient to sit comfortably on the bed or chair.	
5. Wash and dry hands.	To prevent cross-infection.
6. Ensure patients privacy.	To avoid unnecessary embarrassment to the patient.
7. Gently hold the ear upward and backward.	To straighten the ear canal.
8. Gently insert the swab into the outer ear. Rotate the swab gently being alert not to rupture the Tympanic membrane.	
9. Place the swab in a sterile container, label.	
10. Clean and dispose off equipment.	
11. Wash and dry hands.	To prevent cross-infection.
12. Send the specimen to the laboratory with appropriate laboratory forms completed and signed by the doctor.	Note: No antibiotics or other chemotherapeutic agents should have been used in the ear canal 3 hours before taking the swab.
13. Document the procedure appropriately.	

EYE SWAB

Definition

Collection of eye swab for laboratory investigation.

Purpose

Required for microbiological or other laboratory investigation.

Equipment

- Clinically clean tray.
- Sterile swab stick in a sterile container.
- Appropriate laboratory forms.

Procedure (Table 4.17)

Table 4.17: Procedure of collecting eye swab.

Nursing action	Rationale
1. Check the physician's order, progress, notes, and nursing care plan.	To obtain specific instructions/information.
2. Identify the patient. Check identification against the physicians order.	To fulfill legal requirement and hospital policies. To ensure that the right procedure is performed on the right patient.
3. Explain the procedure to the patient. Allow patient to ask questions.	To allay fear and gain patients consent and cooperation. To promote patients education.
4. Wash and dry hands.	To prevent cross-infection.
5. Using a sterile swab stick hold the swab parallel to the cornea and gently wipe the conjunctiva from inner canthus to outer canthus.	To ensure that a swab of the correct site is taken. To avoid contamination by touching the eyelid.
6. Put swab back into the container.	
7. Dispose off equipment.	
8. Wash and dry hands.	To prevent cross-infection.
9. Document the procedure appropriately and dispatch specimen to the laboratory with forms completed and signed by doctor.	

COLLECTING A STOOL SPECIMEN

Laboratory examination and analysis of stool provides useful information about the nature of elimination. Stool specimens are collected to determine pathologic conditions such as tumors, hemorrhage, infection, and malabsorption problems. These conditions can be detected by the presence of blood, bile, urobilinogen, fat, nitrogen content, ova, parasites, protozoa, and bacteria. Single stool specimens are most frequently collected but occasionally stool is collected for a timed period such as 72 hours.

Medical aseptic technique should be followed during collection of any stool specimen. Feces contain a variety of microorganisms that can easily be transmitted, if specimens are handled incorrectly. Often, patients are capable of collecting their own specimens; thus it is important for them to know about aseptic technique. Because of the relative infrequency of defecation, patients should also receive careful instructions about the purpose and technique of stool collection to ensure, specimens are not accidentally discarded or mixed with urine or water.

Equipment

- Wax card board or plastic container with lid or sterile test tube with swab for culture.
- Two tongue blades.
- Paper towel.
- Clean disposable glove.
- Bedpan, specimen container, potty chair, or bed side commode.
- Completed specimen identification label.
- Completed laboratory requisition.
- "Save Stool" signs.

Procedure: Collecting a Stool Specimen (Table 4.18)

Table 4.18: Procedure of collecting a stool specimen.

Steps	Rationale
Assessment	
1. Determine purpose of stool specimen and correct method of obtaining and handling specimen.	Prevents collection of specimen at a time when laboratory cannot test it.
2. Determine if patient should have dietary modifications or restrictions before test.	Prevents invalid test results on stool specimen.
3. Assess understanding of reason for collection of stool specimen.	Reveals patient's ability and willingness to cooperate in the collection of specimen.
4. Determine normal defecation pattern of patient.	Allows for more effective planning. If patient has bowel movement only once every 3–5 days, it may be best to give the patient suppository or enema or have the patient obtain specimen at home.
5. Assess ability to assist in the collection of blood specimen. a. Ability to use toilet facilities. b. Ability to handle specimen container.	Because defecation is a private matter. Most patients prefer to be as independent in collection as possible.
6. Assess patient for discomfort associated with defecation.	Particular type of discomfort might suggest specific elimination problem such as hemorrhoids.
7. Assess patient for gastrointestinal dysfunction, such as abdominal pain, nausea, vomiting, excessive flatus, and diarrhea.	May indicate specific physical problem.
Implementation	
1. If patient is unable to use a bathroom, close the room door or bedside curtains.	Allows patient to relax, promoting defecation.

Contd...

Steps	Rationale
2. Wash hands.	Reduces spread of infection.
3. Assist patient as needed into the bathroom or commode bedpan.	Patient's physical mobility and level of fatigue influence amount of assistance needed.
4. Instruct the patient to void into toilet before defecating (discord urine before collecting specimen in bedpan)	Feces should not be mixed with urine or toilet tissue. Urine inhibits fecal bacterial growth. Toilet tissue contains bismuth, which interferes with test results.
5. Provide patient with clean, dry bedpan and specimen container potty-chair in which to defecate.	Feces should not be mixed with urine or water.
6. Assist patient if needed in washing after toileting and leave in safe, comfortable position after defection.	Promotes comfort and sense of well-being.
7. Take covered bedpan or other container with stool to the bathroom or utility room.	Covering bedpan and removing it from patient's room reduces odor and the patient embarrassment.
8. Put on clean, disposable gloves (optional).	Provides extra barrier between nurse and stool and prevents transfer of bacteria to skin. However, gloves do not substitute for good hand-washing technique.
9. Obtain specimen: a. **For culture:** Remove swab from sterile test tube, gather bean-size piece of stool, and return swab to tube. If stool is liquid, soak cotton swab in it and return to tube. b. **For other tests:** Obtain specimen by using tongue blades to transfer portion of stool to the container. c. **For timed stool specimen:** Place each stool in waxed cardboard or plastic container for specific time ordered and kept in specimen refrigerator.	Stool is touched only by sterile swab to prevent introduction of bacteria. Use of tongue blades prevents transfer of bacteria to hands or other objects. Tests for dietary products and digestive enzymes such as fat content or bile require analysis of all feces over time.
10. For timed tests, place signs stating, "Save all stool" over patient's bed, on bathroom door, above toilet.	Helps prevent accidental disposal of stool.
11. Immediately place lid on container tightly.	Prevents spread of microorganisms by air or contact with other articles.

Contd...

Contd...

Steps	Rationale
12. Wrap used tongue blades in paper towels and dispose off in trash. Remove disposable gloves and discard.	Reduces spread of microorganisms.
13. Empty and clean bedpan or other container used to collect specimen and return it to its place.	Makes them ready for use when needed.
14. Wash hands.	Reduces spread of microorganisms.
15. Attach specimen identification label and label the laboratory requisition with date, time of test and name on it.	Inappropriate identification of specimen can lead to errors in diagnosis and therapy.
16. Send specimen to laboratory immediately or place in specimen refrigerator.	Fresh specimen provides most accurate results.

Evaluation

1. Note character of stool with normal laboratory values; discuss with the physician and the patient.	Certain abnormal constituents such as blood, mucus, parasites, and pus may be seen by the naked eye.
2. Compare patient's laboratory test results with normal laboratory values; discuss with the physician and the patient.	Reveals deviations from normal and indicates if there is a need for intervention.

NASAL SWAB

Definition

Collection of nasal secretion for laboratory examination.

Purpose

Required for microbiological or other laboratory investigations as indicated.

Equipment

- Clinically clean tray.
- Sterile swab in a container with label.
- Sterile water.
- Appropriate laboratory forms.

Procedure: Nasal Swab (Table 4.19)

Table 4.19: Procedure of collecting nasal swab.

Nursing action	Rationale
1. Check the physician's order, progress notes and nursing care plan.	To obtain specific instructions/information.

Contd...

Contd...

Nursing action	Rationale
2. Identify the patient. Check identification against physician's order.	To ensure that the right procedure is performed on the right patient.
3. Explain the procedure to patient. Allow questions to be asked.	To obtain the patient's consent and cooperation. To promote patients education.
4. Wash and dry hands (refer Hand Washing)	To reduce risk of infection.
5. Collect and prepare the equipment.	
6. Ensure the patient's privacy.	To avoid unnecessary embarrassment.
7. Ask the patient to tilt head a bit backwards.	To facilitate visibility.
8. Moist the swab before hand with sterile water.	To prevent discomfort to the patient. The healthy nose is virtually dry and a dry swab may cause discomfort.
9. Move the swab from the anterior nares and direct upwards into the tip of the nose.	To swab the correct site and to obtain the required sample.
10. Gently rotate the swab.	
11. Wash and dry hands.	
12. Put the swab back into the container and dispatch immediately to the laboratory (refer policy on transportation and storage of specimens) with laboratory forms completed and signed by doctor.	
13. Document the procedure appropriately.	

PENILE SWAB

Definition

Collection of specimen from the penis.

Purpose

Required for microbiological or laboratory investigation as indicated.

Equipment

- Clinically clean tray.
- Sterile swab in a container with label.
- Clean gloves.

Procedure: Collection of Specimen from the Penis (Table 4.20)

Table 4.20: Procedure of collecting specimen from penis.

Nursing action	Rationale
1. Check the physician's order, progress notes, and nursing care plan.	To obtain specific instructions/information.
2. Identify the patient. Check identification against the physician's order.	To ensure that the right procedure is performed on the right patient.
3. Explain the procedure to the patient. Allow the patient to ask questions.	To allay fears and gain the patient's consent and cooperation. To promote patient's education.
4. Ensure privacy.	To avoid unnecessary embarrassment to the patient.
5. Wash and dry hands washing.	To prevent cross-infection.
6. Don gloves.	
7. Retract prepuce if appropriate.	To obtain maximum visibility of the area to be swabbed.
8. Rotate swab gently in the urethra meatus.	To collect any secretions.
9. Put the swab in the container and label.	
10. Clean equipment.	
11. Wash and dry hands washing (Hand washing procedure Sec. 13)	
12. Dispatch specimen to the laboratory with appropriate laboratory forms completed and signed by doctor.	
13. Document the procedure appropriately noting the condition of the penis for redness, color of discharge, etc.	

Note: This procedure could be done by the patient, if instructed to do so.

RECTAL SWAB

Definition

Collection of specimen from the rectum.

Purpose

Required for microbiological or other laboratory investigation as required.

Equipment

- Clinically clean tray.
- Sterile swab in a container with label.
- Clean gloves.

Procedure: Collection of Specimen from the Rectum (Table 4.21)

Table 4.21: Procedure of collecting specimen from the rectum.

Nursing action	Rationale
1. Check the physician's order, progress notes and nursing care plan.	To obtain specific instructions/information.
2. Identify the patient. Check identification against physician's order.	To fulfill legal requirements and hospital policies. To ensure that the right procedure is performed on the right patient.
3. Explain the procedure to the patient.	To allay fears and gain consent and cooperation.
4. Ensure privacy.	To avoid unnecessary embarrassment to the patient during the procedure.
5. Request the patient to lie down in a left lateral position with a leg extended up.	To allow easy separation of the buttocks and visibility of rectum.
6. Wash and dry hands	To prevent cross-infection.
7. Don gloves and separate bullocks with one hand.	
8. Pass the swab, with care, through the anus into the rectum.	To avoid trauma. To ensure a rectal and not on anal sample is obtained.
9. Rotate gently.	
10. Put the swab in the container and label.	
11. Clean and dispose off equipment.	
12. Wash and dry hands.	
13. Dispatch specimen to the laboratory with appropriate laboratory forms completed and signed by the doctor.	
14. Document the procedure appropriately noting the condition of the rectum for redness, exudates, etc.	

Note: If the patient is suspected of suffering from threadworms, take the swab from the perianal region. Thread worms lay their ova on the perianal skin.

SEMEN

Definition

Collection of semen specimen.

Purpose

For laboratory investigation as required.

Equipment

- Sterile specimen bottle.
- Appropriate laboratory forms.
(This procedure could be done by the patient)

Procedure: Collection of Semen Specimen (Table 4.22)

Table 4.22: Procedure of collecting semen specimen.

Nursing action	Rationale
1. Check the physician's order, progress notes and nursing care plan.	To obtain specific instructions/information.
2. Identify the patient. Check identification against the physician's order.	To ensure that the right procedure is performed on the right patient.
3. Explain the procedure to the patient (sexual intercourse).	To obtain consent and cooperation.
4. Sexual intercourse should not have taken place for 3–4 days before the specimen is collected.	To ensure the sperm count will be at maximum levels. It takes between 3 and 4 days for the sperm count to return to normal after ejaculation.
5. A fresh masturbated specimen must be collected in a sterile container and delivered to the laboratory within 2 hours of the collection of the sperm.	Sperm will die, if there is a delay in testing. Specimens must not be collected in a condom as sperms die when contacted with materials such as rubber.
6. Send the specimen to the laboratory with appropriate forms filled and signed by the doctor.	

THROAT SWAB

Definition

Collection of specimen from the throat for laboratory examination.

Purpose

Required for microbiological or other laboratory investigations as indicated.

Equipment

- Clinically clean tray.
- Sterile specimen container with label.
- Appropriate laboratory forms.
- Wooden spatula.
- Good source of light.

Procedure: Collection of Specimen from the Throat Swab for Laboratory Examination (Table 4.23)

Table 4.23: Procedure of collecting throat swab.

Nursing action	Rationale
1. Check the physician's order, progress notes and nursing care plan.	To obtain specific instructions/information.
2. Identify the patient. Check identification against the physician's order.	To ensure that the right procedure is performed on the right patient.
3. Explain the procedure to the patient. Allow questions to be asked.	To obtain patient's consent and cooperation. To promote patient education.
4. Ask the patient to sit in such a position that he/she is facing a good source of light. Offer kidney dish to the patient. Depress the patient's tongue with a spatula.	To ensure maximum visibility of the area to be swabbed. The patient might vomit. The procedure is one that is likely to cause the patient to gag and the tongue will move to the roof of the mouth, contaminating the specimen.
5. Wash and dry hands.	
6. Quickly, but gently, rub the swab over the prescribed area, usually the tonsillar fossa or any area with a lesion or visible exudates.	To obtain the required sample.
7. Avoid touching any other area of the mouth or tongue with swab.	To prevent contamination by other organisms.
8. Clean the equipment and wash hands.	
9. Put the swab in the container and immediately dispatch to the laboratory with appropriate laboratory forms completed and signed by the in-charge nurse.	
10. Document the procedure appropriately.	

URINE

Definition

Collection of urine in a sterile or clinically clean container.

Purpose

For microbiological or other laboratory investigations.

Equipment

- Sterile/clean urine specimen container.
- Appropriate laboratory forms.

Procedure: Collection of Urine in a Sterile or Clinically Clean Container (Table 4.24)

Table 4.24: Procedure of collecting urine in a sterile clean container.

Nursing action	Rationale
1. Check the physician's order, progress notes and nursing care plan.	To obtain specific instructions/information.
2. Identify the patient. Check identification against the physician's order.	To ensure that the right procedure is performed on the right patient.
3. Explain the procedure to the patient. Allow questions to be asked.	To obtain patient's consent and cooperation. To promote patient education.
4. Request the patient to void at the time appointed to begin this procedure. Discard this specimen.	To ensure the urine collected is that, which is produced in the 24 hours.
5. All urine passed in the next 24 hours is collected in a large specimen bottle. The final specimen is collected at exactly the same time the bladder was voided 24 hours earlier.	Body chemistry alters constantly. A 24-hours collection will accommodate all the variables within a representative period.
6. Care must be taken to ensure the patient understands the procedure in order to eliminate the risk of an incomplete collection.	A 24-hours collection will not be obtained, if one sample is lost and the results will be invalid, if contacted with materials such as rubber.
7. Send the specimen to the laboratory with appropriate laboratory forms filled and signed by the doctor.	

VAGINAL SWAB

Definition

Collection of specimen from the vagina.

Purpose

Required for microbiological or other laboratory investigation.

Equipment

- Clinically clean tray.
- Sterile swab in a container.
- A selection of sterile speculums (Cuscois, Simis).
- Sterile gloves
- Water-soluble jelly.

Note: This procedure is performed by credentialed nurses only.

Procedure: Collection of Specimen from the Vagina (Table 4.25)

Table 4.25: Procedure of collecting specimen from vagina.

Nursing action	Rationale
1. Check the physician's order, progress notes and nursing care plan.	To obtain specific instructions/information.
2. Identify the patient. Check identification against the physician's order.	To ensure that the right procedure is performed on the right patient.
3. Explain the procedure to the patient. Allow questions to be asked.	To obtain the patient's consent and co-operation. To promote patient education.
4. Collect and prepare equipment.	
5. Instruct the patient to empty bladder.	To ensure comfort during the procedure.
6. Ensure patient's privacy.	To avoid unnecessary embarrassment.
7. Cover the patient and place in a lithotomy position and ask her to relax.	To maintain the patients dignity.
8. Wash and dry hands	To minimize cross-infection.
9. Don sterile gloves.	
10. Lubricate and insert speculum into the vagina to separate the vaginal walls. Take the swab as high as possible in the vaginal wall.	To ensure maximum visibility of the area to be swabbed. To ensure that the swab is taken from the best site. If infection by *Trichomonas* species is suspected a charcoal impregnated swab is recommended as this organisms survives longer in this medium.
11. Put the swab into the sterile-labeled container.	
12. Clean all the equipment.	
13. Wash and dry hands.	
14. Dispatch specimen to the laboratory with appropriate laboratory forms completed and signed by the doctor.	
15. Document the procedure appropriately noting the condition of the vagina for redness, dryness, color of discharge, etc.	

WOUND SWAB

Definition

Collection of specimen from a wound.

Purpose

Required for microbiological or other laboratory investigation as indicated.

Equipment

- Clinically clean tray.
- Sterile swab in a container with label.
- Appropriate laboratory forms.

Procedure: Collection of Specimen from a Wound (Table 4.26)

Table 4.26: Procedure of collecting specimen from wound.

Nursing action	Rationale
1. Check the physician's order, progress notes and nursing care plan.	To obtain specific instructions/information.
2. Identify the patient. Check identification against the physician's order.	To ensure that the right procedure is performed on the right patient.
3. Explain the procedure to the patient.	To obtain patient's consent and cooperation.
4. Ensure the patient's privacy.	To avoid unnecessary embarrassment to the patient.
5. Wash and dry (refer Hand Washing procedure section 13).	To avoid cross-infection.
6. Take swabs required before dressing procedure begins.	To prevent collection of any therapeutic agents that may be present in the dressing procedure.
7. Rotate the swab gently put in the sterile container with label.	To collect samples. It is preferable to send samples of purulent discharge.
8. Clean equipment.	
9. Wash and dry hands	To prevent cross-infection.
10. Send samples to the laboratory with appropriate laboratory forms completed and signed by the doctor.	
11. Document the procedure appropriately noting condition of wound, type of exudates, signs of healing, etc.	

PSYCHOLOGICAL ASSESSMENT

Mood, intelligence, emotions, normal, and abnormal behavior

Psychological test are of different types—Intelligence test, aptitude test, vocational test, attitude test, personality tests.

A psychological assessment can include numerous components such as norm—referenced, psychological test, informal test, and surveys, interview information, school or medical records, medical evaluation, and observation data.

Intelligence

Intelligence test is comprises of mental, verbal, and performance tasks of graded difficulty that have been standardized by the use of a representative sample of the population. Examples of intelligence test include:
- The Stanford-binet intelligence scale
- Wechsler adult intelligence scale

Psychologist, are preferred way to measure intelligence.

Mood Assessment

Mood assessment may be administered retrospectively to the mood state of interest. The method and temporal perspectives used to assess mood status will impact on the nature and precision of the mood.

Mood should include depth, intensity, duration, and fluctuations. Described moods include depressed, despairing, irritable, anxious, angry, expansive, euphoric, empty, guilty, hopeless, futile, frightened, and perplexed.

Assessment of Emotion

Emotions are physical and instantly prompting bodily reactions to threat, reward, and everything in between. The bodily reactions can be measured objectively by pupil dilation, skin conductance, brain activity, heart rate, and facial expression.

Emotional experiences have three components: (1) a subjective experience, (2) a physiological response, and (3) a behavioral or expressive response. Feeling arise from an emotional experience.

Detail Psychological Assessment

Identification Data

Name _____ Age _____

Sex _____ Father/Spouse _____

Education _____ Occupation _____

Income _____ Marital status _____

Religion _____ IP Number _____

Diagnosis _____ Address _____

Informant _____

History of present abnormal behavior

What problem made you to come/bring to hospital _____

When this symptoms started _____ any precipitating factors/aggravating factors _____

_____ was the onset sudden or gradual _____

how often does the problem occurs _____ has the problem occurs before _____

Consider abnormal behavior, associated problem, and disruptive behavior _____

Like suicide/homeside, changes in mood, thought, speech, and abnormal perception _____

_____

Reason for admission _____

Type of admission _____

Past medical history: History of illness-hospitalization, if yes, history of diagnosis and treatment ___

_____

Any medical events, such as head injury, surgery, DM, hypertension, convulsion _____

_____

Personal history: Perinatal history-antenatal period eventful/uneventful _____

Exposure to radiation/drug/infection/ _____

Natal: Birth, premature/normal/delivery/forceps delivery/cesarean section/instrumental delivery.

Birth cry: Immediate/delayed

Bonding: Immediate/delayed

Reaction of parents to childbirth: _____ Separation from mother-yes/no _____

Postnatal complications-Underweight/infection/ separations/underweight/infection/delayed breastfeeding _____

Childhood history:

Parent relationship with the child: Harmonious/disturbed.

Developmental milestone as per age: Normal/delayed

Relationship with family members: Normal/disturbed

Immunization received as per schedule: yes/no

Feeding: Breastfeeding/artificial mode

Weaning: Response to weaning _____

Behavior: Temper tantrum/thumb sucking/stuttering/head banging/nail biting/night mares

Educational history:

Academic achievement: Normal/underachiever

Extracurricular activity: Normal/underachiever

Relationship with teacher: Good/disturbed

Attendance to school: Adequate/frequent absent

Relationship with peers: Normal/not adjusting

Attitude towards schooling: Positive negative

Reason for discontinuing study, if any _____

Play history: Participate in games sports— yes/no— Like to play individual/with group

Relationship with playmates: Good /not adjustable

Puberty: Age _____ Reaction to menarche _____ regularity of cycle _____ duration of flow _____

Occupational history: Job started at what age _____ relationship with superior/colleagues/subordinate/— satisfactory/not satisfactory_____

Sexual and marital history: Type of marriage _____ duration of marriage _____
Relationship with spouse _____ marital disharmony, if any _____

Interest and hobbies: Relationship with neighbors _____ hobbies _____

Pre morbid personality: Predominant mood: anxious/pessimistic/optimistic/stable/fluctuating

Personality: Shy/suspicious/irritable/self-centered/impulsive/unconfidence/obsessional.

Physical examination

- Vital signs: Temperature _____ pulse _____ respiration _____ BP _____
- Any significant changes in CVS System _____
- Any significant changes in respiratory system _____
- Any significant changes in GI system _____
- Any significant changes in musculoskeletal system _____
- Any significant changes in reproductive system _____
- Any significant changes in integumentary system _____

❖ Any significant changes in respiratory system _____

❖ Any other medical problems _____

Personal history:

Level of grooming: Normal/stability dressing/over dressed/idiosyncratically dressed.

Level of cleanliness: Adequate/inadequate/overtly clean

Level of consciousness: Fully conscious and alert/drowsy/stupors/comatose

Mode of entry: Came to hospital willingly/persuaded/brought using physical force

Cooperativeness: Normal/more than so/less than so

Eye to eye contact: Normal/increased/decreased

Psychomotor activity: Normal/increased/decreased

Rapport: Spontaneous/difficult/ not to establish

Gesture: Grimace/tics/mannerism

Posturing: Stereotype/tremors/extra pyramidal

Other movement: Stereotype/tremors/extra pyramidal

Other catatonic phenomena: Automatic obedience/negativism/excessive cooperation/waxy flexibility/echopraxia/echolalia.

Conversion and disassociate sign: yes/no ---**Compulsive act or rituals** -yes/no

Hallucinatory behavior: Yes/no

Speech:

Initiation: Spontaneous/speak when spoken/minimal/mute

Reaction time: Normal/delayed/shortened/difficulty

Rate: Normal/delayed

Tone: Normal variation/monotonous

Others: Rhyming/echolalia/neologism

Mood: Angry/hopeless/retarded/thought block/flight of ideas

Content: Ideas/delusion of worthlessness/helplessness/guilt/bizarre

Obsession compulsive phenomena: Present/absent

Orientation: Time, Normal/impaired

Place: Normal/impaired

Person: Normal/impaired

Attention: Normal/impaired

Concentration: Normally sustained with difficulty

Memory: Immediate: Intact/absent

Recent: Intact/absent

Remote: Intact/absent

Insight: Awareness of abnormal behavior—yes/no

Attribution of physical cause -yes/no

Willingness to take treatment -yes/no

Judgment: Personal—Intact/impaired

Social—Intact/impaired

Reaction to situation—Intact/impaired

UNIT 5

Infection Control

LEARNING OBJECTIVES

After completing this unit, learner will be able to:
- Discuss infection control
  - Nature of infection
  - Chain of infection transmission
  - Defense against infection, natural and acquired
  - Hospital acquired infection (nosocomial infection)
- Explain concept of asepsis
  - Medical and surgical asepsis
  - Isolation precautions, barrier nursing
  - Hand washing, simple hand sepsis, surgical sepsis (scrub)
  - Isolation—source and protection
  - Personal protective equipment, types, use and techniques of wearing and removing
  - Decontamination of unit and equipment
  - Transportation of infected patient
  - Standard safety precautions
  - Transmission-based precautions
- Describe biomedical waste management
  - Importance
  - Types of hospital wastes
  - Hazards associated with hospital waste
  - Decontamination of hospital waste
  - Segregation and transportation
  - Disposal

NATURE OF INFECTION

Nature of Infection—Chain of Infection, Types of Infection

Nature of Infection

Infection, a true pathogen is an infectious agent that causes disease.

Definition

Infection is the entry, development, and multiplication of pathogenic microorganisms in the body. The term infection is used to describe the situation in which organisms reach a vulnerable site in sufficient number to multiply and create an adverse reaction.

Mode of Spreading of Infection

Infection will occur only if there is an imbalance between the agent, the human host, and the environment. In epidemiology, it is known as epidemiological triad.

Agent

Agent is a substance living or nonliving, a force tangible or intangible, the excessive presence of relative lack of which may initiate or perpetuate a disease process.

Disease agents

i. **Biological agents:** Viruses, rickettsiae, fungi, bacteria, protozoa.
ii. **Nutritional agents:** Carbohydrate, vitamins, minerals, and water in excess or deficiency.
iii. **Physical agents:** Heat, cold, humidity, pressure, radiation electricity.
iv. **Chemical agents:**
   - Inside the human body. For example, urea (uremia), serum bilirubin (jaundice), ketones (ketosis), uric acid (gout), calcium carbonate (kidney stone), etc.
   - Outside the human body. For example, allergens, metals, fumes, dust, gases, insecticide.
v. **Mechanical agents:** Continuous friction and mechanical forces which may result in crushing, tearing, sprains, dislocation and even death.
vi. **Social agents:** Poverty, smoking, abuse of drugs and alcohol, unhealthy lifestyle, social isolation, maternal deprivation.

Host factors
- Human beings
- Animals.
- Environment

Environment is all that which is external to the individual human host, living and nonliving and with which he is in constant interaction." This includes all of man's external surroundings such as air, water, food, housing, etc.

Chain of Infection

Development of an infection occurs in a cycle that depends on six elements. A chain of these six elements is called chain of infection. The elements are:

1. An infective agent or pathogen
2. A reservoir or source for pathogen growth
3. A portal of exit from the reservoir
4. A mode of transmission
5. A portal entry to a host
6. A susceptible host

Elements of Infection

1. **Causative agents:** No infection is possible without an infective agent. Hence for any infection an agent is a must. Disease can be avoided by removing agent from the chain of infection.
2. **Reservoir:** Organism cannot survive without a favorable reservoir because for the survival they require air, water, nutrient, etc. Man as a reservoir preserves the organisms inside the body or on the skin. The organisms survive or grow in number within the body. Infection can be prevented by improving the health and health practices of the human being.
3. **Portal of exit:** In the chain, the third element is the portal of exit. The organism cannot spread from one person to another unless it comes from one of the infected persons. Excretion or secretion of the infected person facilitates spread of infection from him or her to a healthy individual. This chain point can be broken to prevent spread of infection by safe disposal of the products from the sick person, such as urine, blood, and sputum and others.
4. **Modes of transmission:** The infection cannot spread in all modes. Each agent requires specific mode of transmission from one individual to the other. For example, typhoid cannot break and be spread through the air or insect, it can only be spread through water. In this case, the chain of infection can be broken by drinking safe water.
5. **Portal of entry:** Organisms always try to invade whenever a suitable entry is available.

   For example, round worm can enter through orofecal route but not through blood; similarly human immunodeficiency virus (HIV) cannot spread through orofecal route. So, each agent requires a special entry point. By blocking this entry point, the chain can be spread of infection can be prevented.
6. **Susceptible host:** It is universally known that health is wealth and no substitute for it is available in the world. A healthy individual is always protected against disease. However, each individual is at risk at times. Core of the risk, susceptible individual can also help to break the chain by paying special attention to one's diet, hygienic practice, and safety measures, etc. So, it can be said that lack of an element in the chain of infection is the ultimate aim of infection control.

Types of Infection

Infection is classified into two groups:
- Endogenous
- Exogenous

Endogenous: Self-infection refers when the microorganisms that exist harmlessly in a part of a person's body that become pathogenic, if transferred to another site of the same person.

Exogenous: Cross-infection occurs, if the bacteria are not of the patient's own but transmitted from another source.

Microorganism Ability to Cause Disease

Varies according to organisms virulence, it is the capacity of the organisms to invade the tissue-overcome defense and damage it through toxin production.

Stages of Infection

1. **Incubation**
2. **Prodromal**
3. **Illness**
4. **Decline**
5. **Convalescence**

Incubation

Incubation is the time elapsed between exposure to a pathogenic organism, a chemical, or radiation, and when symptoms and signs are first apparent.

Prodromal Stage of Infection

The prodromal stage refers to the period after incubation and before the characteristics symptoms of infection occurs. People also transmit infections during the prodromal stage. During this stage, the infectious agents continue replicating, which triggers the body's immune response and mild nonspecific symptoms appear.

Illness

During the illness, persons show the actual symptoms of specific infection, such as a rash in chicken pox or vomiting due to food poisoning.

Convalescence

Final stage of infection is known as convalescence. During this stage, symptom resolves and a person can return to their normal stage, depending on the severity of the infection, some people may have permanent damage even after the infection resolves.

Factors Increasing Susceptibility Person to an Infection

1. **Age:** Infant, children, and older people are more susceptible to infection.
2. **Nutritional status:** Malnourishment
3. Presence of underlying disease, e.g., diabetes mellitus, leukemia (weakens body's natural immunity)
4. Treatment with certain antibiotic, corticosteroid, radiation therapy suppresses the production of lymphocytes and antibodies, so the person is at more risk of developing infection.
5. Patient in poor physical health and hospitalized for a long period.
6. Seriously ill patients those, with burns, in ICU, CCU, etc.
   Many factors which increase, susceptibility to infection are:
   1. Age
   2. Nutritional status
   3. Genetics
   4. Immune status
   5. Existing chronic disease
   6. On medication, immunosuppressive drugs
   7. Exposure to toxic substances
   8. Bad lifestyle practices
   9. Environmental factors
   10. Person not vaccinated to specific disease

Factors Affecting the Severity of Infection

1. The number (the dose) of organisms entering the body
2. The virulence (strength) of the organisms
3. The health of the individuals
4. Immunity (resistance of infection)

Three Blood Borne Pathogens that Nurses could Acquire through Hospital Acquired Infection

When nurse work, they enter a world fraught with dangerous, blood-borne pathogens. They may be exposed to hepatitis B as well as hepatitis C virus (HCV) they may also encounter HIV.

Body defenses against infection, inflammatory response, and immune response. Body defense against infection are local and systemic, nonspecific and specific, and humoral and cellular. The body passive immunity transmitted from the mother, the immunoglobulin's specially IgG from the cord, blood and breast milk from mother responsible for protection of human body against any toxin entering into the body.

Defenses may be as under:

- **Natural immunity:** Natural or innate immunity refers to resistance to infection or toxicity. It depends on genetic and constitutional make up. Intact skin and mucosa in the body act as a barrier against invading microorganism. It acts by the secretion of the body, humoral defense by phagocytic action and natural killing of viruses, and infected cells.
- **Acquired immunity:** Immunity from exposure to the invading agent, bacteria, virus, or toxin. Acquired immunity may be passive or active.
- **Active immunity:** Immune bodies are actively formed against specific antigens, either naturally by having had the disease clinically or subclinically or artificially by introducing the antigen vaccine into the individual. The vaccines are the preparations of live or killed microorganisms or their product. Examples of vaccine are bacterial vaccines, Live, BCG, vaccine for prevention of tuberculosis; Killed TAB vaccine for typhoid.
- **Passive immunity:** Temporary immunity by transfusing plasma proteins either artificially from another human by injecting readymade antibodies, e.g., antitetanus serum, this immunity is short lived. Examples of readymade antibodies are transferred from mother IgG antibodies and immunoglobulins transferred through colostrum from mother breast milk.
- **Antibody:** A protein, found mostly in serum that is formed in response to exposure to a specific antigen. Antibodies are immunoglobulin's (Igs) but all immunoglobulin's are not antibodies, have been divided into five distinct classes namely IgG, IgA, IgM, IgD, and IgE.
- **Antigen:** Antibody formed in response to a toxin (antigen). Substances that can stimulate an immune response in the body are determined by chemical and acid radicals.
- **Toxin:** A poisonous substance, usually produced by the invading microorganisms.
- **Toxoid:** A toxin that has been treated to destroy its toxic properties but retains its antigenic quality.

Immune Response

Primary response: When antigen is administered for the first time, there is a latent period of induction of 3–10 days before antibody appear in the blood and steadily raises and reaches peak.

Secondary or booster response: The response of booster dose shorter latent period production of antibody more rapid.

Immunization is a process by which resistance to an infectious disease is induced or augmented.

Children are immunized against eight [8] identified infectious diseases.

Inflammatory Response

A localized physical condition in which part of the body becomes red, swollen, hot, and often painful, especially as a reaction to injury or infection. Inflammation is a process by which white blood cells protect from infection from invaders such as bacteria and viruses. The cardinal signs of inflammation are redness (rubor), heat (calor), swelling (tumor), and pain (dolor). Redness is caused by the dilation of small blood vessels in the area of injury.

Types of Inflammation
1. Acute inflammation
2. Chronic inflammation

Causes of Inflammation
1. Pathogens, like bacteria and virus, or fungi
2. External injuries
3. Effect of chemicals or radiation

Stages of Inflammation
1. Inflammatory response
2. Repair and regeneration
3. Remodeling and maturation

HOSPITAL ACQUIRED INFECTION (NOSOCOMIAL INFECTION)

Healthcare associated infection or nosocomial infection is greater concern for healthcare providers as the word healthcare associated infection reveals that it is related to the hospital. Hospital-acquired infection is also known as nosocomial infection, i.e., mostly by cross-infection.

Source of hospital-acquired infection includes: Equipment, environment and respiratory droplet

Equipment

Commonly referred as fomites, these include beds, curtains, toys, bedpans, tables, wash bowels, nebulizers, and sphygmomanometer. They can spread infection on hands when performing cleaning tasks such as bed making.

Environment

Environment may act at a source of infection as in the case of *Clostridium difficile,* which are released from the feces of infected patient with diarrhea into the environment and contaminate it in ingestion. Microorganisms can be infected with food or water causing gastrointestinal infection and are excreted in the feces. This is known as the feco-oral route.

Respiratory Droplet

From cases and staffs, sore throat, coughing, sneezing, etc.

Air-borne Spread

Staff's poor technique and discipline
- Long hair and nails
- Dirty apron
- Touching sterile dressing
- Failure to wash hands
- Patients sit on other beds, sharing food.

Hospital-acquired infection

The spread of infection from patient-to-patient, patient to healthcare providers, and healthcare providers to patients during hospitalization is called hospital-acquired infection.

Factors responsible for hospital-acquired infection
- Presence of various types of organisms is in large number.
- Frequent contact with infected patients and infected waste product.
- Presence of large amount of contaminated waste and equipment.

How disease spread indirectly in the hospital?

Indirect contact involves the susceptible host having contact with an intermediate object such as contaminated instruments, needle, dressing that have not been changed and contaminated hands.

Cross-infection occurs in the hospital due to:
- Frequent controls made between people who have or can spread illness and people who are vulnerable to infection.
- Large amount of contaminated equipment and supplies must be processed.
- Some procedures that save lives may increase risk of infection.
- Due to lapses in aseptic technique during procedures.

Source of hospital acquired infection
1. **Cases/patient:** All the patients before diagnosis and after diagnosis with specific disease.
2. **Carrier:** Person who seems to be healthy but carries infection and transmits disease to others.
3. Waste liquid can be drain, fecal matter, patient excretion, urine, blood, etc. Solid: Source, dressings, syringes, needles, etc.

The role of cases, carrier, and waste in hospital-acquired infection is explained below in detail.

Who is a case?
A case is a "person" in the population having a particular disease, health disorders, or condition under investigations. The cases can spread diseases during incubation period, treatment period, or during convalescent period.

Who is a carrier?
A carrier is an infected person or animal that harbors a specific infectious agent in absence of discernible clinical disease and serves as a potential source of infection for others.

Carrier has three elements:
1. Presence of organisms in the body.
2. Absence of recognizable signs and symptoms and disease.
3. Shedding organisms in discharge or excretions.

In which condition carriers can spread disease?
- When they seem to be healthy
- During incubation period
- During convalescent condition

How a carrier can spread disease?
A carrier can spread disease through the excretion of its body such as urine, fecal matter, breathing, and other excretions (discharge from wound and blood).

Mode of entry of organisms into human body
- Inhalation—Air-borne disease
- Ingestion—Worm infestation, etc.
- Inoculation—Blood-borne disease, abscess, etc.

Route of exit or mode of exit of infection
1. Urine
2. Feces
3. Expired air
4. Secretions and body fluids, e.g., sputum, blood, and discharges from wound, vagina, nose, etc.
5. Food and fluids, e.g., contaminated or infected food and fluids by improper handling.
6. Pests and parasites, e.g., flies, lice mosquitoes' may carry disease from one person to the other.

Mode of transmission of disease
Disease can be transmitted by:
- Direct transmission
- Indirect transmission

Direct transmission
Diseases can be transmitted directly through:
- Contact with an infective agent
- Infected droplets coming through sneezing, coughing, and spitting
- Contact with infected soil, etc.
- Inoculation of infective agents into the skin or mucous.

Indirect transmission
It is usually when the infective agent can survive outside the body and is transmitted indirectly to the other person when suitable environment is available.

Indirect transmission can be in a variety of setting.
- **Vehicle:** Water, food, and blood product
- **Vector:** Flies, mosquito, insect, and pets, e.g., dogs, cattle, etc.
- **Air-borne:** Through air, i.e., dust
- **Fomites:** Infected discharges from patient. Uncleaned hands and fingers carry organisms from one person to the other person.

Common hospital-acquired infections
Common hospital-acquired infections are:
- Bacteremia (primary bloodstream)
- Wound infections
- Urinary tract infection
- Chest infections

Bloodstream
Bloodstream infection usually is related to intravascular devices.

Wound infection
Transmitted mainly by the hands of nurses, doctors, or by contaminated equipment.

Urinary tract infection
It is transmitted by the patient's own intestinal bacteria or urinary stasis due to prolonged bed rest but most frequently caused by catheter related or by instruments.

Chest infection
Mainly due to environment pollution (in the ward and hospital). It is common among the people who have breathing difficulties.

The individuals to be considered as infectious:
- All patients before diagnosis the following patients must be considered as high-risk patients until their diagnosis is established
- Drug addict
- Homosexuals
- Renal dialysis patients
- Patients with liver disease
- Hematology patients (thalassemia, hemophiliac)
- Children of HbsAg. HIV-positive mothers

Potential for hospital-acquired infection
- Patients and healthcare workers
- Some groups of healthcare workers are especially vulnerable
- Nurses who have direct contact with many patients
- Laboratory technician
- CSSD technician
- Dentist/Dental employees
- Surgeons/Physicians
- House-keeping personnel
- Laundry workers
- Nurse assistant/Ward assistant

INTRODUCTORY CONCEPT OF ASEPSIS, MEDICAL, AND SURGICAL ASEPSIS

Strategies are otherwise known as standard precautions, aimed at reducing the risk of transmission of microorganism from both recognized and unrecognized sources of infection. Standard precaution can be taken by:
- Universal precaution
- Specific protection
- Standard precautions

Standard precaution **are a set of** precautions designed to prevent transmission of HIV, hepatitis B virus (HBV), and other blood-borne pathogens when providing care or healthcare, which includes:
1. Hand washing
2. Wearing gloves
3. Facial protection (eyes, nose, and mouth)
4. Wearing gown
5. Prevention of needle stick injuries
6. Respiratory hygiene and cough etiquette
7. Environmental protection

Transmission-based Precaution

- Droplet precaution
- Contact precaution
- Air-borne precaution
- Eye protection

Aims

1. Preventing cross-infection from patient to patient, patients to healthcare providers and healthcare providers to patients and relatives during hospitalization.
2. To ensure that the risk of transmissions of infection is minimized and if it occurs, it is controlled quickly and effectively as far as possible.
3. Providing a consistent approach to the prevention of transferable infection from both known and unknown sources of infection.
4. To protect high-risk group of patients, healthcare practitioners as well as other care takers from known and unknown risk of hospital-acquired infection.

Hand Washing

Hands are a common source where organisms come in contact frequently during any activities. So hand-washing is one of the most important elements of infection control in general and in patient care.

Objective

To prevent spread of nosocomial infection in the hospital or prevent cross-infection through hands.

Principle: Hands must be washed thoroughly

- Prior to and after handling patients
- Prior to and after performing aseptic technique and any procedure

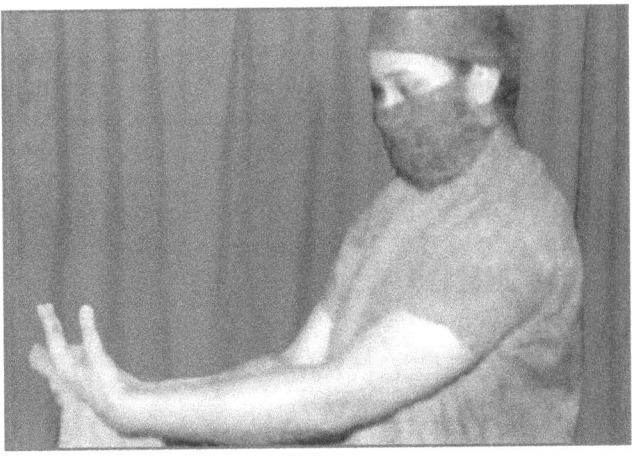

Fig. 5.1: Drying hand after scrubbing.

- After handling contaminated materials (after being in contact with blood and body fluids and secretions)
- On arrival for and prior to departure from duty
- After using the toilet
- Before preparing and serving food
- After touching hair, nose, mouth and handkerchief
- During care when the nurse moves from the contaminated site to clean area, priority should be given to washing hands with cleaning agents (**Fig. 5.1**).

Methods

- Cut nail short
- Wet hands and take sufficient quantity of solutions in the hands
- Lather hands using friction and ensure that all parts of the hands and wrist are covered, it should not be less than 1 minute
- Attention to be given to the palm, back of finger, and between fingers
- Rub backward forward thoroughly
- Rinse hands with running water
- Use water-less antiseptic hand rub for 30 seconds
- Dry with sterile/laundered towel.

Protective Clothing

All healthcare workers should routinely use appropriate barrier precautions to prevent skin mucous membrane exposure during contact with patients' blood or body fluids that require universal precautions.

Purpose

To prevent cross-infection during and after care of patients.

Protective clothing includes:
 i. Gown
 ii. Cap
 iii. Face mask
 iv. Gloves
 v. Other special protective barrier

Gown principles
- After the hands are scrubbed with an antiseptic lotion, washed, and dried with a sterile towel, gown is to be put on. This allows nurses to participate in patient care activities, while maintaining a state of asepsis in a practical way as far as possible.
- Use nontouch technique while wearing the gown, if you are preparing for sterile procedures.

Cap principles
- Select the correct size cap to ensure adequate fit and complete coverage of all hair.
- Separate the elastic band with hands and pull the cap over the crown of the head so that the hand is pulled below the ear lobe.
- Tuck all hair completely inside the elastic band, to prevent contamination of desired sterile field's with hair.
- Change after care and dispose in the labeled container for disposal.

Face mask principles
- Select a mask and locate the edge.
- Hold the mask by the top 2 loops or strings and place in front of the face.
- Place the tap strings over the tops of the ear and then behind the head.
- The bottom is to be tied behind the neck drawing the lower edge of the mask under the chin.
- Adjust the plastic or metal bridge piece securely over the bridge.
- Change after each patient care and any spillage in between the procedures.

Gloves
Gloves are to be used while coming in contact with blood and body fluids while attending sterile procedures.

Principles of wearing
- After hands are washed with antiseptic solution and drying, gloves are put on (gown cap to be worn as required)
- Outer side should not be touched
- Use dry gloves
- Check for any tear or leakage
- Use appropriate size
- For handling items or surfaces soiled with blood and body fluids to which universal precautions apply
- Use gloves when healthcare is provided to cut on their skin.

Principles of changing gloves
Gloves should be changed:
- After contact with each patient.
- Wash hands after removing gloves.
- Gloves should be removed before leaving patient area.
- If gloves are contaminated by infected blood and body fluids during procedures they should be changed immediately.

- In case of scarcity of gloves, it is important to use non-touch technique for all procedures and wash hands with waterless hand rub.

Other protective barriers as part of universal precautions
- All healthcare workers should routinely use other appropriate barrier to prevent exposure of skin and mucous membrane while handling blood or body fluids as universal precautions.
- Other protective barriers which are used in case of specific precautions are plastic aprons, and shoes.

Plastic apron
- The plastic apron must be used while coming in contact with blood and body. It should be changed and disinfected in between the care of the patient.
- The plastic apron is to be changed, if the care taker has to go from infected side to the clean area.

Shoes
- Personal shoes have to be removed outside the patient area and the unit shoes have to be used while in the care area.
- There is least importance of shoe cover, as it does not prevent transmission of microorganisms.

Goggles or eye shields
The eye is a sensitive and vital organ, it is necessary to use goggles or eye shields when there is a chance of splashing of the patient product, i.e., body fluids or blood into the eyes of the care giver.

Sharp
The word "sharp" indicates dangers of getting injuries. Common sharp items of the hospital include scalpel blades, needles, broken glass pieces, and other instruments and devices.

Precautions
While handling sharp objects care should be taken to avoid injuries by the following measures:
- Needle should not be recapped, bent, broken, and removed by hands.
- Disposal of syringes and needles scalpel blades and other sharp items should be placed in a puncture resistance container for disposal.
- The puncture resistance or sharp disposal should be located close to the use area.
- Before giving injection the needle port should never be touched, after procedure.

Sharp disposal bin can be used for:
- Syringes, needles, glass ampoules, blade, disposal, razors, contaminated broken glass, small broken glasses, and small cannula.
- Unbroken glass bottle containing body fluids.
- Aerosol cons.
- Batteries (aerosol and batteries must not be sent for incineration as there is an explosion hazard.

- ❖ Large items of uncontaminated broken glasses must be well-wrapped and podded.
- ❖ Small amount of broken glasses must be disposed off in a sharp bin.
- ❖ Change when two-third is filled with waste.

Clinical Waste

Clinical waste is a waste generated in any healthcare setting or patient care area. It is a potential infection risk to staff and patients, if not handled or disposed off correctly. The key to safe disposal of waste is the responsibility of all the staff to confirm clear identification of clinical waste and appropriate disposal.

Principles to be followed during collection of waste

In collection of waste, the waste can be classified into:
- ❖ **Clinical waste:** Dressings, sanitary items, disposable, intravenous tubing, sharp syringes, glass ampoules, blades, small cannula, etc.
- ❖ **Domestic waste:** Nonclinical waste paper containing patient information.
- ❖ **For incineration:** Blood bags, catheter, and stoma bags, disposable drainage bottle.
- ❖ **Glass waste:** A clearly labeled plastic bin must be provided in each ward and department, they are to be collected weekly or when filled.

Collection of waste

- ❖ Use color-codes system for clear identification of type of clinical waste
- ❖ Must be labeled the neck with the ward and department of origin
- ❖ Do not over fill the bags and ensure that complete sealing takes place
- ❖ Ensure complete sealing take place, when 3/4th is filled.

Transportation of waste

- ❖ Must be transported by a responsible person
- ❖ Must be trained with protective clothing vehicle and equipment used for transport, must have smooth impermeable surface, which are easy to clean
- ❖ It should be transported in a close wheel bar
- ❖ All the waste should be sent for disposal once a day, whereas food waste needs to be sent twice a day from the wards.

Disposal

It is according to the institutional policy.

Spillage

Avoid spilling by careful handling. If any spillage occurs, it should be mopped up immediately with a paper towel and a disinfectant should be used for infective material and undiluted Milton in the case of viral infection and labeled as biomedical hazard.

Linen

- ❖ Used linen must be handled with care at all times
- ❖ Used linen must be put into the appropriate container
- ❖ Clean linen must be delivered to the patient care area in a way which maintains a clean state.

Categories of linen

- ❖ Used linen (soiled and fouled).
- ❖ Soiled.
- ❖ Fouled—is contaminated with urine feces, sputum, vomits, blood, or other body fluids.
- ❖ Collected linen used for a patient with known infection.
- ❖ Heat-liable linen—used by patient with known infection.
- ❖ Heat-liable linen—used by patient infected with hazardous group.

Principles

- ❖ Infected linen must be put into designated bags and sealed immediately
- ❖ Contaminated woolen blankets can be decontaminated by exposure to formaldehyde vapors or autoclaving.
- ❖ Matters and pillows must be enclosed with plastic cover, washed with detergent frequently.

References

- ❖ Hospital-Infection Program
- ❖ National Center for Infectious Disease, Center for Disease Control.

Specific Protection

In child-birth process

The delivery of a child is more or less a crisis management, thus the person conducting delivery may get splashes of potentially infected blood and amniotic fluid and even cuts, the chances of exposure to blood-borne infection are much higher. The following guidelines may be useful:
- ❖ All instruments, equipment, and material used for delivery, must be sterile and should be decontaminated after use, for all the deliveries.
- ❖ The surface including table top sand floor, which have been contaminated, must be decontaminated.
- ❖ Protective barrier is recommended for all activities.

The Personnel to be protected

i. Healthcare providers who have exudates lesion. And sweeping dermatitis to be excluded from providing care.
ii. If anyone has abrasions and cuts, it must be covered with water-proof dressing.

Immunization

All healthcare providers must be specially protected with following immunization:
- ❖ Influenza varicella (chickenpox) for susceptible employees with direct contact
- ❖ Tetanus/diphtheria vaccination is given to who have not had booster in 10 years

Protection against infected materials

A procedure that can achieve killing of vegetative microorganisms and reduction of microbial load to safe levels, spores will not usually be destroyed is known as disinfection. It is essential for all the infected materials. The effective use of disinfecting, antiseptics and sterilization procedures constitutes important factors in preventing cross-infection or hospital-acquired infection.

Principles
- Thorough cleaning with water and detergent must be carried out before any method of disinfecting.
- Disinfecting must be done at recommended concentration.
- Disinfecting should be freshly prepared.
- The choice of method of disinfecting depends on the risk of the patient and healthcare workers, microorganisms involved.
- Chlorine-based agents required for disinfecting contaminated bedding.

Disinfection of infected linen
- The contaminated linen must be disinfected by chemical disinfectant or autoclaving at low pressure of steam.
- Contaminated soiled woolen blankets can be decontaminated either by exposing to formaldehyde vapors or autoclaving.
- It is advisable to cover all matters with water-proof materials.

Disinfection of frequently used equipment such as bed-frame and cot, cradles, IV stand, lockers, etc.
- Daily wash with detergent and dry.
- For infected patients wash with Milton solution or locally recommended solution.

Disinfection of bedpans/urinals
- Heat infect in washer disinfector (if available)
- If washer disinfector is not available add phenolic disinfectant and leave for 5 minutes before emptying
- Wash with detergent
- Disposable gloves and disposable plastic apron must be used in handling bed pans and urinals
- Weekly scrubbing is recommended to remove the scum on stainless steel equipment.

Disinfection of equipment
- Decontamination between patients essential
- Normal decontamination procedures are sufficient
- Thoroughly decontaminate before it is inspected or repair it.

Accidental inoculation of injury includes:
- Precautions injury, e.g., needle pricks, injury with any contaminated sharp object
- Contamination of nonintact skin conjunctiva or mucous membranes with blood and any other body fluids example CSF peritoneal, plural, pericardial synovial and amniotic fluids, unfixed tissues organs and ports of bodies, etc.

Action after accidental injury
- Squeeze the wound to make it bleed
- Wash the injury site for 5 minutes in running water
- Splashes on eyes are thoroughly irrigated with water or normal saline
- Splashes on the mouth should be washed with water.

Isolation Precautions
The aim of isolation precaution is to prevent the risk of transmission of microorganisms; certain care measures can be taken to decrease the risk of transmission.

Essentials of isolation precautions
- Handwashing
- Wearing gloves
- Wearing protective clothing
- Patient placement
- Disposal of linen
- Clinical waste
- Decontamination of equipment and other articles
- Routine and terminal cleaning

Above essential isolation precautions are explained under universal precaution except terminal cleaning.

Routine and terminal cleaning
After the patient has been discharged or shifted to another room following isolation, the room should be:
- Thoroughly cleaned before another patient's use.
- Cleaned, bed rails, lockers, tables, chairs, door handles, sinks, taps, etc.
- Curtain should be replaced and washed.

MEDICAL ASEPSIS

Definition
Medical asepsis refers to all the practices that help to reduce the number and spread of microorganisms **(Table 5.1)**.

Medical Aseptic Practices

Table 5.1: Medical asepsis practices.

Practices	Rationale
When to wash hands	
Hand washing	
1. Wash hands thoroughly using plenty of soap and water:	To reduce number of transient bacteria present on hands.
a. On arrival at the hospital.	To prevent cross-infection.
b. Before, between, and after all physical contacts with the patient.	
c. Before entering and leaving the patient's unit.	
d. Before and after performing any procedure.	
e. Before preparing and after serving the food.	
f. Before and after performing any bodily function such as eating, blowing the nose, use of toilet, combing hair, etc.	

Contd...

Contd...

Practices	Rationale

g. After handling any contaminated items, e.g., used sputum cups, urinals, bed pan, etc.
h. Before and after collection of specimens.
i. When hands are obviously soiled.
j. On completion of duty, etc.
2. Cleaning
a. Clean the least soiled areas and articles first and then the most soiled ones.
b. Use damp dusting always.
c. Rinse the articles first with cold water (Contaminated with organic material such as blood, pus, etc.)
d. Wash the articles with plenty of soap and water.
e. Dry and replace the articles.
f. Ensure that the floors and surfaces are cleaned with detergent solution and water.
g. Use practices of personal grooming. Example: shampooing the hair, taking bath daily, etc.
3. Avoid
a. Shaking the linen.
b. Soiled items and equipment from touching the uniform.
c. Placing the soiled bed linen or any other items on the floor.
d. Talking, coughing, or sneezing directly on others.
e. Cuts or lesions on the skin.
4. Sterilization and Disinfection
a. Ensure that all the articles are cleaned thoroughly before sending for sterilization or disinfection.
b. Sterilize all the instruments using steam under pressure.
c. Disinfect
  i. The articles that cannot be sent for sterilization.
  ii. The articles, including soiled linen, contaminated articles, etc., before it is sent out of the unit.
	
	To prevent soiling of the clean areas and articles. To prevent contamination.
	To prevent scattering of dust. Cold water prevents coagulation of organic material.
	
	To remove organic material easily. Soap lowers the surface tension and removes dirt easily. Presence of moisture promotes growth of microorganisms.
	
	To maintain cleanliness.
	
	To inhibit the growth of microorganisms. To prevent harboring of microorganisms.
	To prevent scattering of duct and microorganisms.
	To prevent contamination.
	
	To prevent contamination of the floor.
	
	To prevent droplet infection.
	
	To prevent microorganisms entering the skin.
	
	To remove dirt, grease or debris from the instruments.
	
	To reduce the number of pathogenic microorganisms from the article.
	To kill pathogenic and nonpathogenic microorganisms including spores.
	To destroy the pathogenic organisms. To prevent cross-infection.

Contd...

Practices	Rationale

5. Use of Masks
i. Wear disposable masks while caring for patients in isolation units.
ii. Ensure that the mask:
  a. Covers the mouth and nose completely.
  b. Snugly fits in around the face.
iii. Avoid touching the part of the mask that comes in contact with the nose.
iv. Change the mask—
  a. Every 1–2 hours.
  b. When it is wet.
6. Use of Gown
Wear gown when:
a. Articles contaminated by the feces or wound discharges.
b. Bodily discharges such as faces, urine, pus or any other discharges from the wound.
c. Change the gloves after each contact with bodily discharges and between the two activities, e.g., gloves used for the cleaning of the patient should be changed before feeding the patient.
7. Isolation
1. Isolate all the infected cases in a separate room or cubicle.
2. Wear gown, gloves and mask while caring for patients in isolation unit.
3. Wash hands thoroughly before and after attending each patient and procedure.
4. Use disposable articles as far as possible.
5. Keep only the essential equipment, instrument, and supplies required for that patient.
6. Restrict visitors and personnel attending on the patient.
7. Treat instruments with antiseptic solution after cleaning and before sending it to CSSD.
	To filter the microorganisms from exhalations.
	
	To prevent the spread of microorganisms to and from the patient.
	
	To prevent escape of microorganisms from the sides. To prevent contamination.
	To ensure effective filtering of microorganisms. A moist mask is a poor filter.
	
	To prevent contamination.
	
	To prevent contamination.
	
	To prevent spread of infection.
	
	To protect the nurses uniform from contamination.
	
	To prevent cross-infection.
	
	To prevent spread of cross-infection. To minimize infection.
	To reduce infection.
	
	To minimize chances of spreading of infection.
	
	To prevent spread of infection.

Contd...

Contd...

Practices	Rationale
8. Dispose soiled or used items directly into appropriate containers. a. Wrap items that are moist from body discharge in water proof containers such as plastic bags, before discarding into the waste container. b. Pour liquid wastes such as bath water, mouth rinse, urine, and any other secretions directly into the drain.	To avoid contamination while handling.
9. Clean the isolation unit daily, including the floors using disinfectant solution, e.g., Dettol, Lysol, Savlon, etc.	To prevent splattering in the sink and on you.
10. Perform terminal disinfection of patient's unit with all the articles used on discharge, transfer or death of a patient with infectious disease.	To prevent cross-infection.

SURGICAL ASEPSIS (STERILE TECHNIQUE)

Definition

It refers to all the practices used to keep the objects or areas sterile or free from all microorganisms (**Table 5.2**).

General Principles of Surgical Asepsis

Table 5.2: Surgical asepsis practices.

Practices	Rationale
1. Use all sterile equipment and supplies for any surgical procedure.	To prevent cross-infection.
2. Wear sterile gloves or use sterile forceps while handling sterile supplies and equipment.	To prevent contamination.
3. Put on surgical cap mask and gown for any sterile surgical procedure.	To prevent contamination.
4. Always face a sterile field. a) Avoid turning your back or side on a sterile field. b) Always pass back to back when passing a scrubbed person or non-sterile area.	Sterile objects which are out of vision are considered questionable and their sterility cannot be guaranteed. To avoid contamination of sterile surfaces and areas.
5. Hold sterile objects above the waist level.	To ensure keeping the sterile articles within eyesight.

Contd...

Contd...

Practices	Rationale
6. Never cough, sneeze or talk over a sterile field. **Note:** If it is necessary to do so, turn your head away from the sterile field.	To prevent accidental contamination. To prevent droplet infection.
7. Plan to assemble and handle all the needed sterile equipment and supplies from the sterile area at time.	To avoid unnecessary contact with sterile field. To avoid contamination.
8. Never reach across a sterile field.	To prevent falling of microorganisms into the sterile field due to gravity when a non-sterile object is held above the sterile field.
9. Prevent excessive air currents around the sterile field, e.g., air currents can be caused by moving fast, flopping the clothes and drapes and closing the doors, etc.	To prevent travel of microorganisms through air currents.
10. Place the unsterile objects separate from the sterile field.	To prevent transfer of microorganisms from unsterile field to the sterile field.
11. Keep sterile field dry, e.g., avoid drapes or wrappers becoming wet while pouring lotions, etc.	To prevent transfer of microorganisms from sterile field to unsterile field through capillary action due to moisture.
12. Consider any article as unsterile if there is any doubt about its sterility.	To ensure safety.
13. The edge of the sterile field is considered as unsterile.	Proximity to a contaminated area makes sterility doubtful.
14. Place the sterile pack in such a way that the wrapper is opened away from you.	To avoid the possibility of a sterile surface touching the unsterile clothing.
15. Discord unused sterile supplies or resterilize if it can be used again.	To prevent contamination of sterile stock. To ensure sterility.
16. Sterile surfaces or articles may touch other sterile surfaces or articles and remain sterile.	Both the surfaces and articles are sterile.
17. All sterile objects used for one patient are sterile only for that patient and cannot be used for another patient.	To ensure safety.
18. Label each sterile supply with regard to its contents, date and time of sterilization.	To ensure sterility of sterile supplies.

Principles of Surgical Asepsis in Relation to Handling/Transfer Forceps/Cheatle Forceps (Table 5.3)

Table 5.3: Principles of Surgical Asepsis in Relation to Handling/Transfer Forceps/Cheatle Forceps.

Practices	Rationale
1. Sterilize the transfer forceps and the container daily.	To ensure sterility. To reduce chance of contamination due to frequent and varied use.
2. Hold the transfer forceps pointing downwards.	To prevent the solution from flowing onto the contaminated area (the handle of the forceps) and then back to the sterile area (the tip of the forceps).
3. Never allow the tip of the transfer forceps touch the top or surface of the container above the disinfectant level when removing the forceps from the container.	The tap of the container and surface of the bottle which is above the level of the disinfectant solution are considered unsterile.
4. Tap the prongs together gently over the container to remove excess solution.	To keep the sterile field dry. To avoid contamination of sterile field from capillary action due to moisture.
5. Keep the prongs (tip) of the forceps within the eye view and at or above the waist level.	To prevent sterile objects which are not of vision touching the unsterile field accidentally
6. Drop the sterile article gently on the sterile field without touching the tip of the transfer forceps.	To prevent contamination of the transfer forceps.

Principles of Surgical Asepsis in Relation to Handling of a Sterile Container (Table 5.4)

Table 5.4: Principles of surgical asepsis in relation to handling of a sterile container.

Practices	Rationale
1. Remove the lid only when necessary and only for a short period of time.	To prevent possibility of contamination of the lid through air currents.
2. Lift the lid of the container in such a way that the inside of the lid is pointing downwards.	To prevent contamination of inside part of the lid with air currents.
3. Invert the lid only when it is necessary to place it down.	To prevent contamination of the sterile lid with an unsterile surface.
4. Never return the unused sterile objects to the sterile container once they have been taken out.	To prevent contamination of the sterile container.

Principles of Surgical Asepsis in Relation to Pouring of Sterile Solutions (Table 5.5)

Table 5.5: Principles of surgical asepsis in relation to pouring of a sterile solutions.

Practices	Rationale
1. Open the lid of the bottle without touching the inner surface of the lid.	The cap and outer space of the bottle are unsterile.
2. Pour a small amount of solution into the sink or kidney tray.	To clean the tip of the sterile bottle.
3. Hold the bottle outside the edge of the sterile field and pour the solution carefully into the sterile bowel without spilling the solution.	To prevent contamination of sterile field.
4. Ensure that the tip of the bottle does not touch the sterile container or dressing.	To prevent contamination.

AIMS OF STANDARD PRECAUTIONS AGAINST HOSPITAL-ACQUIRED INFECTION

Strategies are otherwise known as standard precautions, aimed at reducing the risk of transmission of microorganism from both recognized and unrecognized sources of infection. Standard precaution can be taken by:
- Universal precaution
- Specific protection

Universal Precaution

"Universal Precautions" as defined by Center for Disease Control (CDC) are a set of precautions designed to prevent transmission of human immunodeficiency virus (HIV), hepatitis B virus (HBV), and other blood-borne pathogens when providing fresh air or healthcare.

Aims

1. Preventing cross-infection from patient to patient, patients to healthcare providers and healthcare providers to patients and relatives during hospitalization.
2. To ensure that the risk of transmissions of infection is minimized and if it occurs, it is controlled quickly and effectively as far as possible.
3. Providing a consistent approach to the prevention of transferable infection from both known and unknown sources of infection.
4. To protect high-risk group of patients, healthcare practitioners as well as other care takers from known and unknown risk of hospital-acquired infection.

Elements of Universal Precautions
a. Hand washing
b. Protective wears (clothing)
c. Sharp
d. Clinical waste
e. Spillage
f. Linen

BIOMEDICAL WASTE MANAGEMENT

Types of Hospital Waste

The WHO defines medical waste as waste generated by healthcare activities including a broad range of materials, from used needle and syringes to soiled dressings, body parts, diagnostic samples, blood chemicals, pharmaceutical medical devices, and radioactive materials.

Types of Medical Waste

1. Human anatomical waste like tissues, organs, and body parts
2. Animal wastes generated during research from veterinary hospitals
3. Microbiology and biotechnology waste
4. Sharps like hypodermic needles, syringes, scalpels, and broken glass
5. Discarded medicine
6. Discarded medicine and cytotoxic drugs

Waste Segregation and Hazards

The waste must always be segregated into different fractions based on their potential hazard and disposal route **(Tables 5.6 and 5.7)**.

Table 5.6: Categories of biomedical waste.

Categories	Waste categories	Treatment and disposal
1.	Human anatomical waste	Incineration/deep burial
2.	Animal waste (animal tissue, organs, body parts, and waste)	Incineration/deep burial
3.	Waste from laboratory	Autoclaving/incineration
4.	Sharp waste (needles, syringes, scalpel, blades, glass)	Mutilation/shredding
5.	Drugs, outdated, contaminated	Destruction, disposal in secured landfills
6.	Solid waste. Material contaminated with blood, fluid, including cotton dressings, soiled plaster casts, linen	Incineration
7.	Liquid waste. Waste generated from laboratory and washing, cleaning, housekeeping and disinfecting activities	Disinfection by chemical treatment and discharge into drains

Table 5.7: Color coding and type of container for disposal of biomedical wastes.

Color coding	Type of container	Waste category
Yellow	Plastic bag	1, 2, 3, 6
Red	Disinfected container/plastic bag	3, 6, 7
Blue/white translucent	Plastic bag/puncture proof container	4, 7
Black	Plastic bag	5, 9, 10

UNIT 6

Therapeutic Nursing Care

LEARNING OBJECTIVES

After completing this unit, learner will be able to:
- Deep breathing and coughing exercise
- Oxygen inhalation
- Dry and moist inhalation
- Oronasal suctioning
- Explain care of patient with altered body temperature—hot and cold applications
- Describe care of patients with fluid and electrolyte imbalance
- Explain care of unconscious patient
- Discuss care of the bed ridden patient (traction, fracture, etc.)
- Explain care of patient with pain
- State care of patient with body elimination deviation

PATIENTS WITH UPPER RESPIRATORY AIRWAY INFECTION

Assessment

The nurse obtains a complete history of the patient's problems. The health history focuses on the physical and functional problems.

Signs and symptoms may include:
- Headache
- Sore throat
- Pain around the eyes and on either side of the nose
- Difficulty in swallowing
- Cough
- Hoarseness
- Fever
- Stuffiness
- Generalized discomfort and fatigue

The nurse determines the time of onset of the symptoms, what relieves them and what aggravates them.

Physical Examination

1. The nurse inspects the nose, she/he looks for:
   - Swelling lesions
   - Bleeding or discharge
   - Abnormal mucosa, reddened color, asymmetry
2. The throat is observed by having the patient open his/her mouth and take a deep breath. The tonsils and pharynx are inspected for the abnormal findings or reddened color or evidence of drainage, ulceration or enlargement
3. The trachea is palpated for any lumps or deformities. The lymph nodes also are palpated for associated enlargement and tenderness.

Diagnostic Tests

1. Culture of nose or throat for causative organism
2. Radiographs of sinuses are used to determine the presence and extent of the problem

Nursing Diagnoses

Based on the analysis of patient's data, the patient's major nursing diagnoses may include the following:
1. Ineffective airway clearance related to excessive secretions secondary to an inflammatory process.
2. Pain related to upper airway irritation secondary to an infection.
3. Impaired verbal communication related to upper airway irritation secondary to infection.
4. Fluid volume deficit related to increased fluid loss secondary to diaphoresis associated with a fever.

5. Knowledge deficit regarding prevention of upper respiratory infections due to lack of exposure to information or misinterpretation of information.

Planning

Goals: The major goals for the patient may include:
- Maintenance of a patient airway
- Relief of pain
- Maintenance of effective means of communication
- Absence of fluid volume deficit
- Knowledge of how to prevent upper airway infections

Nursing Interventions

Airway clearance

An accumulation of secretions can block the airway in many patients with an upper airway infection. Changes in the respiratory pattern result and the work of breathing required to get beyond the blockage is increased.

Measures to loosen thick secretions are:
a. Increasing fluid intake to provide systemic hydration, which is an effective expectorant.
b. Humidifying the environment by steam inhalation or room vaporizers also to loosen secretions and reduce inflammation of the mucous membranes.
c. Instructing the patient about the bed position to assume for facilitating drainage. For example, drainage of sinusitis or rhinitis is achieved in the upright position.
d. Administering medications as prescribed to relieve nasal or throat congestion.

Comfort measures

Upper respiratory tract infections usually produce localized discomfort:
- In sinusitis, pain may occur in the area of the sinuses or the patients may experience a headache.
- In pharyngitis, laryngitis or tonsillitis, a sore throat occurs.

Measures to relieve discomfort:
a. Administer analgesics as prescribed
b. Hot packs help relieve the congestion of sinusitis and promote drainage
c. Warm water gargles or irrigations relieve the pain of a sore throat
d. An ice collar is applied in the immediate postoperative period after tonsillectomy and adenoidectomy to reduce swelling and decease bleeding.
e. Bed rest will help relieve the generalized discomfort or fever that accompanies many upper airway conditions.
f. Instruct the patient in general oral and nasal hygiene techniques to help relieve localized discomfort and to prevent the spread of infection.

Communication:

Upper airway infections may result in hoarseness or loss of speech.

Measures to improve communication:
a. Instruct the patient not to try to speak, but instead, to communicable in writing if appropriate.
b. Placing objects close to the patient minimizes unnecessary use of the voice to request items as additional strain on the vocal cords may further delay return of full voice.

Fluid intake

In upper airway infections, the work of breathing, and the respiratory rate increase as inflammation and secretions develop. This in turn may increase insensible fluid loss. An associated fever increases the metabolic rate, which results in diaphoresis and increased fluid loss.

Measures to maintain fluid volume:
Encourage the patient to drink 2-3 liters of fluid per day during his upper airway infection, unless contraindicated. Liquid (hot or cold) may be soothing, depending on the illness.

Patient education

The prevention of most upper airway infections is difficult because there are many potential causes. The responsible pathogen usually cannot be identified and vaccines are unavailable except in rare cases. Allergies, pathologic conditions of the sputum, emotional problems, and various systemic illnesses may be predisposing factors in some cases:

The nurse instructs the patient about the following hygienic measures:
a. **Practice good health measures:** Nutritious diet, appropriate exercise, adequate rest and sleep and handwashing.
b. Correct air dryness by proper home humidification.
c. Avoid irritants (dust chemicals, tobacco and smoke) and allergens when possible
d. Avoid unnecessary chilling of this skin-chilling lowers resistance
e. Avoid crowded area during flu season
f. Maintain adequate dental hygiene
g. Obtain influenza vaccination if advised by a physician. This is usually recommended for the elderly and that chronic illness.

Evaluation-expected outcomes:
1. **Maintaining a patent airway by managing secretions:**
   a. Reports decreased congestion
   b. Uses room humidifier
   c. Assumes best position to facilitate drainage of secretions for the condition
   d. Verbalizes familiarity with use of medication (oral or nasal) to relieve nasal congestion.

2. **Is comfortable:**
   a. States that use of analgesics helps relieve localized pain or headache
   b. Demonstrates the application of hot packs for sinusitis, warm water gargles for a sore throat, and an ice collar after tonsillectomy an adenoidectomy
   c. Verbalizes an understanding of the need for rest at this
   d. Demonstrates adequate oral hygiene
3. **Is able to communicate:**
   a. Demonstrates ability to communicable needs, level of comfort
   b. Uses paper and pencil as a method of communication
   c. Uses voice minimally
4. **Maintains an adequate fluid balance:**
   a. States rationale for drinking plenty of fluids
   b. Demonstrates no significant weight loss
   c. Shows no sign of dehydration
5. **Identifies strategies to prevent upper airway infections and allergic reactions:**
   a. Eat a balanced diet daily
   b. Practices good handwashing
   c. Does not smoke
   d. Avoids enclosed areas polluted with smoke
   e. Stays away from crowded areas during flu season
   f. Uses room humidifiers when necessary
   g. Wears protective clothing to keep warm and avoid chilling
   h. Verbalizes understanding of irritants/allergens that precipitate upper airway reactions
   i. Contacts physician/clinic to receive a flu shot.

PATIENTS WITH PULMONARY DISEASES

Assessment

History

The health history focuses on the physical and functional problems experienced by the patient and the effect of these problems on the patient's life and lifestyle.
1. Identify the chief reason why the patient is seeking healthcare. It may be related to one of the followings:
   a. Dyspnea
   b. Pain
   c. Accumulation of mucous
   d. Wheezing
   e. Hemoptysis
   f. Edema of the ankles and feet
   g. Cough
   h. General weakness
2. Determine when the health problem or symptom started, how long it lasted, if it was relieved at any time, how relief was obtained.
3. Collect information on precipitating factors, duration, severity and associated factors or symptoms.

Factors that may contribute to the patient's respiratory conditions may include:
   a. Smoking
   b. Previous personal or family history of lung diseases
   c. Occupational history
   d. Allergens and environmental pollutants
   e. Hobbies
4. Evaluate psychological factors that may affect the patient's life, e.g., anxiety, role changes, family relationships, financial problems and employment or unemployment.

Physical Assessment

Physical assessment of the chest provides objective data that along with information obtained about the health history, forms the database necessary to formulate nursing diagnoses appropriate to the individual.

Inspection: Inspection of the thorax provides information about the musculoskeletal structure, nutrition and the status of the respiratory system.

The patient is observed for:
General appearance
- Skin color
- Evidence of loss of subcutaneous tissue
- Position assumed
- Mucous membrane
- Nail beds
- Asymmetry

Rate and breathing pattern
Observation of the rate and depth of respirations is also important (The adult normal respiratory rate is 12-18 breathes per minute. It is regular in depth and rhythm).

Examples of abnormal findings are:
a. **Tachypnea:** An increase in the rate of respiration
b. **Bradypnea:** Respiration that are regular in rhythm, but slower than normal in rate
c. **Hyperpnea:** An increase in depth of respiration
d. **Hyperventilation:** An increase in both and in depth that results in a lowered arterial PCO_2.
e. **Apnea:** Total absence of breathing
f. **Cheyne-Stokes respiration:** Cyclical deeper and shallower breaths followed by periods of apnea-associated with heart failure and damage to the respiratory center.
g. **Paradoxical:** Portion of chest wall moves in during inhalation, resembling the blowing of wind, due to obstruction of air passages.

Note: Although the nurse may not recognize the specific pattern and its association with a disease state, she is expected to be able to describe abnormal patterns of breathing and their deviation from normal.

The major signs and symptoms of respiratory diseases are:
1. **Dyspnea:** Dyspnea is difficult breathing and may be a result of a cardiac or respiratory disease. The circumstances that

produce the patient's dyspnea must be determined. It is important to ask the patient:
- How much exertion triggers shortness of breath?
- Is there an associated cough?
- Is dyspnea related to other symptoms?
- Was the onset of shortness of breath sudden or gradual?
- Is the shortness of breath worse when the patient is flat in bed?
- Does the shortness of breath occur at rest? With exercise? Running? Climbing stairs?
- Is the shortness of breath worse while walking? If so, when walking how far?

2. **Cough:** Cough results from irritation of the mucous membrane anywhere in the respiratory tract.
   Areas of assessment are:
   - The character of the cough. Is it dry? Wheezing? Loose? Severe?
   - The time of coughing *night* or *morning*?
   - A cough at *night* is associated with left-sided heart failure
   - A cough in the *morning* with sputum production is indicative of bronchitis
   - A cough after food intake may indicate aspirated material into the tracheobronchial tree
   - A cough of recent onset is usually from an acute infectious process
   - A cough that worsens when the patient is supine may indicate sinusitis.

3. **Sputum production:** Sputum production is the reaction of the lungs to any constantly recurring irritant.
   Areas of assessment are:
   The amount and the color or change in color of sputum:
   - Rusty sputum indicated bacterial infections
   - A thin, mucus sputum results from viral infections
   - A gradual increase may indicate the presence of chronic bronchitis or bronchiectasis
   - Sputum with bad breath may indicate the presence of a lung abscess or bronchiectasis.

4. **Chest pain:** Chest pain associated with pulmonary conditions may be sharp, stabbing and intermittent or dull, aching or persistent.
   Areas of assessment are:
   - The quality, intensity, and radiation of pain
   - The factors that precipitate the pain: Posture, phases of respiration

5. **Wheezing:** It is often the major finding in a patient with air way narrowing. It is heard with or without a stethoscope.

6. **Clubbing of fingers:** It is found in patients with chronic hypoxic condition. Chronic lung infections and malignancies of the lungs.

7. **Hemoptysis:** Coughing up blood from the respiratory tract.
   Areas of assessment are:
   - *Onset:* Sudden, intermittent or continuous
   - Associated factors/causes
   - *Character:* Pure hemorrhage or mixed with sputum, amount
   - *Determine the source of bleeding:* Gums, nasopharynx or stomach.

8. **Cyanosis:** Cyanosis is a bluish by room lighting, patient's skin color, and depth of vessels from the surface of the skin.
   Central cyanosis: Central cyanosis refers to cyanosis found on the central parts of the body including the mouth, head and torso.
   Assessment of central cyanosis: Cheeks, nose, ears, and oral mucosa are the best areas to assess cyanosis as the skin on these area is thin, blood supply is good. The prime sites of the bluish discoloration in central cyanosis are lips, tongue, hands, feet and mucous membranes of the oral cavity. The depth of the color usually correlated with the amount of desaturated hemoglobin and hence the severity of cyanosis.
   Peripheral cyanosis: Peripheral cyanosis is the bluish discoloration of the distal extremities (hands, fingertips, toes) and can sometime involve circumoral and periorbital areas. Mucous membranes are generally not involved, peripheral cyanosis is rarely a life-threatening medical emergency. Peripheral cyanosis affects the extremities and the skin around the lips but not the mucous membrane. Peripheral cyanosis has a normal systemic arterial oxygen saturation. However, inhaled oxygen extraction results in a wide systemic arteriovenous oxygen difference and inhaled deoxygenated blood on the ventral side of the capillary bed.

Assessment of Breathing Abilities

Tests of the patient's breathing abilities are easily assessed at the bedside by measuring.
- **Respiratory rate:** Normal 12–18 breaths/min
- **Tidal volume:** The volume of each breath, and it is measured by the Wright respirometer.
  Normal 5–8 mL/kg of body weight
- **Minute volume:** It is the volume of air expired per minute. It is measured directly using a respirometer.

It may be decreased by a variety of conditions, such as:
1. Spinal cord trauma, or tumors, which limit impulses, transmitted from the brain to respiratory muscles.
2. Anesthesia or narcotic overdose leads to depression of respiratory centers in the medulla.
3. Kyphoscoliosis, pleural effusion, pneumothorax lead to limitation of thoracic movement.
4. Chronic pulmonary diseases lead to reduction of lung function.

Vital capacity: Vital capacity is the maximum volume of air that is exhaled after a full inspiration.

Oxygen Inhalation

Factors Affecting Oxygenation

1. **Physiological factors:** Any cardiopulmonary disorders affect the oxygen demand of the body, anemia, any

infection, pregnancy, toxic inhalant, high altitude, dehydration, and pulmonary disease.

2. **Developmental factors:** Infants and toddlers are risk for upper respiratory tract infection, unhealthy diet, lack of exercise, stress, substance abuse.
3. **Lifestyle factors:** Acquiring healthy behavior reduces the risk for developing respiratory problems. Malnourished children experience respiratory problems, children who are obese, children are encouraged to have healthy food practice high in potassium, calcium, fruit, vegetables protein, and fiber rich diet. Physical exercise program has many benefits.
4. **Environmental factors:** The environment also influences oxygenation, pollution, dust, airborne fibers creating lung diseases.

Oxygen Therapy

A deficiency of oxygen leads to a lowered oxygen tension of blood plasma **(Table 6.1)**.

Table 6.1: Procedure: Oxygen therapy.

Steps	Rationale
1. Explain to the client and family, what procedure entails and purpose of oxygen therapy	Decreases client's anxiety and oxygen consumption, increases cooperation
2. Place "oxygen in use" signs at door at client's room and overhead bed	Provides client and staff safety. Oxygen is combustible and can fuel a fire, even from cigarette sparks
3. **Implementation** Wash hands	Reduces transmission of microorganisms
4. Attach nasal cannula to oxygen tubing and to humidified oxygen source	Humidification prevents drying of nasal and oral mucous membranes and airway secretions. Humidification might not be used for <3 minute
5. Adjust oxygen flow rate to prescribed dosage usually between 1 and 6 liter/min. Observe that water in humidifier is bubbling	Oxygen flow rate > 6 L/m, may irritate nasal mucosa
6. Place tips of cannula into client's nares and adjust elastic headband or plastic slide until cannula fits snugly and comfortably. Allow sufficient slack on oxygen tubing and secure to client's cloths	Directs flow of oxygen into client's upper respiratory tract. Client is more likely to keep cannula in place, if apparatus fits comfortably
7. Check cannula every 8 hours, keeping humidification jar filled at all times, if used	Ensures patency of cannula and oxygen flow and prevents inhalation of dehumidified oxygen
8. Encourage physician to obtain ABGs 10–15 minutes after initiating oxygen therapy or changing oxygen flow rate	ABGs provide objective data regarding blood oxygen
9. Wash hands	Reduces transmission of microorganisms
10. Observe for decreased anxiety, improved level of consciousness and cognitive abilities, decreased fatigue, absence of dizziness, decreased pulse with regular rhythm, decreased respiratory rate, return to normal blood pressure, improved color	Determines that hypoxia is corrected or reduced
11. Observe clients nares and superior surface of both ears for skin breakdown	Oxygen therapy can cause drying of nasal mucosa. Pressure on ears from cannula tubing or elastic can cause skin irritation
12. Observe pulse oximetry for oxygen saturation	Documents arterial oxygen saturation
13. Assess adequacy of oxygen flow through nasal cannula each shift	Documents patent nasal cannula
14. Unexpected outcomes that may occur include: client experiences nasal irritation, irritation to posterior surfaces of ear, drying of nasal mucosa, sinus pain, and epistaxis	One or more of these signs indicate adverse response to method of oxygen delivery

Indications for Administering Oxygen

1. Correct hypoxemia (anoxemia)
2. Increase the oxygen tension
3. Restore the oxyhemoglobin in the red blood cells

Oxygen given in higher concentration than it present in the air. Usually, it is given in concentrations from 40 to 60%, although even 100% may be given through the face mask technique.

Oxygen should be warmed to room temperature and humidified before it is given to prevent chilling of the child and drying of secretions in the respiratory tract.

Method of Oxygen Administration in Children

Oxygen can be administered by following methods (Tables 6.2 and 6.3):

1. **Oxygen mask:** It can be simple face mask, and venturi mask or partial rebreathing mask, which can be simple face mask permits easy access to the child mobility of the

Table 6.2: Performance checklist: Applying a nasal cannula.

Steps	S	U	Comments
Implementation			
1. Washed hands			
2. Attached nasal cannula to oxygen tubing and to humidified oxygen source			
3. Adjusted oxygen flow rate to prescribed dosage			
4. Placed tips of cannula into clients' nares and adjusted cannula to clients comfort. Allowed sufficient slack on oxygen tubing and secured to clients clothing			
5. Check cannula every 8 hours keeping humidification jar filled at all times			
6. Followed the advice of the physician if ABGs were necessary			
7. Washed hands			
Evaluation			
1. Reassessed client to determine response to oxygen administration via nasal cannula			
2. Observed clients nares and ears for skin breakdown			
3. Checked physician order each shift			
4. Assessed adequacy of cannula each shift			
5. Identified unexpected outcomes			
Recording and reporting			
Record in nurses notes respiratory assessment. Findings before and during oxygen therapy, method of oxygen therapy, delivery, flow rate, patency cannula, clients response, adverse reaction and any change in physician order			

child, and high consistent flow rate of oxygen. Children may not cooperate when this technique is used.

2. **Nasal cannula:** A nasal cannula is a simple, comfortable device for delivering oxygen to a client. The two tips of the cannula about 1.5 cm (0.5 inches) long, protrude from the center of a disposable tube and are inserted into the nostrils. Oxygen is delivered via the cannula with a flow rate up to 5–6 L/min. Higher flow rates dry airway mucosa and do not increase inspired oxygen concentration. The nurse must know what flow rate produces a given percentage of FiO_2, these oxygen percentage will vary, depending on the rate and depth of the client breathing.

A nasal cannula is an effective mechanism for oxygen delivery. It allows the client to breath through the mouth or nose, and is available for all age groups, and adequate for short-term or long-term use. Cannula is inexpensive, disposable, generally comfortable, and easily accepted by most clients.

Traditional nasal cannula commonly effectively provide only up to 4 to 6 liter per minute of supplemental oxygen.

3. **Oxyhood or face tent:** It permits easy access to the child without loss of oxygen and efficient delivery of oxygen. Children generally accept an oxyhood without loss of oxygen and efficient delivery of oxygen should not blow directly on the child face. The edges of the hood should not rub against the child's chin, neck or shoulder. Some oxygen hoods may be open at the top.

4. **Invasive method:** By orotracheal or nasotracheal or tracheostomy route and nasopharyngeal catheter or nasal cannula or prong.

5. **Oxygen tent or canopy:** Comfortable for children beyond the age of infancy, when a child has facial injuries or for any other reason cannot tolerate an oxygen mask, then this method can be used. The tent is first flooded with oxygen and then flow of 4–5 liters per minute is given. This will maintain a service of 40–50% in the tent. A tent is a most uneconomical and inefficient method of giving oxygen because of leakage loss of oxygen whenever the tent is opened, and a high liter flow needed to provide the required concentration. A cooling mechanism is used to maintain a comfortable temperature level within the tent.

Table 6.3: Performance checklist: Applying an oxygen mask.

Steps	S	U	Comments
Implementation			
1. Washed hands			
2. Attached face mask to appropriately sized oxygen tubing			
3. Attached oxygen tubing to humidified oxygen or gas source			
4. Adjusted oxygen flow rate to prescribed dosage and verified that water in humidifier was bubbling			
5. Placed face mask or tent on client and adjusted to snug comfortably fit			
6. Observed for proper functioning of nonbreathing mask, partial rebreathing mask, venturi mask or face tent			
7. Observed for presence of moisture in reservoir bag or oxygen tubing			
8. Assessed humidity source every 4 hours and changed container every 24 hours			
9. Observed for pressure necrosis with tightly fitting mask every 2 hours			
10. Followed up with verifying need for ABGs			
11. Checked physician order every 4 hours			

Contd...

Contd...

Steps	S	U	Comments
12. Observed for gagging, vomiting and removed mask when necessary			
13. Washed hands			

Evaluation
1. Reassessed client to determine response to administration of oxygen by nasal cannula
2. Observed the client's nose and ears for skin breakdown
3. Identified unexpected outcomes

Recording and reporting
Recorded in nurses notes respiratory assessment findings before and during oxygen therapy, method of oxygen delivery, flow rate, patency of airway, client response any adverse reactions or side effects, change in physician's orders

Safety Alert

Oxygen in high concentration has a great combustion potential and readily fuels fire.

- Place an "oxygen in use" sign on the client door and in the client room
- Keep oxygen delivery system away from any open flames
- No smoking should be allowed on the premises
- When using oxygen cylinder secure them so that they will not fall over
- Check that all electrical equipment in the room/ward is functioning properly grounded. An electrical spark in the presence of oxygen can result in a serious fire
- Check the oxygen cylinder level of portable tanks before transporting a client to ensure that there is enough oxygen in the cylinder
- Hospital oxygen cylinder usually connects the regulator to the oxygen source

CARE OF PATIENT WITH ALTERED BODY TEMPERATURE

Factors Affecting Body Temperature

Nurse should be aware of the factors that can affect a client's body temperature so that they can recognize the normal temperature variations and understand the significance of body temperature measurements that deviate from normal.

- **Age:** The infant is greatly influenced by the temperature of the environment and must be protected against extreme changes. Elderly people are also particularly sensitive to extremes in the environmental temperature due to decreased thermoregulatory controls.
- **Diurnal variations:** Body temperatures normally change throughout the day, varying as much as 2.0°C (1.8° between the early morning and the late afternoon).
- **Exercise:** Hard work or strenuous exercise can increase body temperature to as high as 38.3–40°C (101–104°F) measured orally.
- **Hormones:** In women, progesterone secretion at the time of ovulation raises body temperature. Thyroxin, norepinephrine, and epinephrine also affect body temperature.
- **Stress:** Stimulation of the sympathetic nervous system can increase the production of epinephrine and norepinephrine, thereby increasing the metabolic activity and heat production.
- **Environment:** Extremes in environmental temperatures can affect a person's temperatures regulatory systems.

Alterations in Body Temperature

Pyrexia: A body temperature above the usual range is called pyrexia, hyperthermia, or fever. A very high temperature, e.g., 41°C (105°F) is called hyperpyrexia.

Common Types of Fevers

- **Intermittent fever:** During intermittent fever, the body temperature alternates at regular intervals between periods of fever and periods of normal temperatures.
- **Remittent fever:** During a remittent fever, a wide range of temperature fluctuations occurs over the 24 hour period, all of which are above normal.
- **Relapsing fever:** In a relapsing fever, short febrile periods of a few days are interspersed with periods of 1–2 days of normal temperature.
- **Constant fever:** During a constant fever, the body temperature fluctuates minimally but always remains elevated.

Clinical Signs of Fever

- The clinical signs of fever vary with the onset, course, and abatement stages of the fever.
- *Onset (cold or chill stage)*
- Increased heart rate and respiratory rate and depth
- Shivering due to increased skeletal muscle tension and contraction
- Cold skin due to vasoconstriction
- Complaints of feeling cold
- Cessation of sweating
- Rise in body temperature

Course
- Skin feels warm
- Increased pulse and respiratory rate
- Increased thirst
- Mild to severe dehydration
- Drowsiness, restlessness, or delirium and convulsions due to the irritation of the nerve cells
- Loss of appetite with prolonged fever
- Malaise, weakness, and aching muscles due to protein breakdown.

Abatement stage
- Skin that appears flushed and feels warm
- Sweating
- Decreased shivering
- Possible dehydration.

Nursing Interventions for Patients with Fever

Nursing interventions for a patient who has a fever are designed to support the bodies, normal physiologic processes, provide comfort, and prevent complications.

Following are the examples of nursing interventions for patients with fever:
- Monitor vital signs
- Assess skin color and temperature
- Monitor white blood cell count and other pertinent laboratory records
- Remove excess blankets when the patient feels warm, but provide extra warmth when the patient feels chilled
- Provide adequate food and fluids (e.g., 2,000–2,500 mL/day) to meet increased metabolic demands and prevent dehydration
- Measure intake and output
- Maintain prescribed intravenous fluids
- Reduce physical activity to limit heart production
- Administer antipyretics (drugs that reduce the level of fever) as ordered
- Provide a tepid sponge bath to increase heart loss through conduction
- Provide cool circulating air by using a fan to increase heart loss through convection.

CARE OF PATIENT WITH FLUID AND ELECTROLYTES IMBALANCE

Disturbances in Fluid Volume

Deficit
Deficient fluid volume is also known as fluid volume deficit (FVD), hypovolemia is a state or condition where the fluid output exceeds the fluid intake. It occurs when the body loses both water and electrolytes from the extracellular fluid (ECF) in similar proportions.

Hypovolemia
There are two fundamentally different disorders of water balance—(1) dehydration and (2) overhydration. Depending on the extracellular sodium concentration, one can distinguish hypotonic, isotonic and hypertonic dehydration and overhydration.

Hypotonic dehydration
Fluid and sodium are lost but sodium loss is more. Serum sodium low leads to low serum osmolarity. The low osmolarity of the extracellular space produces a reduction of extracellular volume and in the intracellular volume.

Isotonic dehydration
Sodium and fluid proportionate, with normal serum sodium. The extracellular volume is reduced with a normal serum osmolarity while the intracellular volume is normal.

Hypertonic dehydration
Sodium and fluid both are lost, but fluid losses more and serum is high, water deficiency with elevation of serum osmolarity and reduction of extracellular volume.

Hypotonic overhydration
This is the condition where there is excess of water with elevation of extracellular and intracellular volume.

Isotonic overhydration
In this condition both water and sodium are lost, but losses more water and serum sodium is high, excess of water and sodium. The serum osmolarity is normal.

Hypertonic overhydration
Sodium and fluid are in excess, but sodium disproportionately more than fluid. Serum osmolarity and extracellular volumes are increased.

Causes, Symptoms and Treatment of Dehydration
The causes, symptoms, and treatment of dehydration are described in **Table 6.4**.

Electrolyte Balance
Electrolytes are substances formed ions. There is a distinction between positively and negatively charged ions (cations and anions). The most important cations and anions are discussed here.

Sodium
The total body sodium of an adult is 4,200 mmol (60 mmol/kg body weight).

Normal range	Mean value	Daily requirements
132–152 mmol/L	142 mmol/L	1–3 mmol/kg body weight per day

Hypo- and hypernatremia (Electrolyte imbalance)
Hyponatremia is defined as a serum sodium concentration <132 mmol/L and hypernatremia is concentration 152 mmol/L **(Table 6.5)**.

Nursing intervention monitor:
- Fluid loss and gain, containing sodium
- Changes in behavior
- Look for elevated temperature
- Sodium intake and level

Potassium
The total body potassium of on adult is about 3,500 mmol (50 mmol/kg body weight), decreasing with age. Potassium is quantitatively the most important cation in the intracellular

Table 6.4: Causes, symptoms and treatment of dehydration.

Disorder	Causes	Symptoms	Treatment
Hypotonic dehydration	Inadequate sodium, vomiting, and diarrhea, sweating. Increased sodium losses due to adrenal failure. Chronic diuretic therapy loss due to fistula	Hypotonia, muscle cramps, fever, rapid pulse, vomiting, depressed conscious level, fainting, and collapse	Treat the primary disorder Administration of NaCl 0.9%, NaCl 5.8%
Isotonic dehydration	Isotonic fluid losses through vomiting, diarrhea, diuretics. Drainage of ascites with peritonitis, burns, sedatives, and carbon monoxide intoxication sunstroke	Tiredness, thirst, fainting, collapse, vomiting, hypotonia, muscle cramps rapid pulse	Treat the primary cause. Administer Ringer's solution and Hartmann solution (compound sodium lactate)
Hypertonic dehydration	Inadequate water intake or increased water losses due to sweating, somatic diuretics, hyperventilation. Chronic nephropathy, polyuric phases of acute renal failure, diabetic insipidus	• Thirst • Fever • Restlessness • Delirium • Coma	Treat the primary cause Administration of glucose 5% (10–20%)
Hypotonic overdehydration	Excessive administration of salt free solution, gastric lavage with water, increased ADH activity	Weakness, vomiting, dyspnea, and loss of consciousness	Treat the primary cause, Fluid restriction, possible dialysis if tendency to alkalosis NaCl 5.85%
Isotonic overhydration	Excessive administration of isotonic infusions, cardiac failure, nephritic syndrome, chronic uremia, acute glomerulonephritis, cirrhosis of liver	• Edema • Effusion • Dyspnea	Treat the primary cause Restrict salt and fluid, diuretics, osmofundin 20% Renal dose of dopamine 5 mEq/mL
Hypertonic overhydration	Excessive administration of salt Overactive adrenal cortex in Conn's and Cushing syndrome. Administration of steroids, cerebral salt retention syndrome	• Vomiting, Diarrhea and • Liable blood pressure • Pulmonary edema • Restlessness • Changes in central venous pressure	Treatment of the main cause Salt and fluid restriction, salt depletion diuretics. Osmofundin 20%

Table 6.5: Hyponatremia.

Causes	Symptoms	Treatment
• Insufficient water intake, sweating, gastrointestinal losses, diuretics over dose • Major blood losses • Terminal cardiac failure • Cirrhosis of liver	• Loss of appetite • Nausea and vomiting • Muscle weakness, cramps • Fits, altered conscious state	• Treatment of primary disorder • Sodium restriction • Stop diuretics • If water deficiency administration of glucose 5%.

space. Normal range and daily requirement of potassium in adults:

Normal range	Mean value	Daily requirements
3.5–5.5 mmol/L	4.4 mmol/L	1–2 mmol/kg body weight

Hypo- and hyperkalemia

Hypokalemia is said to exit when the serum potassium concentration falls below 3.0 mmol/kg and hyperkalemia when the concentration rises above 5.5 mmol/L **(Tables 6.6 and 6.7)**.

Alkalosis is associated with increased potassium losses and acidosis often with potassium retention.

Nursing intervention

❖ Potassium should always be diluted and infused. If, K^+ is infused without dilution patient may have sudden cardiac arrest due to arrhythmia
❖ Urine output (rule: think twice before giving potassium to a patient in renal failure) should be monitored
❖ Repeat serum K^+ level while on intravenous (IV) potassium
❖ Be careful while administering intravenous potassium in a patient as it may result in ventricular arrhythmia

Table 6.6: Hypokalemia.

Causes	Symptoms	Treatment
• Inadequate intake • Gastrointestinal losses from drain, fistulae, diarrhea, enteritis • Insulin treatment • Excessive diuretics • Cushing's syndrome • Steroid therapy	• Reduced muscle tone, apathy • Stomach and bowel atony with constipation • Hypotension, arrhythmias • Sudden cardiac arrest • Increased sensitivity to digitalis	• Treat the primary cause • Oral potassium replacement • Parenteral replacement of potassium • Serum potassium should be raised slowly to avoid arrhythmias

- ❖ Preferably infuse in a central or big vein
- ❖ If there is facility, monitor ECG
- ❖ Administer potassium only after adequate urine flow.

Table 6.7: Hyperkalemia.

Causes	Symptoms	Treatment
• Reduced renal potassium clearance • Renal failure • Treatment with aldosterone antagonists • Insulin deficiency • Potassium release from inside the cells • Burns • Hypercatabolism	• Confusion • Coma • Bradycardia • Arrhythmias • Ventricular fibrillation • Diastolic cardiac arrest	• Treatment of primary disorder, sodium bicarbonate 10% or 20% intravenous or calcium gluconate 10%, 10–20 mL IV, Glucose 20% + 10 units soluble insulin • Dialysis

Nursing intervention

- ❖ Avoid administration of potassium sparing diuretics
- ❖ Watch for ECG changes
- ❖ Be familiar with treatment of hyperkalemia

Calcium

The total body requirement of calcium is from 22,500 to 29,900 mmol.

Normal range	Mean value	Daily requirements
Total 2.15–2.8 mmol/L	Total 2.45 mmol/L	0.2–0.5 mmol/kg body weight/day
Ionized 1.35–1.55 mmol/L	Ionized 1.45 mmol/L	

Hypercalcemia: Higher then normal level of calcium in the blood. Mild hypercalcemia: 10.5–11.9 mg/dL.
Hypocalcemia: Low calcium level in the blood serum.

Table 6.8: Hypocalcemia.

Causes	Symptoms	Treatment
• Insufficient intake of vitamin D or exposure to sunshine • Hyperparathyroidism • Magnesium deficiency • Renal failure • Acute pancreatitis • Massive transfusion of citrated blood • Alkalosis and diuretics	• Paresthesia or tetany • Spasm of smooth muscle • Epileptic form attack • Depression • ECG findings: Prolongation of QT interval by lengthening of ST segment	• Treatment of primary cause • Oral calcium replacement • Parenteral administration of calcium as gluconate 10% in the event of Hypocalcemia with severe tetany • Slow IV calcium gluconate 10% • Rapid administration may produce sensation of palpitation and collapse

Magnesium

An adult has magnesium storage of 1,000 mmol (**Table 6.9**).

Normal range	Mean value	Daily requirements
0.8–1.0 mmol/L	0.9 mmol/L	0.05–0.1 mmol/kg/body weight

Table 6.9: Hypomagnesemia and Hypermagnesemia.

Causes	Symptoms	Treatment
• Excessive administration of magnesium containing antacids and enemas • Treatment of eclampsia • Renal failure	• Nausea, vomiting and constipation • Muscle weakness • Danger of coma • Respiratory and cardiac arrest	Treat the primary disorder LV. Calcium gluconate 10% 10–20 mL, slowly or with infusion

Phosphate

The total body phosphate of an adult amounts to 27,000 mmol (**Tables 6.10 and 6.11**).

Normal range	Mean value	Daily requirements
0.9–1.5 mmol/L	1.2 mmol/L	0.2–0.5 mmol/kg/day

Table 6.10: Hyperphosphatemia.

Causes	Symptoms	Treatment
• Phosphate binding antacids • Vomiting and diarrhea • Insufficient intake associated with high calorie carbohydrate intake and with insulin treatment of diabetic coma • Diuretics, hyperparathyroidism	• Diffuse pains, general weakness, nausea, vomiting, anorexia • Cardiac arrhythmias • Disturbance of respiratory function	• Treat the primary cause "Parenteral" phosphate administration of sodium phosphate or potassium phosphate • Treatment of diabetic coma and metabolic disturbance in diabetes

Table 6.11: Hypophosphatemia.

Causes	Symptoms	Treatment
Excessive transfusion of old blood, reduced excretion in renal failure and increased reabsorption, hyperparathyroidism and metabolic disturbance in diabetes	Precipitation of calcium phosphate particularly in metabolically inactive tissue	Treatment of primary cause

Chloride

An adult has a total body chloride of 2,800–3,500 mmol. Chloride is the most abundant ion in the extracellular space.

Normal range	Mean value	Daily requirements
97–110 mmol/L	103 mmol/L	1.3 mmol/kg/day

During the administration of IV fluids, the chloride intake may vary with a considerable range without clinical consequences.

Water and Electrolyte Balance in Children

Infant and children have greater requirements for water in proportion to their body weight as compared to adult. The capability of the kidney to excrete electrolyte excess without generous quantities of water is less in infant. Excessive administration of water and electrolytes, in pediatrics therefore particularly important to maintain exact balance of water and electrolytes.

Acid-base Imbalance

Metabolic Acidosis

Metabolic acidosis results because of the high acid content of the blood, which also causes a loss of sodium bicarbonate, the alkaline half of the carbonate buffer system, resulting in a bicarbonate deficit. Severe diarrhea or renal disease causes metabolic acidosis.

Metabolic Alkalosis

Metabolic alkalosis is the result of the heavy loss of acid from the body or an increase in levels of bicarbonate. The most common causes are vomiting and gastric suction and use of thiazide therapy.

Respiratory Acidosis

Respiratory acidosis is a combination of increased arterial carbon dioxide concentration, excess carbonic acid and increased hydrogen ion concentration. Respiratory acidosis is the result of hypoventilation. With respiratory acidosis, the cerebrospinal fluid and brain cells become acidic causing neurologic changes. To manage for this acidosis, the kidney conserves bicarbonate and releases hydrogen ions in the urine.

Respiratory Alkalosis

Respiratory alkalosis is resulted from decreased $PaCO_2$ and increased pH >7.45, like respiratory acidosis respiratory alkalosis begins outside the respiratory system, e.g., anxiety with hyperventilation or within the respiratory system, e.g., asthma attack. The body does not usually compensate for respiratory alkalosis because the pH returns to normal before the kidneys can respond.

CARE OF UNCONSCIOUS PATIENT

Unconsciousness

A state of complete or partial unawareness lack of response to sensory stimuli as a result of hypoxia resulting from respiratory insufficiency or shock from metabolic or chemical brain depressants such as drug, poisons, ketones or electrolytes imbalance or from brain pathology such as trauma, seizures, cerebrovascular accidents, brain abscess, hemorrhage, infections and brain lesions, etc.

Coma

A state of profound unconsciousness characterized by the absence of spontaneous eye movement, response to painful stimuli, and vocalization. The person cannot be aroused, coma may be the result of trauma, hematoma, toxic conditions, acute infectious diseases such as encephalitis, vascular, diseases, poisoning diabetes and intoxication.

Causes and Risk Factors

Three kinds of disorders produce sustained unconsciousness:

Structural Lesions

- Brain tumors
- Brain abscess (rare)
- Cerebral hemorrhage
- Epidural hematoma
- Subdural hematoma

Metabolic Disorders

- Fluid electrolytes or acid-base imbalance
- Infection, metabolic encephalopathy
- Nutritional deficiencies
- Hypoglycemia, diseases of the organs, e.g., liver, lungs, endocrine, and kidney
- Anoxia or ischemia—anoxia poison alcohol and drug
- Temperature regulation disorders.

Psychogenic causes

- Hysteria
- Catatonia

Pathophysiology

Masses within the brain alter the functioning of the brain in many ways. Masses or lesions may place a pressure on the brain is encase in the cranium, there is no space within the skull for the expending brain, pressure slows as its blood and cerebrospinal fluid flow out of the brain and reduces cerebral function. The level of consciousness and the ability to move purposefully are affected. When pressure reaches the brainstem it affects the vital organs especially respiration.

Initial Assessment of the Comatose Patient

It includes:
- Level of consciousness
- Pattern of respiration
- Pupil's size and reactivity
- Deep and superficial reflexes
- Responses to painful stimuli
- Ruptured eardrum and otorrhea
- Determination of serum oxygenation, blood alcohol, blood urea nitrogen ammonia and glucose level if manifestation suggests metabolic disorders
- Glasgow coma scale assessment

Clinical Manifestation of Unconsciousness

- Decreased level of consciousness
- Confusion and decreased attention
- Headache
- Sensory motor deficit
- Aphasia
- Visual loss
- Seizures
  Specific manifestations are related to specific area of brain that is affected.

Diagnostic Procedures

- Lumbar puncture (LP)
- Computed tomography (CT)
- Electroencephalography (EEG)
- Magnetic resonance imaging (MRI)

Laboratory Tests

- Blood glucose
- Electrolyte
- Serum ammonia
- Blood urea nitrogen (BUN) level
- Calcium level
- Prothrombin time (PT)
- Serum ketones and alcohol

Emergency Care

Initial care of an unconscious patient includes:
- Clearing the airway immediately and loosening all tight clothing especially around the neck. Never move freshly injured or unconscious patient without cervical collar until confirming the cervical injury
- Remove and store any dentures, these could cause airway obstruction or could be broken and swallowed
- Remove the cause of obstruction
- Place the patient in semi-prone or lateral position to facilitate drainage of pulmonary secretion and prevent tongue falling back
- Maintain airway, ventilation, and circulation. A nasal or oral airway may be inserted for a short time, or endotracheal intubation
- If required patient may be put into ventilator to reduce partial pressure of arterial carbon dioxide ($paCO_2$)

Immediate intervention includes:
- Treatment of common causes of coma
- KVO (Keep Vein Open) and start follow IV fluids as per instruction
- Assessment of neurological status
- For alcohol abuse commonly given thiamine (as per instruction or follow institutional policies)
- If the patient is having repeated seizures, intravenous diazepam or lorazepam is given as per the order, to avoid complications such as brain damage and coma
- If the patient is not intubated closely monitor the airway
- Patient's level of acid-base balance should be reported quickly
- Fluid imbalance should be reported
- Culture of the blood, throat, nose, and wounds should be obtained, before starting antibiotics (as per instruction and policies of the institution)
- Drug overdose induced coma may be reversed by specific antidotes

Nursing Management (Tables 6.12 and 6.13)

- Establish an adequate airway and ensure ventilation. Obstruction of the airway is a risk for unconscious patient as the epiglottis and tongue may relax occluding the oropharynx or the patient may aspirate vomitus or nasopharyngeal secretions.
- Elevate the head of the bed to a 30° angle, helps to prevent aspiration of secretions.
- The patient requires frequents suctioning and oral hygiene.
- The nurse must maintain the patency of endotracheal tube or tracheotomy.
- Monitor ABG and maintain ventilator setting accordingly.
- Chest physiotherapy and postural drainage are initiated to promote pulmonary hygiene.
- Frequent systematic and objective nursing assessment, including neurological status is essential.
- Periodically assess the entire body, observing laceration, bruises, ulcerations, fractures, dislocation, and contractures and also note skin color, texture, and temperature.
- Inspect dressing frequently for purulent drainage.
- Follow interventions appropriate for all unconscious patients regardless of the cause of the unconsciousness or coma, as below.

Easy access to:
- Ambubag with valve and mask or intubation and tracheotomy equipment
- Neurological observation tray, thermometer, and sphygmomanometer.

Table 6.12: Nursing care of unconscious patient.

S. No.	Nursing action	Rationale
1.	The room or ward area should be warm and well ventilated. Adequate light should be there for easy access to the patient	To facilitate comfort to the patient as well as the care giver to assess the patient at a glance, e.g., • Skin color, which is cherry red after carbon monoxide poisoning, frost in uremia, yellow in hepatic failure, blue in cyanosis • Smell, which is "toasted almonds" after cyanide poisoning the sickly sweet of diabetic ketoacidosis and alcohol
2.	Nurse the patient in a bed with a firm base, a detachable bed head and side railings	To facilitate cardiac massage and incubations if required and to prevent accidental fall
3.	Insert a bed cradle if required	To allow unhampered limb movements. To enhance vision of limbs if leg is in plaster or on traction as in multiple injuries
4.	Place patient in lateral or semiprone position if condition allows	To prevent occlusion of airway by tongue falling back against the pharyngeal wall. To encourage drainage of respiratory secretions and to prevent pooling of secretion in throat
5.	Pass nasogastric tube	To empty gastric contents in regular intervals. To prevent paralytic ileum. To avoid aspiration of stomach contents, which may give rise to respiratory complications
6.	Place the patient as follows: • Head: Put the patient's head on a pillow	To promote comfort and maintain proper alignment of the body
	• Trunk: Keep the spine straight and place the pillow at the patient's back for support	To prevent edema by inappropriate pressure on venous flow
	• Upper limbs: Bring the uppermost arm forward in front of the patient. Bend the elbow slightly, but keep the wrist extended. Support the arm on a pillow and bring the bottom arm alongside the face facing upward	To prevent internal rotation of the hip
	• Lower limbs: Flex the uppermost leg and bring it forward. Support it on pillows. Keep the lower leg extended straight and in line with the spine. Make sure the patient's uppermost leg does not rest on the lower leg	To avoid pressure ulcers
	• Consult with physiotherapist and anesthetist about positioning and exercise to enhance pulmonary function	To effort optimal respiratory function and gaseous exchange.
	• Institute passive physiotherapy exercises and observe, color temperature and pulse of limbs	To prevent deep vein thrombosis formation To recognize early signs of limb deformity
	• Apply antiembolism stockings as ordered	To aid venous return to the heart
7.	• Remove all dental prostheses and note caps, loose teeth, bleeding gums, etc. • Clean patient's nostrils • Insert an airway (either oral or nasal) as appropriate	To obtain and maintain clear airway
8.	Perform neurological assessment as physician order or patient's condition dictates	To note changes in condition and action changes as appropriate
9.	Strict asepsis must be maintained when carrying out procedures involving puncture site of cannula or sterile ends of intravenous infusion sets	To prevent local or systemic infections
10.	Maintain feeding regime by nasogastric tube, if the condition permits	To maintain metabolic stasis. To prevent weight loss
11.	Call the patient by his/her name. Introduce yourself, explain each procedure before starting and tell the patient date and time, etc.	Hearing often remains intact in unconscious patient. To prevent sensory deprivation
12.	Touch the patient gently and describe boundaries and environment, e.g., place patient's hand on the bedside, blankets, locker and explain what each item is, and describe the room also	Through touch, individuals establish (and maintain) their body boundaries and relationships with others and their environment. Being denied opportunities to touch can impair physiological, psychological and social development

Contd...

Contd...

S. No.	Nursing action	Rationale
13.	Give the patient daily bath (as per the order)	To maintain the hygiene
14.	Carry out eye care. The eye may be cleansed with cotton balls moistened with sterile normal saline to remove debris and discharge	The blink reflex is absent during unconsciousness (or the patient's eyes may be open all the time). This may lead to corneal drying, irritation and ulceration
15.	Carry out mouth care. Inspect for dryness, infection and presence of crusting. Apply thin coating of petroleum on the lips	To maintain clean moist mouth, to prevent the accumulation of oral and postnasal secretions and infection. Petroleum protects the lips from drying and cracking
16.	Observe the patient for signs of bladder distention. If nursing measures fails to empty the bladder, catheterization to be performed as per order. Perform catheter care regularly	• To prevent urinary complications such as infection and rupture bladder • To avoid ascending infection
17.	Carry out bowel care. Inspect for bowel sounds and any distention.	To early detection and treatment of complications (e.g., paralytic ileum), and to prevent constipation
18.	Change the patient's position every two hours or as directed	To relieve pressure areas. To prevent respiratory complications by allowing postural drainage and to equalize the compression to both sides of the chest and to aid in free expansion
19.	Keep relatives and friends informed of changes in the patient's condition and involve them in care	To help family and friends adjust to the situation and to facilitate anticipatory grief (Pension, 1988)

Table 6.13: Nursing care plan.

S. No.	Problem	Causes	Suggested action
1.	Restlessness or confusion	A degree of restlessness may indicate that the patient is regaining consciousness During this time, there may be a clouding of consciousness with confusion, aggression, uncooperative behavior and disorientation.	Try to rectify the cause for discomfort, wherever possible. Try to get help to control the patient whenever he becomes violent and aggressive.
		Restlessness may also indicate brain damage, cerebral anoxia (when there is a partially obstructed airway), and discomfort or pain with full bladder	Ensure the safety of the patient to protect him from inflicting self-injury
2.	Seizures	An unconscious patient is potential candidate for seizures	Maintain a clear airway. Protect the patient from self-injury. Observe the patient during the seizure and record observations on the chart. Administer prescribed drugs
3.	Cerebrospinal fluid leakage through nose or ears	• Head Trauma • Tumor at the skull base • Abnormalities of the skull base or inner ear	Place sterile swab against nose and ears to collect fluid and test fluid for sugar. If it is positive, then it is proved that the leakage is CSF fluid. Inform medical staff immediately
4.	Vomiting	Unconscious patient is prone to paralytic ileus, or regurgitation of stomach contents due to indigestion	Maintain a clear airway. Keep stomach empty until problem resolves
5.	Distended bladder	See procedure for urinary bladder catheterization	
6.	Inability to maintain own nutritional intake	See procedure— nasogastric intubations	

Contd...

Special Considerations

❖ Padded side rails are provided and raised at all times.
❖ Physical restrains should be avoided if possible.
❖ Fluids are never given by mouth to the patient who cannot swallow.
❖ The patient is assessed for hydration status. Mucous membranes are examined and the skin is assessed for tissue turgor.
❖ Correct body position to be maintained to prevent contractures and pressure sores.
❖ Use of foot board and splints, aids in prevention of foot drops.

CARE OF THE PATIENT IN TRACTION

Definition

- **Traction:** Traction is the application of a pulling force to a part of the body.
- **Counter traction:** The force pulling in the opposite direction is called the counter traction. This is used to balance the force of pulling.

Purposes of Traction

- To maintain muscle spasms and to relieve pain
- To reduce, align and immobilize fractures
- To correct dislocations
- To correct, lessen or prevent deformity

Classification of Traction

1. **Skin traction:** Using patients' body weight as counter traction. Application of a pulling force to the skin and soft tissues by means of adhesive plaster and bandages.
2. **Skeletal traction:** Application of a pulling force directly to the bone by the use of a metal pin or wire, e.g., Steinmann pin, Kirschner wire. It is used in the treatment of fracture of the femur, the humerus, the tibia and the cervical spine.

Both skin and skeletal traction can be:

- **Fixed traction:** This is pulling force between two fixed pints.
- **Balance traction:** In this, the metal weights are used as the traction and the patients' body weight as the counter traction.

Principles of Effective Traction and the Role of the Nurse

- Counter traction must be maintained. This principle should be observed by the nurse for effective traction
- Traction must be continuous

So the nurse should:
 i. Never interrupt skeletal traction
 ii. Not remove the weight unless the traction is prescribed intermittently
 iii. Maintain the line of pull

To achieve this, the nurse should:
Be sure that the patient is centered in bed in good body alignment when traction is applied.

Observe that the:
a. Weights hang free and not rest on the bed or floor
b. Ropes should be unobstructed in straight alignment
c. Knots in the rope should not touch the pulley or the foot of the bed.

Skin Traction (Tables 6.14 and 6.15)

Definition

Traction is a process whereby a force is exerted on a part or parts of the body as a method of treatment. When traction is applied to a limb the necessary counter traction which is a force exerted in the opposite direction of the traction should be maintained.

Table 6.14: Process of skin traction.

S. No.	Nursing action	Rationale
1.	Check the physician's order, progress notes and nursing care plan	To obtain specific instructions and/or information
2.	Explain the procedure to patient and check	To allay fears and obtain patient's confidence and cooperation
3.	Ensure privacy	To avoid unnecessary embarrassment to the patient during the procedure
4.	Wash and dry hands	To prevent cross-contamination
5.	Place the protective sheet under the affected limb	To protect the bed from soiling
6.	Expose the affected limb. Check if the skin is clean and intact	Any abrasion on the skin must be cleaned and covered to prevent infection
7.	Assess the neurovascular status of the limb	To make a baseline record for later comparison
8.	Shave and clean both sides of the limb	To ensure that the adhesive sticks to the skin not to the hair to prevent hair being pulled when traction is removed
9.	Apply tincture benzoin compound to the shoved area of the limb	To reduce moisture through perspiration. To increase the adhesive quality of the material used. To act as a barrier to adhesive in the event of the patient developing contact dermatitis
10.	The patient's foot should be held firmly in dorsiflexion by one nurse. Leave the knee 10–15 off full flexion	To ensure that the correct anatomical alignment of the limb is maintained. To prevent limb deformity, foot drop, and joint stiffness
11.	The second nurse unrolls the extension plaster, measures correct length and cuts at the level of upper third of thigh	
12.	Hold firmly the spreader with foam padding inward at a distance of 2 inches from the sole	To allow full dorsi and plantar flexion of the ankle. To prevent the development of pressure sores from friction
13.	Carefully pull of the protective covering at the same time smoothing the adhesive surface of the extension plaster firmly up to the limb. In the same way apply the other length of the extension plaster to the opposite side of the limb	To ensure extension plaster sticks to the skin firmly. To prevent discomfort and skin deterioration under the skin from fold; and creases of the plaster

Contd...

Contd...

S. No.	Nursing action	Rationale
14.	Apply elastocrepe bandage from just above the malleoli to thigh just below the knee. Apply second elastocrepe just above knee to thigh	To ensure extension plaster firmly to the skin, allow for free movement of limb and ovoid pressure on the common perennial and subsequent foot drop
15.	Place the pillow underneath the whole length of the limb (Do not place under the calf only as this could increase the risk of deep vein thrombosis)	To provide comfort and prevent complication
16.	Elevate the foot of the bed (Use bed elevator, if required) to prevent patient toward the foot end of the bed	To achieve counter-traction
17.	Run the cord over the pulley system and correct it to the weight as ordered by the doctor	
18.	Make the patient to be comfortable and clear away the equipment	
19.	Clean and dispose of equipment	
20.	Wash and dry hands	
21.	Evaluate and document procedure	

Table 6.15: Follow-up care.

S. No.	Nursing action	Rationale
1.	Check neurovascular status of the limb at regular intervals	To identify any neurovascular complication
2.	Remove the elastocrepe bandage daily prior to bed bath and reapply	To check the skin for rashes, sores excoriation, etc.
3.	Encourage active exercise to the joints and muscles, e.g., ankle, toes and quadriceps muscles	To prevent muscle wasting and joint stiffness
4.	Ensure pulley system runs freely and weights are securely attached to the cord and hang freely	To ensure the desired effect

Purposes

- To relieve pain and/or muscle spasm
- To restore and maintain correct anatomical alignment of a limb or a bone following a fracture
- To ensure rest for a limb or part of the skeletal system that may be diseased or broken
- To reduce dislocation of joints
- To correct deformity
- To immobilize a fractured limb as a preoperative measure prior to internal fixation.

Equipment

Adhesive type
- Clean trolley
- Disposable razor
- Protective sheet
- Gauze swabs
- Forceps
- Tincture benzoic compound
- Skin traction kit
- Extension plaster
- Elastocrepe bandage
- Spreader
- Soft foam lining
- Traction cords
- Pillow
- Bed elevator if required
- Pulley system and weight as ordered by doctor.

Procedure

Two nurses may be required to carry out this procedure.

General Nursing Care of the Patient with Traction

- Shave the leg or arm before applying the traction
- Observe for record and report
  - **Circulation:** Skin color, joint mobility, numbers, coldness or swelling of the extremity. Avoid pressure in the popliteal space.
  - **Skin condition:** Check areas over heel, dorsum of the foot and sacral area for pressure sores.
  - **Body alignment:** Observe for body alignment and position for the extremity whether traction being maintained.
  - **Counter traction:** Whether or not balanced traction is achieved.
  - **Position of bandages:** Check for the position of bandages, pins, cards supporting pads and slings.
  - **Supporting pads and slings:** Are they correctly positioned?
  - **Prevention of deformity:** Whether measures are taken to prevent foot drop or hip flexion in the sitting position.
  - **Complications:** Observe for hypostatic pneumonia
- Avoid using a pillow under the extremity in traction unless specifically ordered by the physician
- Inspect pulleys and ropes daily (the ropes can slip out of their grooves)
- Report to physician if the foot piece is touching the floor
- Follow the physician's order for the exact amount of weight to be used
- Be sure that weights are hanging freely
- Maintain the patient's body alignment
- Keep the patient clean and comfortable
- Assist the patient in feeding and elimination

- ❖ Treat pressure areas daily to prevent pressure sores
- ❖ Encourage deep breathing and coughing to prevent hypostatic pneumonia
- ❖ Provide diversional activities (therapy) to relieve boredom
- ❖ Physiotherapy:
  - ◆ Give exercises (according to doctor's orders) to the joints and muscles to prevent joint stiffness and muscle wasting
  - ◆ Use sand bags and foot board to support the foot
  - ◆ Encourage the patient to exercise the feet periodically to prevent foot drop.

Special Nursing Care of the Patient with Different Types of Traction

Fixed Traction

The ring of the splint can cause pressure sores. So the nurse should:
a. Provide pressure area care to the skin beneath the ring every 2 hours
b. Place the patient in an upright position
c. Teach the patient to ease the tissue gently under the ring to a different position every hour if he feels discomfort.

Balanced Traction

The nurse should:
a. Nurse the patient in supine position
b. Raise the foot of the bed to create counter traction
c. Allow the cords connected to the traction to run freely over the pulley to reduce friction
d. Avoid extra use of pillows as this increases friction and reduces traction
e. Maintain body alignment at all times
f. Keep the weight to hang freely
g. Avoid the patient to slip toward the head or foot of the bed
h. Teach the patient to move himself up the bed as and when required.

Skin Traction

The nurse should:
a. Make sure that the bandage should not be too tight or too loose
b. Check the extension plaster is in place. If not reapply again
c. Observe for record and report:
   i. Allergy to extension plaster such as redness, rash, pain and irritation
   ii. Altered sensation
   iii. Peripheral pulse, color and temperature of fingers or toes
   iv. Tenderness in the calf muscle (indicate thrombophlebitis).
d. Special back care every 2 hours to prevent pressure sores
e. Encourage active, hourly foot exercises
f. Maintain proper positioning and counter traction.

Skeletal Traction

Infection may develop in and around the pin site. So, the nurse should:
a. Clean and dress the pin site daily
b. Observe for signs of infection
c. Follow strict surgical aseptic precautions to prevent infection.

Care of Patient in a Cast

Definition

A cast is a rigid external immobilizing device that is molded to the part of the body to which it is applied. Cast application is a process of applying plaster of Paris to a body part for immobilization, or to align malpositioned tissues such as club foot, congenital hip dislocation, etc.

Purposes

- ❖ To immobilize a body part in a specific position
- ❖ To immobilize a reduced fracture
- ❖ To correct a deformity
- ❖ To apply uniform pressure to underlying soft tissue
- ❖ To provide support and stability for weakened joints
- ❖ To support and rest a part after surgical intervention until healing occurs.

Types of Casts

The condition being treated influences the type and thickness of the cast applied:
- ❖ Short arm cast—extends from below the elbow to the palmar crease
- ❖ Long arm cast—extends from the upper level of the axillary fold to the proximal palmar
- ❖ Short leg cast—extends from below the knee to the base of the toes
- ❖ Long leg cast—extends from the junction of the upper and middle third of the thigh to the base of the toes
- ❖ Body cast—encircles the trunk
- ❖ Spica cast—incorporates a portion of the trunk and one or two extremities
- ❖ Shoulder spica cast—a body jacket encloses the trunk, shoulder and the elbow.
- ❖ Minerva cast—applied around the neck and trunk of the body.

CARE OF PATIENT WITH PAIN

Pain disables and distresses more people than any single disease entity. It is probably the most common reason for a person to seek health care. Most medical-surgical problems are associated with pain, resulting either from:
1. Disease process
2. Diagnostic tests
3. Treatment modalities

Pain has **three components:**
1. A **stimulus,** physical or mental.
2. A **bodily sensation** of hurting.
3. The **reaction** of the person experiencing it.

The nurse spends more time with the patient with pain than any other members of the healthcare team and therefore the nurse has the opportunity to make a significant contribution toward increasing the patient's comfort and relieving pain.

Definition

Pain is a subjective, unpleasant, and emotional experience associated with actual or potential tissue damage. Pain is whatever the patient says it is, existing whenever the patient says it does.

Types of Pain

Acute Pain

Acute pain is a very common occurrence. It indicates that some degree of damage has occurred within the body that requires some form of treatment or intervention. Healing may also be accompanied by acute pain. As healing progresses, the pain subsides and gradually disappears. Acute pain is accompanied by muscle tension and anxiety (**Table 6.16**).

Chronic Pain

Chronic pain is sometimes defined as pain lasts for 6 months for or longer. An episode of pain may assume the characteristics of chronic pain long before 6 months have elapsed, or some types of pain may remain primarily acute in nature for longer than 6 months. Nevertheless, after 6 months the majority of pain experiences are accompanied by problems associated with chronic pain.

Table 6.16: Comparison of acute and chronic pain.

Acute pain	Chronic pain
Mild to severe	Mild to severe
• Sympathetic nervous	• Parasympathetic
• System responses:	• Nervous system responses:
➤ Increased pulse rate	➤ Vital signs normal
➤ Increased respiratory rate	➤ Dry, warm skin
➤ Elevated blood pressure	➤ Pupils normal or dilated
➤ Diaphoresis	➤ Continues beyond healing
➤ Dilated pupils	➤ Client appears
• Related to tissue injury:	➤ Depressed and withdrawn
➤ Resolves with healing	➤ Client often does not mention pain unless asked
➤ Client appears restless and anxious	➤ Pain behavior often absent
➤ Client reports pain	
➤ Client exhibits behavior	
• Indicative of pain:	
➤ Crying	
➤ Rubbing area	
➤ Holding area	

Referred Pain

Referred pain is felt in areas other than those stimulated. It may occur when stimulation is not perceived in the primary areas. For example, the person having a heart attack may complain only of pain radiating down the left arm when in fact, the tissue damage is occurring in the myocardium.

Referred pain occurs most often with damage or injury to visceral organs, and the pain is referred to coetaneous surfaces.

Psychogenic Pain

The term "psychogenic" has been used to describe pain where no physical pathology has been found or where the pain appears to have a greater psychology basis than a physical one. A caution here is that diagnostic tests are not definitive measures and may not be sophisticated enough to detect path physiologic chances. Distinguishing between physical and emotional components of pain is difficult and it is important to remember that all pain is real.

Clinical Manifestations of Pain

The patient's responses to the pain may be any one or a combination of possible reactions. These may include:
1. Physiologic manifestations
2. Verbal statements
3. Vocal behaviors
4. Facial expressions
5. Body movements
6. Physical contact with others
7. Alterations in response to the environment
8. Adaption of physiological and behavioral response

These behaviors vary greatly from one person to another and may differ within the same person from one time to the next.

The objective signs of pains are described in **Table 6.17** and factors that influence responses to pain are given in **Box 6.1**.

Table 6.17: Objective signs of acute pain.

Physiologic signs	Behavioral signs
Pulse: Increased rate	Rigid body position
Respirations: Increased depth and frequency	Restlessness
Blood pressure: Increased systolic and diastolic	Frowning
Diaphoresis, Pallor	Clenched teeth
Dilated pupils	Clenched fists
Muscle tension: Face, body	Crying
Nausea and vomiting: If pain is severe	Moaning

Guidelines for the Assessment of the Patient with Pain

Assess the characteristics of the patient's pain:
a. Severity of pain
b. Quality, location, duration, and rhythm city of pain
c. Tolerance for pain
d. Harmful effects of pain on patient's recovery
e. Strategies that patient believe will help relieve pain
f. Concerns that patient has about his pain

> **Box 6.1:** Factors that influence responses to pain.
>
> - Meaning of pain to individual person
> - Degree of pain perception
> - Past experience
> - Cultural values
> - Social expectations
> - Physical and mental health
> - Parental attitudes toward pain
> - Setting in which pain occurs
> - Fear, anxiety
> - Usual way of responding to stressors
> - Age
> - Preparation for pain context
> - Health professional responses

Assess the patient's behavioral responses to the pain experience:
a. Determine if the pain is acute or chronic
b. Observe for the following behavioral responses:
  1. Physiologic manifestations (change in pulse, blood pressure, respiratory rate, etc.)
      i. Verbal statements
      ii. Vocal responses
      iii. Facial expressions
      iv. Body movements
      v. Alteration in response to the environment
      vi. Physical contact with others
      vii. Adaptation of physiological and behavioral responses
      viii. Effect of pain on ability to communicate and carry out usual activities of daily living.
  2. Assess factors that influence responses to pain:
      i. Ethnic and cultural factors
      ii. Previous pain experience
      iii. Patient's responses to pain relief strategies

Nursing Diagnosis for the Patient with Pain

Acute pain related to psychological distress. When writing the diagnostic statement, the nurse may further specify the type or location of the pain (e.g., postoperative, chest, abdominal, back). Etiologic factors, when known, must be part of the diagnostic statement.

Because the pain experience affects so many facets of human functioning, pain itself may be the etiology of other nursing diagnoses. Examples of such nursing diagnoses are also discussed here.

- Ineffective airway clearance related to postoperative incisional chest pain.
- Anxiety related to past experience of poor control of pain and to anticipation of pain.
- Ineffective breathing pattern related to postoperative abdominal pain.
- Ineffective individual coping related to prolonged continuous back pain, ineffective pain management, and inadequate support systems.
- Fear related to anticipated pain after surgery. Health maintenance related to chronic pain and fatigue.
- Hopelessness related to ineffective pain management strategies.
- Knowledge deficit (pain control measures) related to lack of exposure to information resources.
- Impaired physical mobility related to arthritic pain in knee and ankle joints.
- **Self-care deficit:** Bathing/hygiene, dressing/grooming, toileting related to pain in the joints.
- Sleep pattern disturbance related to increased pain perception at night.

PLANNING

The nurse identifies nursing interventions that will assist the client in achieving the overall client goals of preventing, modifying, or eliminating pain so that the clients able partially or completely to resume usual daily activities and be able to cope more effectively with the pain experience.

When planning, nurses need to choose pain relief measures appropriate for the client. Nursing inventions may include a variety of pharmacologic and non-pharmacologic interventions.

Implementation

Pain management is the alleviation of pain or a reduction in pain to a level of comfort that is acceptable to the client. It includes two basic types of nursing interventions:
1. Pharmacologic
2. Nonpharmacologic interventions

Generally speaking, a combination of strategies available for the client in pain. Sometimes strategies need to be tried and changed until the client obtains effective pain relief.

General Strategies for Pain Management

1. Assess patient's pain status based on patients past experience.
2. Incorporate the following factors in the assessment of patient's pain status:
   - Locality/characteristics
   - Onset
   - Frequency
   - Intensity
   - Quality
   - Precipitating factors
   - Effective pain control measures
   - Pain expression style (verbal, crying, moaning)
   - Impact on quality of life
   - Effect of pain on daily activities
   - Effect on sleep/wake pattern
   - Effect on energy level
3. Apply previous strategies that have controlled pain.

4. Explore strategies that have been successful in the past.
5. Assess patient's willingness to incorporate no pharmaceutical pain control measures.
6. Administer medication as per physician's orders.
7. Immobilize or rest affected area.
8. Relieve pressure areas with turning or pressure reduction devices such as air-fluidized support systems.
9. Suggest and instruct patient in relaxation techniques: short simple techniques with
10. Encourage patient's attention to proper posture and alignment.
11. Provide therapeutic positioning.
12. Rest affected area.
13. Provide distraction.
14. Use hypnotic strategies as prescribed.
15. Provide music therapy.
16. Use counter stimulation: Pressure, massage, vibration, heat/cold, external analgesics, and transcutaneous nerve stimulation.
17. Provide a supportive environment.
18. Help patient identify activities that may enhance pain.
19. Discuss strategies to reduce enhancement of pain.
20. Discuss strategies to avoid these activities within patient's lifestyle.
21. Provide touch, especially for infants or for disoriented or unresponsive patients.

Evaluation

Example of evaluative statements indicating goal achievements are given here:

Evaluative statements indicating goal achievements:
1. Reports lower intensity of pain.
2. Accepts pain medications as prescribed.
3. Exhibits decreased physical and behavioral signs of pain and discomfort.
4. Identifies effective pain relief strategies.

CARE OF PATIENTS WITH BODY ELIMINATION DEVIATION

Common Alterations in Urinary Elimination

Altered Urine Production

Polyuria

Polyuria or diuresis refers to the production of abnormally large amounts of urine by the kidneys, about 2500 mL or more/day. Polyuria can be the result of (a) excessive fluid intake, (b) ingestion of substances containing caffeine and alcohol; and also in diabetes mellitus, hormone imbalances, [e.g., deficiency of antidiuretic hormone (ADH)] or in chronic kidney disease.

Oliguria

It refers to voiding scanty amount of urine such as 100–500 mL/day. Oliguria may result from—(a) extremely low fluid intake, (b) excessive fluid loss, e.g., burns, diarrhea, etc., (c) renal failure. Oliguria may also accompany fever and heavy perspiration.

Anuria

It refers to voiding <100 mL/day. The terms complete kidney shutdown. Renal failure and urinary suppression have the same meaning. Anuria can result from (a) kidney diseases, (b) severe heart disease, (c) burns and (d) shock.

Altered Voiding Pattern

Frequency

It refers to voiding at frequent intervals, that is, more often than usual. Normally with an increased intake of fluid there is some increase in the frequency with which a person voids. Frequency without an increase in fluid intake may be the result of—(a) cystitis, (b) stress, (c) pressure on the bladder, e.g., in pregnancy. In frequency, the total amount of urine voided may be normal. This is because the amount of urine voided each time is usually about 50–100 mL only.

Nocturia: It is an increased frequency at night that is not the result of an increase in fluid intake. It is expressed in terms of the number of times the person gets out of bed to void. For example, "Nocturia × 4".

Urgency

Urgency is the feeling of urge to void at once. There may or may not be a great deal of urine in the bladder, but the person feels a need to void immediately. Often the person hurries to the toilet with the fear of being incontinent. Urgency accompanies psychological stress and irritation of the trigone and urethra.

Dysuria

It means voiding that is either painful or difficult. It can be caused by: (a) stricture of the urethra, (b) urinary infection, (c) injury to the bladder or urethra.

Enuresis

It is defined as repeated involuntary urination in children beyond 4 or 5 years of age, when voluntary bladder control is normally acquired. Enuresis can be nocturnal (night time) and diurnal (day time) or both.

Hesitancy

It is defined as delay or difficulty in initiating voiding. It may be due to:
1. Urethral stricture
2. Prostatic enlargement
3. Surgical procedures in perinea area
4. Post catheterization
5. Cystitis/Urethritis

Urinary incontinence

It is inability to control the passage of urine. Incontinence is a symptom, not a disease. Incontinence may be caused by stress, neurological impairment, injury to urethral sphincter and physical mobility.

Urinary retention

Urinary retention is the accumulation of urine in the bladder associated with inability of the bladder to empty itself. Because urine production continues, retention distends the bladder. An adult urinary bladder normally holds 250–450 mL of urine when the urination reflex is triggered. With urinary retention, some adult bladders may distend to hold 3,000 mL of urine. Prolonged retention leads to stasis (a slowing of the flow of urine) and stagnation of urine, which increases the possibility of urinary tract infection. Distention also causes reduce blood flow to the bladder, making it less resistant to invading gram positive organisms and thereby increases the chances of urinary tract infections.

Retention may occur due to several factors:
1. After surgical procedures on perineal and anal regions.
2. Prostatic enlargement and urethral strictures.
3. Acute illness or chronic bed ridden state.
4. Anxiety and aging process.
5. Drugs such as atropine, phenothiazines, actifed and propranolol.

Facilitating Urine Elimination: Assessment, Types, Equipment, Procedures, and Special Considerations

Assessing Urinary Elimination

Assessment of urinary elimination includes: (a) taking a nursing history, (b) performing a physical examination of the kidneys, bladder, urethral meats, skin integrity and hydration, (c) examination of the urine. The nurse should also (d) review any data obtained relevant diagnostic tests and procedures.

Nursing History

The nurse determines the client's normal voiding pattern and amount, frequency, appearance of the urine and to any recent changes, any past or current problems with urination, the presence of an ostomy, and factors influencing the elimination pattern.

Examples of interview questions to elicit this information are given here. The number of questions asked depends on the individual and the responses to the first three categories.

Examples of interview questions
Voiding pattern
- How many times do you void during a 24-hour period?
- Has this pattern changed recently?
- Do you need to get out of bed to violating in night? How often

Description of urine and any changes
- How would you describe your urine in terms of color, clarity (clear, transparent, or cloudy), and odor (faint or strong)?
- Have you had or do you now have with passing your urine passage of large amounts of urine problems
- What are the problems of urine elimination?

Passage of small amounts of urine voiding at more frequent intervals. **Trouble getting to the bath room in time or feeling of urgency to void or painful voiding. Difficulty in starting urine stream: Frequented robbing of urine or feeling of bladder fullness associated within small amount to urine.**

Reduced force of stream and accidental leakage of urine: If so, when does this occur (e.g., when coughing, laughing, or sneezing; at night; during the day). Past urinary tract illness such as urinary tract infection of the kidney, bladder or urethra; urinary calculi; urinary tract surgery of kidney, ureters or bladder.

Presence and management of urinary diversion/ostomy
- What is your usual routine with your ostomy?
- What problems, if any do you have with it?
- How can the nurse help you manage it?

Factors Influencing Urinary Elimination

- **Medications:** Have you taken any medications that could increase urinary output (e.g., diuretic) or cause retention of urine (e.g., anticholinergic – antispasmodic, antidepressant, and antihistamines, antihypertensive)? Note specific medication and dosage.
- **Fluid intake:** What amount and kind of fluid do you take each day (e.g., 6 glasses of water, 5 cups of coffee, 3 cola drinks with or without caffeine)?
- **Environmental factors:** Do you have any problem with toileting (mobility, toilet seat tool low, facility without grab bar)?
- **Presence of long-term catheter:** How do you care for your catheter? Do you have any discomfort with it or other problems? How can the nurse help you manage it?
- **Stress:** Are you experiencing any long-term or short-term stress? If so, what are the stressors?
- **Disease:** Have you had or do you have any illnesses other than urinary tract disease that may affect urinary function, such as hypertension, heart disease, neurologic disease (e.g., multiple sclerosis), cancer, prostatic enlargement, diabetes mellitus, or diabetes insipidus?
- **Diagnostic procedures:** Have you recently had a cystoscopy or spinal anesthesia?

Physical Examination

Complete physical assessment of the urinary tract usually includes percussion of the kidneys to detect areas of tenderness and palpation for contour, size tenderness, and lumps. During examination of the genitals, the urethral meatus of both male and female clients is inspected for swelling, discharge, and inflammation. Because problems with urination can affect the elimination of wastes from the body, it is important for the nurses to assess the skin for color, texture, and tissue turgor as well as the presence of any waste products (e.g., crystals on the skin). In addition, the skin of the perineum should be inspected for irritation because contact with urine can excoriate the skin. This is particularly evident in the incontinent client.

Examination of Urine

Normal urine consists of 96% water and 4% solutes. Organic solutes include urea, ammonia, creatinine, and uric acid. Urea is the chief organic solute. Inorganic solutes include sodium, chloride, potassium sulfate, magnesium and phosphorus. Sodium chloride is the most abundant inorganic salt. Assessment of urine involves measuring the volume of urine; comparing the output of the client's intake; inspecting the urine for color, clarity, and odor; testing urine for specific gravity, glucose, ketones bodies, blood and pH; and reviewing of data obtained from diagnostic tests. The **Table 6.18** summarizes the characteristics of normal and abnormal urine and possible causes.

Maintaining Normal Voiding Habits

Positioning

❖ Assist the client to a normal position for voiding—standing for males, for females, squatting or leaning slightly forward

Table 6.18: Characteristics of normal and abnormal feces.

Characteristics	Normal	Abnormal	Possible cause
Color	Adult: Brown	Clay or White	Absence of bile (infant): Yellow pigment (bile obstruction): Diagnostic study using barium
		Greenish/Black	Drug (e.g., iron) bleeding from upper gastrointestinal tract (e.g., stomach, small intestines): diet high in red meat and dark green vegetables (Spinach)
		Red	Bleeding from lower gastrointestinal tract (e.g., rectum), some food (e.g., beetroots)
		Pale	Malabsorption of fats. Diet high in milk products and low in meat
		Orange/Green	Intestinal infection
Consistency Laxative abuse	Formed, soft, semisolid, moist	Hard, dry, constipated stool fiber in diet, lack of exercise,	Dehydration Decreased intestinal motility resulting from lack of emotional upset
		Diarrhea	Increased intestinal motility (e.g., irritation of the colon by bacteria)
		Rice water stools	Characteristics of cholera
		Pea-soup stools	Characteristics of typhoid
Shape	Cylindrical (contour of rectum) about 2.5 cm (1 inch) in diameter in adults	Narrow, pencil shaped or string like stool	Obstructive condition of the rectum
		Sheep droppings	Spastic colon little hard knob by bits of feces passes through spastic colon
Amount	Varies with diet (about 100 to 400 g per day)	Ribbon-like Grooved shape	Presence of growth in the colon Show definite growth in the colon wall
Odor	Aromatic, affected by undigested food and person's own bacterial flora	Pungent Sour smell	Infection, blood, digestive disorder
Constituents	Small amounts undigested roughage sloughed dead bacteria and epithelial cells fat; protein; dried constituents of digestive juice (e.g., bile pigment in organic matter (e.g., calcium, phosphates)	Pus, Mucus, Parasites, Blood, Large quantities of fat, Foreign objects, Worms	Bacterial infection, inflammatory condition gastrointestinal bleeding Malabsorption, Accidental ingestion Intestinal Worms, e.g., Pinworm, Roundworm, Hookworm, Tapeworm Ameba
Urge	Normal urge	Urgency Pain tenesmus Urge to evacuate the bowel without result	Diarrhea Dysentery

when sitting. These positions enhance movement of urine through the tract by gravity.

- Use bedside commodes as necessary for females and urinals for males standing at the bedside.
- Encourage the client to push over the pubic area with the hands or lean forward to increase intra-abdominal pressure and external pressure on the bladder. Elevate the head of the client's bed to Fowler's position, place a small pillow or rolled towel at the back to increase physical support and comfort, and have the client flex the hips and knees. This position stimulates the normal voiding position as closely as possible.

Relaxation

- Provide privacy for the client. Many people cannot void in the presence of another person.
- Allow the client sufficient time to void.
- Suggest the client to read or listen to music.
- Provide sensory stimuli that may help the client relax. Pour warm water over the perineum of a female or have the client sit in a warm bath to promote muscle relaxation. Applying of hot-water bottle to the lower abdomen of both men and women may also faster muscle relaxation.
- Turn on running water within hearing distance of the client to mask the sound of voiding for persons who find this embarrassing.

Most interventions to maintain normal urinary elimination are independent nursing functions. These include:
1. Promoting fluid intake
2. Maintaining normal voiding habits
3. Strengthening muscle tone
4. Assisting with toileting

Promoting fluid intake

- Increasing fluid intake increases urine production, which in turn stimulates the urination reflex. A normal, average daily intake of 1,200–1,500 mL of measurable fluids is adequate for most clients.
- Additional amounts are required for clients whose fluid demands are great, such as those who have abnormal fluid losses other routes (e.g., excessive perspiration, vomiting, diarrhea, wound drainage and burns).
- Immobilized clients who are susceptible to calculi (kidney stone) formatting require daily intakes of 2,000–3,000 mL/day (unless medically contraindicated). Dilute urine helps prevent urinary tract stones and infection.
- Fluid intake can also be increased by encouraging the client to eat plenty of raw fruits and vegetables, which have high water content.
- Increased fluid intake as contraindicated in clients who require fluid restrictions, such as those with renal impairment or congestive heart failure.

Alteration in Bowel Elimination

There are five common problems of fecal elimination:
1. Constipation
2. Fecal impaction
3. Diarrhea
4. Fecal incontinence
5. Flatulence

Constipation

Constipation refers to the passage of small, dry hard stool or the passage of no stool for a period of time. Constipation occurs when the movement of feces through the large intestine is slow, thus allowing time for additional reabsorption of fluid from the large intestine. Constipation is often accompanied by abdominal distension and discomfort, nausea, headache and diminished appetite.

Causes

- Age
- Irregular defecation habits
- Inappropriate diet
- Insufficient fluid
- Insufficient exercise
- Increased psychological stress
- Disease process: Refer to the explanation under factors affecting bowel elimination

Fecal Impaction

Fecal impaction is a mass or collection of hardened feces in the folds of the rectum.

Causes

- Prolonged retention and accumulation of fecal material
- Poor defecation habits and constipation
- Medications
- Barium used for diagnostic purposes
- Poor fluid intake, insufficient bulk in the diet, lack of activity, weak muscles.

In severe cases, the feces accumulate and extend up into the sigmoid colon and beyond.

Symptoms

- Passage of liquid fecal seepage and no normal stool.
- Liquid portion of the feces seeps out around the impacted mass. Generalized feeling of illness, anorexia, distended abdomen, nausea and vomiting.
- Hardened mass can be palpated by digital examination of the rectum.

Diarrhea

Diarrhea refers to the passage of liquid/feces and an increased frequency of defecation or it is discharge of frequent loose stool to the rapid passages of content through the intestines.

Causes

Rapid passage of chyme reduces the time available for the large intestine to reabsorb water and electrolytes. Diarrhea is a symptom of various conditions that include:

- Irritation of inflammation of the gastrointestinal tract, due to pathogenic causes.
- Infection, highly spiced foods, or medications that increase intestinal motility.
- Disorders of digestion or absorption.
- Disorders that affect secretion and utilization of bile or pancreatic juice, obstructive jaundice.
- Emotional stress such as anxiety or stress.

Symptoms

- Increased frequency, uniformed and excessive liquid stools
- Unable to control the urge to defecate
- At times, piercing abdominal cramps associated with diarrhea
- Stools with mucous and blood at times
- Nausea and vomiting
- If diarrhea persists, irritation of the anal region
- Fluid electrolyte loss leading to fatigue, weakness, malaise.

Fecal Incontinence

Fecal incontinence refers to loss of voluntary ability to control fecal and gaseous discharge through the anal sphincter or inability to control the expulsion of feces.

Fecal incontinence is an emotionally distressing problem that can lead to social isolation. Affected persons withdraw into their homes or, if in the hospital, they confine to their room to minimize the embarrassment associated with soiling. People prefer easily with washable night garments to street cloths. Therefore, the area around the anal region should be kept clean and dry and be protected with zinc oxide or other ointment.

Causes

Incontinence occurs at specific times like after meals or irregular impaired functioning of the anal sphincter. Spinal cord trauma, tumors of the external sphincter muscle.

Flatulence

Flatulence is the presence of excess flatus in the intestines and leads to stretching and inflation of the intestines (intestinal distention). Air or gas in the gastrointestinal tract is called "flatus".

Causes

Large amounts of air gas collection in the interesting resulting in gastric distention. An adult usually form 7 to 10 liters of flatus in the intestines every 24 hours. Some gases are swallowed with food and fluid and others are formed through the action of bacteria on the chyme in the large intestine.

The gases swallowed are expelled through the mouth by eructation (belching). The gases formed in the large intestine are chiefly absorbed, through the intestinal capillaries, into the circulation. Flatulence can occur in the colon, however, from a variety of causes, such as abdominal surgery, anesthetics, or narcotics. If this gas cannot be expelled through the anus, it may be necessary to insert a rectal tube or provide are turn flow enema to remove it.

Other common causes are:

- Constipation
- Drugs that decrease intestinal motility: Codeine or Barbiturates Anxiety
- Consumes gas-forming foods such as beans, cabbage, due to anesthesia, narcotics, reduction inactivity.

Facilitating Bowel Elimination: Equipment and Procedures

Assessment

Assessment interview form-bowel elimination

1. **Defecation pattern:**
    - Frequency _____ Any pain/Tenesmus Time
    - Any change in pattern Yes/ No
2. **Description of feces and any changes:**
    - Color: Clay or White/Greenish/Black or Tarry/Red/Pale/Orange
    - Consistency: Formed/Hard/Soft/Watery
    - Shape: Cylindrical/Narrow/Pencil-shaped/String-like/Sheep droppings/Ribbon-like
    - Odor: Aromatic/Pungent/Sour smell
3. **Problems:** Constipation/Diarrhea/Excessive Flatulence/Seepage or Incontinence
    How often _____
    What causes _____
    Food/Fluid/Emotions/Medications/Disease/Surgery
    What methods did you use for remedy _____
    _____
    Was it useful: Yes/No
4. **Factors influencing elimination:**
    Diet:
    Do you take meals at regular times? Yes/No
    Foods typically eat:
    Foods typically avoid:
    Fluid:
    Amount of fluid: Number of glasses:
    Cups of tea/Coffee:
    Exercise:
    Usual daily exercise pattern: _____
    Medications: Any drugs affecting GI tract (Iron-antibiotics)
    Stress: Long term/Short term stressors
    Use of any elimination aids:
    Routine followed
    Taking natural acids—Lemon juice, water
    Laxatives—Yes/No
    Enemas—Yes/No

5. **Physical examination:**
   Abdomen : Inspection
   : Auscultation
   : Percussion
   : Palpation examination of rectum and anus
6. **Characteristics feces:**
   Inspect the stools : Color
   : Consistency
   : Shape
   : Amount
   : Odor
   : Presence of any abnormal constituents

Role of the Nurse in Bowel Elimination

Assessment of fecal elimination includes taking a nursing history, performing a physical examination of the abdomen, rectum and anus and inspecting the feces.

Nursing History

A nursing history for fecal elimination helps the nurse ascertain the patient's normal pattern. The nurse elicits a description of usual feces on any recent changes and collects information about past or current problems with elimination and factors influencing the elimination pattern.

Physical examination of the abdomen:

- **Inspection**—observe contour, any masses, scars, or distension
- **Auscultation**—listen for bowel sounds in all quadrants
  - Note frequency and character, audible clicks, and flatus
  - Describe bowel sounds as audible, hyperactive, hypoactive, or inaudible
- **Percussion**—expect resonant sound or tympany
  - Areas of increased dullness may be caused by fluid, mass, or tumor
- **Palpation**—note any muscular resistance, tenderness, enlargement of organs, masses.
- **Percussion** is necessary to access the size of liver and nature of an abdominal mass.
- **Physical assessment of the anus and rectum**
  - Inspection and palpation
  - Examine anal area for cracks, nodules, distended veins, masses or polyps, fecal mass
  - Insert gloved finger into anus to assess sphincter tone and smoothness of mucosal lining
  - Inspect perineal area for skin irritation secondary to diarrhea

Inspecting the Feces on the Basis of:

- **Color**—varies from light to dark brown foods and medications may affect color
- **Odor**—aromatic, affected by ingested food and person's bacterial flora
- **Consistency**—formed, soft, semi-solid; moist
- **Frequency**—varies with diet (about 100 to 400 g/day)
- **Constituents**—small amount of undigested roughage, sloughed dead bacteria and epithelial cells, fat, protein, dried constituents of digestive juices (bile pigments); inorganic matter (calcium, phosphates).

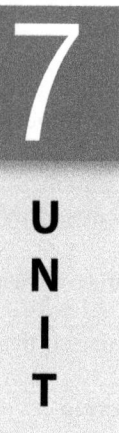

UNIT 7
Introduction to Clinical Pharmacology

LEARNING OBJECTIVES

After completing this unit, learner will be able to

- Administration of medication: Discuss general principles, considerations
  - Purpose of medication
  - Principles: Rights, special considerations, prescriptions, safety in administering medications and medication errors
  - Drugs forms
  - Routes of administration
  - Storage and maintenance of drugs and nurses responsibility
  - Broad classification of drugs
  - Therapeutic effect, side effect, toxic effect, allergic reaction, reaction, drug tolerance, drug interactions
  - Factors influencing drug actions
  - Systems of drug measurement, metric system, house hold measurements
  - Converting measurements units, conversion within one system, between systems, dosage calculations. Terminologies and abbreviations used in prescription of medications
- Explain oral drug administration: Oral, sublingual, buccal, equipment and procedure
- Describe parenteral administration
  - General principles
  - Types of parenteral therapies
  - Types of syringes, needles, cannula and infusion sets
  - Protection from needle stick injuries, giving medications with a safety syringe
  - Routes of parenteral therapies
  - Purposes, site equipment, procedure and special considerations in giving intradermal, subcutaneous, intramuscular and intravenous medications
  - Advanced techniques: Epidural, intrathecal, intraosseous, intraperitoneal, intrapleural, intra-arterial.
  - Roles of the nurse
- Explain topical administration: Purpose, site, equipment, procedure, special considerations for applications to skin and mucous membrane.
- State direct application
  - Gargle, throat swab
  - Insertion of drug into body cavities, nasal pack, suppositories/medicated packing in to rectum/vagina
  - Installations, ear, eye, nasal, bladder and rectal
  - Irrigations: Eye, ear, bladder, vaginal and rectal, spray, nose and throat
- Explain Inhalations
  - Nasal, oral, endotracheal (steam, oxygen, and medications): Purposes, types, equipment, procedure and special considerations
- Recording and reporting of medications administered

ADMINISTRATION OF MEDICATION: GENERAL PRINCIPLES, CONSIDERATIONS, PURPOSE OF MEDICATION

Nurses utilize much more time to administer medication and taking responsibilities. The nurse also ensures clients are adequately prepared to receive medication by following basic general principles, because medication administration and evaluation are essential to nursing practice.

GENERAL PRINCIPLES

1. The nurse administering medication does not have sole responsibilities, but she is accountable for knowing which medications are prescribed, their therapeutic and side effects and related nursing responsibilities
2. Before administering medication, the nurse obtains review of the client medical history
3. She should be familiar with indication
4. She should be able to give education on medication usage
5. Nurse utilize the knowledge learned from many disciplines when administering medication
6. Nurse understand why a particular medication has been prescribed for the patient how this medication will alter the client physiology
7. Administering medication safely to clients some medication administering skills are essential
8. Verify history of allergy
9. Confirm medication order is complete, which includes patient full name, medication name, dosage, route, time and frequency of administration, date of order written, and signature of physician.
10. The nurse accepts full accountability and responsibilities for all action that are taken
11. Nurse should be familiar with dosage, side effects
12. Most of the errors that are made by nurses are medication errors. A medication error is any events that could cause or lead to a client receiving inappropriate medication
13. The nurse is the essential link in the prevention of medication error
14. The type of dosage of medication vary from institute to institute
15. To ensure safe medication administration nurse should be aware of nursing standards.

Nurses play an essential role in medication preparation and administration, teaching and evaluating client responses to medications on clients' health status.

PURPOSE OF MEDICATION

1. Medication is used to prevent, diagnose or treat disease
2. Restore or maintain clients health
3. Medications are the primary treatment for restoration of health
4. Clients with acute or chronic alterations in their health use many modalities of treatment to restore or to maintain their health. A medication is a substance used in diagnosis, treatment, cure, relief or prevention of health alterations. In fact, medications are the primary modality associated with restoration of health. No matter where clients receive their healthcare either hospitals, clinics, or home the nurse plays an essential role in medication administration.
5. Administration of medication: Medication administration is a basic nursing function that involves skillful technique and consideration of patient development, health status and safety. The nurse administering medication needs to have knowledge base about drugs.

Knowledge Base for the Nurses

Medication administration and evaluation are essential to the nursing practice; nurses need to have knowledge about the action and effects of the medications they deliver to the clients. This cannot be done if the nurses do not have an understanding of the life sciences. Moreover to safely and accurately administer medications to the clients, the nurses must have an understanding of the pharmacokinetics (the movement of medications in the human body), growth and development, human anatomy, nutrition, and mathematics. The nurse's previous learning is important and is often applied to medication administration.

DRUG NOMENCLATURE

Drug Names

Medications may have as many as three different names. The chemical name of a medication provides an exact description of the medication's composition and molecular structure. Chemical names are rarely used in clinical practice. The generic name is approved by the manufacturer who first developed the medications. The trade name/brand name is the name under which a manufacturer markets a medication.

Rights of Drug Administration

The *10 rights of drug administration* as described in **Table 7.1**.

Medication Orders and Prescription and Safety in Administering Medications

The nurse does not bear sole responsibility for drug administration. The physician and pharmacist play the key roles in ensuring that the right medication gets to the right client. However, administering medication bears responsibility and accountability for accuracy of the rights.

Table 7.1: 10 rights of drug administration.

1.	**Right drug**	As many drugs have similar form and name, clarify patient receive right drugs, patient diagnosis make sense for the right to have this medication
2.	**Right reason**	As nurses administering medication for many patient and many disease condition, they are familiar with patient symptoms did the patient condition and symptoms give rationale for this medication
3.	**Right dose and route**	Verify right route of medication, read the label of medication this medication for IV, IM, or oral preparation is the correct dose being prepared and administered (check the prescribed dose against the range specified in a reliable reference) and what route medication ordered verify before administration
4.	**Right patient**	Verify the identity of the patient, by checking ID band with clarification from patient and patient chart or ask the patient to state his/her name. Confirm, is this right patient to receive this medication
5.	**Right time**	Depends on frequency of medication administration, administer medication according to due schedule
6.	**Right route**	Is the order is for oral, IM, IV, or other route administer as per route prescribed
7.	**Right education**	Knowledge deficit will arise, before patient receive medication nurse should educate, purpose of this medication, dosage, and duration, side effect if he experiences any side effect immediately report to the ward nurse
8.	**Right documentation**	After administration immediately write the name of the drug, dosage, route in nurse's notes and proper signature with date and time
9.	**Right evaluation**	Monitor the patient after administration, immediately and after 15 minutes if you suspect drug reaction frequently monitor
10.	**Right reporting**	Any untoward incidence after administration report to the concerned

Physician's Role

1. The physician prescribes medications.
2. The physician writes an order on a designated form in the client medical records.
3. Students cannot carry out medication orders.
4. No medication should be given without an order.
5. Common abbreviation is used while writing orders.
6. The abbreviation indicates dosage, frequencies or times, route of administration, and special information for the nurse to follow in giving the drug.

Standing order

A standing order is carried out until the physician cancels it by another order or until a prescribed number of days elapsed.

PRN order

The physician may order a drug on a PRN basis (when a client requires it).

Single (one time) orders

A physician may order a drug to be given only once at a specified time.

State orders

A state order signifies that a single dose of a medication is to be given immediately and only once. Often state orders are written for emergencies when a client condition changes suddenly.

Nurse's Role

The nurse is the most appropriate health care worker to administer medication, spending most of the time with the client. This puts nurses in an ideal position to monitor clients response to medications, provides education to the client and the family about the medication regimen. When medications are effective, ineffective or no longer effective or no longer necessary. Hence, to determine the need for a potential response to drug therapy, the nurse assesses many factors.

Medical history provides indications or contraindications for drug therapy. Disease or illness may place clients at risk for adverse drug effects. For example, if a client has a gastric ulcer or bleeding tendency, compounds containing aspirin or anticoagulants will increase the likelihood of bleeding.

History of allergies

If the client has a history of allergy to medication, the nurse informs other members of the healthcare team. All allergies should be noted on the nurse's admission notes, medication records, and physician's history.

Drug data

The nurse assesses information about each drug, including action, purpose, normal dosage, route, side effects, and nursing implications for administration and monitoring, often several resources must be consulted to gather needed information, pharmacology, textbook, nursing journals, the physician reference, drug package inserts, and the pharmacist are valuable resources. The nurse is responsible for knowing as much as possible about each drug given.

Medication Delivery

Preparation and administration of medication requires accuracy by the nurse. The nurse must pay full attention in preparing medication and must not attempt to do other tasks simultaneously. The nurse must use the "10 rights" of drug administration to ensure safe drug administration.

Medication Errors

Errors in Medication Administration

A medication error is any event that could cause or lead a client receiving inappropriate drug therapy or failing to receive appropriate drug therapy. Medication error can occur by anyone involved in prescribing, preparation, dispensing, and administering of medication.

Nurse manager, the physician may decide to counteract the effects of the error by administering an antidote. When the wrong drug is given, withholding a dose when a previous medication has been given too soon, or monitoring the effects when an unusual high dosage is given. Attempt should not be made to hide the medication error. There should be a system in the client record as to what was administered to the client, the notification to the physician, the observed side effects in the client as a response to the error and the events under taken to counter act the drugs, e.g., administration of antidote.

Special Consideration for Administering Medications to Specific Age Groups: Infants and Children

Children vary in age, weight, body surface area, the ability to absorb, metabolize, and excrete medications. Children dosages are lower than those of adults, so special caution is needed in preparing medications for them.

Older Adult

Older adults require special consideration during drug administration. In addition to the physiological changes of ageing, behavioral and economic factors will also influence an older person's use of drugs.

DRUGS FORMS

Forms of Medication

The different forms of medication are described in **Table 7.2**.

Table 7.2: Forms of medication.

Form	Description
Capsule	Solid dosage form for oral use, medication in powder, liquid or oil forms and encased by gelatin shell, capsule colored to aid in product identification
Elixir	Clear fluid containing water and/or alcohol, designed for oral use, usually has sweetener added
Enteric coated tablet	Tablet for oral use coated with materials that do not dissolve in stomach, coating dissolve in intestine where medication is absorbed
Liniment	Preparation usually containing alcohol, oil or soapy emollient that is applied to skin
Lotion	Medication in liquid suspension applied externally to protect skin
Ointment	Semisolid, externally applied preparation usually containing one or more medication
Paste	Semisolid preparation, thicker and stiffer than ointment, absorbed through skin more slowly than ointment

ROUTES OF ADMINISTRATION OF MEDICATION

The route chosen for administering a drug depends on its properties and desired effect as well as the client's physical and mental condition. Because the nurse is constantly involved in caring the clients, he or she is frequently involved in judging the best route for a medication in collaboration with physicians.

Routes of Drug Administration

1. Oral Route

The oral route: It is the easiest and the most commonly used route. Medication is given by mouth and is swallowed. Orally administered medications are less expensive than many other preparations. They have as lower onset of action and a more prolonged effect. Clients generally prefer the oral route **(Table 7.3)**.

Table 7.3: Procedure: Oral drug administration.

Steps	Rationale
1. Assess for contraindications to client receiving oral medication, including difficulty in swallowing, nausea or vomiting, bowel inflammation or reduced peristalsis, recent gastrointestinal surgery, reduced or absent bowel sounds, gastric suction, decreased level of consciousness	Alterations in gastrointestinal function interfere with drug distribution, absorption, and excretion. When gastric suction in place, medication can be suctioned out before it can be absorbed, clients with lowered consciousness are prone to aspiration
2. Prepare needed supplies and equipment ➢ Medication cards, records form ➢ Medication cart or tray ➢ Medication cups ➢ Glass of water, juice or preferred liquid ➢ Pill crush device (optional)	
3. Check physician written order. Check clients' name and drug name, dosage, route of administration, and time for administration	Physician order is most reliable source of information.

Contd...

Contd...

Steps	Rationale

4. Prepare drug
  a. Wash hands
 	
  b. Arrange medication tray
  c. Prepare medications for one client at a time
  d. Select correct drug from stock supply. Compare label of medication with medication form, card
  e. Calculate correct drug dose
 	
  f. To prepare tablet or capsule from bottle, pour required numbers into bottle cap and transfer to medication cup do not touch with fingers. Extra tablets or capsules may be returned to bottle
  g. If client has difficulty in swallowing, grind tablets in pill crusher do not crush enteric coated or sustained action medications
	a. Reduce transfer of microorganisms from hands to medication and equipment
	b. Save time and reduce error
	c. Prevents preparation errors
	d. Reduce error
	
	e. Calculation is more accurate when information from drug label is at hand
	f. Maintains cleanliness of drugs
	
	g. Larger tablets can be difficult to swallow. Verify that medication can be crushed before doing so. Enteric-coated medication is not designed to be absorbed in stomach

5. Prepare liquids:
  1. Thoroughly mix before administering. Check and discard those that have turned cloudy or changed color
  2. Remove bottle cap from container and place cap upside-down
  3. Hold bottle with label against palm of hand while pouring
  4. Hold medication cup at eye level and fill to desired level on scale
  5. Discard excess liquid in cup into sink wipe lip of bottle with paper towel
  6. Compare medication form with prepared drug and container.
  7. Do not leave drugs unattended
	1. Prevent drug adverse effect
	
	2. Prevents contamination of inside of cap
	3. Spilled liquid will not soil or fade label
	4. Ensure accuracy of measurement
	
	5. Prevents contamination of bottles contents and prevents bottle cap from sticking
	6. Reading label second time reduces errors
	7. Nurse is responsible for safekeeping of drugs

6. Administer medication
  1. Take medications to client at correct time
  2. Identify client by comparing name on card, form or ask client to state full name
	1. Medications are given within 30 minutes before or after the prescribed time to ensure intended effect
	2. Avoid errors

7. Administer drug properly
  a. Ask if client wishes to hold-solid medication in hand or cup before placing in mouth
  b. Offer full glass of water or juice with drugs to be swallowed
  c. For sublingual administered drugs, have client place medication under tongue and allow it dissolve completely. Caution client against swallowing
  d. Mix powdered medication with liquids at bedside and give to client to drink
  e. Caution client against chewing or swallowing lozenges
 	
  f. If client is unable to hold medications, place medication cup to lips and gently introduce each drug into mouth, one at a time. Do not rush
  g. Stay with client until each medication has been swallowed. If uncertain whether medication has been swallowed, ask client to open mouth
  h. For highly acidic medication (e.g., aspirin) offer snack
  i. Assist client in returning to comfortable position
  j. Dispose of soiled supplies and wash hands
  k. Record actual time that each drug was administered on medication record. Include initial or signature
  l. Return within 30 minutes to evaluate response to medication
	a. Client can become familiar with medications by seeing each drug
	b. Choice of fluid promotes comfort and can improve fluid intake
	c. Drug is absorbed through blood vessels of undersurface of tongue. If swallowed, the drug is destroyed by gastric juice or is so rapidly detoxified by liver that therapeutic blood levels are not attained
	
	e. Drug acts through slow absorption through oral mucosa, not gastric mucosa
	f. Administering single tablets or capsule cases swallowing and prevents aspiration
	
	g. Nurse assumes responsibility for ensuring that client receives ordered dosage. If left unattended client may not take dose or may save drugs, causing risk to health
	h. Reduces gastric irritation
	i. Maintains comfort
	j. Reduces transmission of microorganism
	k. Prompt documentation prevents errors such as repeated doses. Signature establishes accountability for administration
	l. Assess drug therapeutic benefits and detect on set of side effects or allergic reactions

2. Sublingual Route

Sublingual drugs are designed to be absorbed readily after being placed under the tongue to dissolve. A drug given sublingually should not be swallowed because the desired effect will not be achieved. Nitroglycerin is commonly given sublingually. The client should not take liquids until the drug is completely dissolved.

3. Buccal Route

Administration of a drug by the buccal route involves placing the solid medication against the mucous membranes of the cheek until the drug dissolves. Clients should be taught to alternate cheeks until with each subsequent dose to avoid mucosal irritation. Clients are also warned not to chew or swallow the drug or to take liquids with it. A buccal medication acts locally on the mucous or systemically as it is swallowed with saliva (dissolved in saliva).

4. Oral–Sublingual and Buccal Routes

The most desirable way to administer medications is by mouth; unless the client has impaired gastrointestinal functioning or is unable to swallow but an oral medication is the safest and easiest method of administration.

PARENTERAL ADMINISTRATION

Parenteral administration involves giving a drug through injection into body tissues. Parenteral administration of medication involves the following four major types of injection.

1. **Subcutaneous (SC):** Injection into tissues just below the dermis of the skin.
2. **Intradermal (ID):** Injection into the dermis just under the epidermis.
3. **Intramuscular (IM):** Injection into a muscle body.
4. **Intravenous (IV):** Injection into a vein.
5. **Intraspinal or intrathecal injections:** Medication when introduced into the spinal cavity is called intraspinal or intrathecal injections.
6. **Epidural:** Drugs are administered in the epidural space via a catheter, which has been placed by a nurse anesthetist or an anesthesiologist. This technique of drug administration is most commonly used for the administration of analgesics postoperatively.
7. **Intraperitoneal injection:** Medicine when introduced into the peritoneal, cavity, it is called intraperitoneal injection.
8. **Intrapleural:** Drugs are administered through the chest wall and directly into the plural space. This may be done directly into the pleural space. Through an injection or through a chest tube.
9. **Infusions:** When a large quantity of medicine or fluids is to be introduced into the body, it is called infusions. Usually these are given intravenously.
10. **Venesection or cut down:** Opening a vein and introducing a tube or wide bore needle and introducing medicines and fluids or taking out blood is called venepuncture venesection. This is done in emergencies.
11. **Intra-arterial:** This method calls for drugs to be administered directly into the arteries. Intra-arterial infusions are common in clients who have arterial clots.
12. **Transfusions:** It is the introduction of whole blood or plasma into a vein or artery to supply actual volume of blood or to introduce constituents as clotting factors or antibodies, which are deficient in the patient.
13. **Hypo spray:** The hypo spray permits drugs to be sprayed through the skin without a needle. Pressure of about 125 pounds is created in a device, which forces the drug into the tissues without pain and without a visible mark.
14. **Intraosseous:** This method of drug administration involves the infusion of medication directly into the bone marrow. It is most commonly used in infants and toddlers that have poor access to their intravascular space.

Other methods of drug administration that are usually limited to physician administration such as intracardiac, injection of a drug directly into cardiac tissue, and intra-articular, injection of a drug into a joint.

Introduction to Parenteral Administration of Drugs

Administering an injection is an invasive procedure that must be performed using aseptic technique. After a needle pierces the skin, the risk of infection exists. The nurse administers drugs parenterally by SC, IM, ID and IV routes. Each type of injection requires certain skills to ensure that the drug reaches the proper location. The effects of parenterally administered drug can develop rapidly, depending on the rate of drug absorption.

Preventing Infection During an Injection

1. To prevent contamination of solution, draw medication from ampoule quickly. Do not allow it to stand open.
2. To prevent needle contamination, avoid letting needle touch contaminated surface (e.g., outer edges of ampoule or vial outer surface of needle cap, nurses' hands countertop, and table surface).
3. To prevent syringe contamination, avoid touching the length of plunger or inner part of barrel. Keep the tip of syringe covered with needle cap.
4. To prepare skin, wash skins soiled with dirt, drainage or feces with soap and water and dry. Use friction and a circular motion while cleaning with an antiseptic swab. Swab from center of site, and move outward in a 2-inch radius **(Table 7.4)**.

Table 7.4: Procedure: Administering subcutaneous, intramuscular, and intradermal injections.

Steps	Rationale
1. Assess indications for proper route for medication	Ensures proper drug absorption through tissue to enhance drug action. Ensures proper route appropriate for client as per physician order
2. Assess medical history and history of allergies	Alerts nurse to any precautions to observe during administration. History of allergies may cancel order for drug
3. Wash hands	Reduces transmission of microorganisms
4. Prepare needed equipment and supplies: ➢ Proper size syringe ➢ Proper size needle ➢ Antiseptic swab (betadine or alcohol) ➢ Disposable gloves ➢ Medication ampoule or vial ➢ Medication card, forms or printouts.	
5. Check medication order.	Ensures accuracy
6. Prepare correct medication dose from ampoule or vial, check carefully. Be sure all the air is expelled (for IM medication that is particularly irritating to tissues). Ensure that medication is sterile, preparation techniques differ for ampoule and vial	
7. Identify client and ask name	Ensures that correct client is receiving prescribed medication
8. Explain procedure to client and proceed in calm, confident manner. Helps client anticipate actions. Calm approach minimizes anxiety	
9. Close room curtains or door	Provides for privacy
10. Keep sheet or gown draped over body parts not requiring exposure	Proper selection of injection site may require exposure of body parts
11. Select appropriate injection site. Inspect skin surface over sites for bruises, inflammation, or edema a. SC: Palpate site for masses or tenderness, for daily insulin, rotate site daily, be sure needle is of correct size by grasping skin fold at site with thumb and forefinger, measure fold from top to bottom. Needle should be one-half of this length b. IM: Note integrity and size of muscle and palpate for tenderness or hardness. If injections are given frequently, rotate sites c. ID: Note lesions or discoloration of forearm, select site three to four finger width below antecubital space and hand width above wrist	Injection sites should be free of anomalies that may interfere with drug absorption. Site used repeatedly can become hardened from lip hypertrophy (increased growth in fatty tissue). ID site should be tested clear so that results of skin can be seen and interpreted correctly
12. Assist client to comfortable position: a. SQ: Have clients relax arm, leg, or abdomen, depending on site chosen	Relaxation of site minimizes discomfort
b. IM: Have client lie flat, on side, or prone or have client sit, depending on site chosen	Reduces strain on muscle and minimizes discomfort of injections
c. ID: Have clients extend elbow and support it and forearm on flat surface. Talk with client about subject of interest	Stabilizes site for easiest accessibility. Distraction reduces anxiety
13. Relocate site using anatomical landmarks	Accurate injection requires insertion in correct site to avoid injury to underlying tissues, blood vessels, nerves, or bone
14. Cleanse site with antiseptic swab. Apply swab at center of site and rotate outward in circular direction for about 5 cm (2 inch)	Mechanical action of swab removes secretions containing microorganisms
15. Keep swab close to hand	Swab remains readily accessible when needle is withdrawn
16. Remove cap from needle by pulling it straight off	
17. Hold syringe correctly between thumb and fore finger of dominant hand	Quick smooth injection requires proper manipulation of syringes parts

Contd...

Contd...

Steps	Rationale

18. Administer injection:
   a. Subcutaneous
     1. For averag**e** client use nondominant hand to spread skin tightly across injection site or grasp tissue creating a roll of 1/2 inch
     2. Inject needle quickly and firmly at 45–90° angles. (Then release skin, if pinched)
 	
     3. For obese client, pinch skin at site and inject needle below tissue fold
     4. Grasp the lower end of syringe barrel with nondominant hand to end of plunger. Avoid moving syringe while slowly pulling back on plunger to aspirate drug. If blood appears in syringe, remove needle, discard medication and syringe, and repeat procedure. *Exception:* Do not aspirate when giving heparin
     5. Inject medication slowly
 	
   b. Intramuscular
     1. Position nondominant hand at proper anatomical landmarks and spread skin tightly. Inject needle quickly at 90° angle into muscle
     2. If clients muscle mass are small, grasp body of muscle between thumb and other fingers
     3. Aspirate as step 18-4
 	
     4. Inject medication slowly
 	
   c. Intradermal Injection
     1. With nondominant hand, stretch skin over site with forefinger or thumb
     2. With needle almost against clients' skin insert it slowly at 5–15° angles until resistances felt
     Then advance needle through epidermis to approximately 3 mm below surface. Needle tip can be seen through skin
     3. Inject medication slowly (it is normal to feel resistance, if not, needle is too deep and should be withdrawn)
     4. While injecting medication, a light-colored bleb resembling a mosquito bite approximately 6 mm in diameter forms at site and then disappears
	Needle penetrates tight skin easier than loose skin. Pinching skin elevates SC tissue and may desensitize area
	
	Quick, firm insertion minimizes discomfort (injecting medication into compressed tissue irritates nerve fibers). Obese clients have fatty layer of tissue above SQ layer. Pinching skin elevates the SQ tissue for injection
	Properly performed injection requires smooth manipulation of syringe parts. Movement of syringe may displace needle and cause discomfort
	Aspiration of blood into syringe indicates
	
	IV placement of needle. SQ and IM injection are not for IV use (dermis is relatively vascular)
	
	Aspiration of heparin injection may cause the needle to move creating tissue damage and bleeding. Speed insertion reduces discomfort
	Ensures that medication reaches muscle mass
	
	Needle pierces tight skin more easily. Ensures that needle tip is in dermis
	Dermal layer is tight and does not expand easily. It is not necessary to aspirate, since dermis is relatively a vascular
	
	Indicates medication is deposited in dermis

19. Withdraw needle while applying alcohol swab gently above or over injection site	Supports tissues around injection site to minimize discomfort during needle withdrawal.
20. For SC or IM injections, massage skin lightly. Do not massage after SQ injection of heparin or insulin	Stimulate circulation and improves drug distribution. Massage of site after heparin injection may cause bleeding and may increase absorption rate of insulin. Massage of ID site may disperse medication into underlying tissue layers and after test results (e.g., tuberculin test)
21. Assist client to comfortable position	Gives client sense of well-being
22. Discard an uncapped needle or needle enclosed in safety shield and attached syringe in appropriately labeled container	CDC and OSHA mandate that needles not be recapped for prevention of needle-sticks and disease transmission
23. Remove disposable gloves. Wash hands	Reduces transmission of microorganisms
24. For ID injection, draw circle around perimeter of injection site with pencil or ink pen	Site must be read at various intervals to determine test results.

Contd...

Steps	Rationale
25. For SC and IM injections, chart dose, route, and site and time and date given in medication record. Correctly sign according to institutional policy	Timely documentation prevents administration errors
26. For ID injections, record area of injection, amount and type of testing substance, and date and time on medication record	Timely documentation prevents administration errors and allows for follow-up assessment
27. Return to room and ask if client feels acute pain, burning, numbness, or tingling at injection site. Observe for allergic reaction after ID injection	Continued discomfort may indicate injury to underlying bones or nerves. Anaphylactic reaction may occur suddenly after ID injection because of drug toxicity
28. Return to evaluate response to medication in 10–30 minutes	IM medication absorbs quicker than SQ undesired effects might also develop rapidly. Observations determine efficacy

Subcutaneous Injection

Subcutaneous injections involve placing medication into the loose connective tissue under the dermis, because SC tissue is not as richly supplied with blood as the muscles. Drug absorption is somewhat slower than with IM injections. However, drugs are absorbed completely if circulatory status is normal. Because subcutaneous tissue contains pain receptors, the client may experience some discomfort. The best sites for SC injections include vascular areas around the outer aspect of the upper arms, the abdomen from below the coastal margins to the iliac crests, and the anterior aspect of the thigh. These areas are easily accessible especially for clients with diabetes who self-administer insulin. The injection site chosen should be free of infection, skin lesions, scars, bony prominence, and large underlying muscles or nerves. Clients with diabetes should regularly rotate daily injection sites to prevent hypertrophy (thickening) of the skin. No injection site should be used more than every 6 to 7 weeks.

The SC route should give only small doses (0.5–1 mL) of water-soluble medication. SC tissue is sensitive to irritating solutions and large volumes of medication. Collection of medication within the tissue can cause sterile abscesses, which appear as hardened pain full umps under the skin.

Body weight indicates the depth of the subcutaneous (SQ) layer. Therefore, the nurse must choose the needle length and angle of insertion based on the clients weight generally 25-gauge 5/8-inch needle inserted at a 45-degree angle.

To ensure that the insulin reaches SQ tissue, the nurse follows this simple rule: if 2 inches of tissue can be grasped the needle should be inserted at a 90-degree angle, and if 1 inch of tissue can be grasped the needle should be inserted at a 45-degree angle.

Intramuscular Injection

The intramuscular route provides faster drug absorption than the SQ route because of greater muscle vascularity. The danger of causing tissue damage is less when drugs enter deep muscle, but there is the risk of inadvertently injecting drugs directly into blood vessels. The nurse uses a longer and larger gauge needle to pass through SC tissue and penetrate the deep muscle tissue. However, weight influences selection of needle size. For example, a client weighing 100 pounds may only require a needle 1¼ to 1½ inches long, whereas a child weighing 50 pounds usually requires a 1 inch needle. The angle of insertion for an IM injection is 90 degrees. Muscle is a less sensitive to irritating and viscous drug. A normal, well-developed client can safely tolerate as much as 3 mL of medication in larger, more developed muscles such as the dorsogluteal or vastus lateralis. Smaller muscles can tolerate only smaller amounts of medications without severe muscle discomfort. Children, older adults, and thin clients tolerate <12 mL of medication.

The nurse assesses the integrity of muscle before giving an injection. The muscle should be free of tenderness. Repeated injections in the same muscle can cause considerable discomfort. By asking the client to relax, the nurse can palpate the muscle to rule out the presence of hardened lesions. Normally a muscle feels soft when relaxed and firm when tense. The nurse can minimize discomfort during an injection by helping the client assume a position that will help reduce the strain on the muscle.

Sites

When selecting an IM site, the nurse assesses the following:
1. Is the area free of infection or necrosis?
2. Are there local areas of bruising or abrasions?
3. What is the location of underlying bones, nerves arid major blood vessels?
4. What volume of medication is to be administered?

Vastus Lateralis Muscle

The thick, well-developed vastus lateralis muscle is a preferred injection site for adults, children, and infants. The muscle is located on the anterior lateral aspect of the thigh and extends in an adult from a hand breadth above the knee to a hand breadth below the greater trochanter of the femur. The middle third of the muscle is the best site for the injection. In width the site extends from the midline of the thigh's top to the midline of the thigh outer side.

Ventrogluteal Muscle

The ventrogluteal muscle involves the gluteus medius and minimus. The client lies on either side with knee bent and the nurse locates the muscle by placing the palm of the hand over the greater trochanter and index finger on the anterior superior iliac spine of the client's hip. The right hand is used for the left hip and the left hand is used for the right hip. The nurse points the thumb toward the client groin and fingers toward the client's head. The injection site becomes exposed while spreading the middle finger back along the iliac crest toward the buttock. The index finger, the middle finger, and the iliac crest form a triangle, and the injection site is the center of it. The client may lie on his or her side or back. Flexing of the knee and hip helps the client relax this muscle.

Dorsogluteal Muscle

The dorsogluteal muscle has been a traditional site for IM injections. However, accidental insertion of a needle in to the sciatic nerve can cause permanent or partial paralysis of the involved leg. Major blood vessels and bone are also near the site. In client with flabby, sagging tissues, this site is difficult to locate.

The dorsogluteal site is located in the upper outer aspect of the upper outer quadrant of the buttock, approximately 5-8 cm (2-3 inches) below the iliac crest. Clients may lie in the prone position with toes turned medially or in a side lying position with the upper leg flexed at the hip and knee. To locate the nurse palpates the poster superior iliac spine and the greater trochanter of the femur. An imaginary line is drawn between the two anatomical landmarks. The sciatic nerve runs parallel and below the line. The injection site is above and laterals to the line. Nurses may use the injection site in adults and children with well-developed gluteal muscle.

Deltoid Muscle

In some adults, infants, and most children, the deltoid muscle is not well developed. The radial and ulnar nerves and the brachial artery lie within the upper arm along the humerus. The nurse rarely uses the deltoid site unless other injection sites are inaccessible because of dressing, cast, or other obstructions.

To locate the deltoid muscle the nurse asks the client fully expose the upper arm and shoulder. The nurse should not try to roll a tight-fitting sleeve. The nurse asks the client to relax the arm at the side and flex the elbow. The client may sit, stand, or lie down. The nurse palpates the lower edge of the acromion process, which forms the base of a triangle in line with the midpoint of the lateral aspect of the upper arm. The injection site is in the center of the triangle, about 2.5-5 cm (1-2 inch) below the acromion process. The nurse may also locate the site by placing four fingers across the deltoid muscle, which the top fingers along the acromion process. The injection site is then three finger-breadths below the acromion process.

Intradermal Injection

The nurse typically gives intradermal injections for skin testing (e.g., tuberculin screening and allergy tests). Because these medications are potent, they are injected into the dermis, where the blood supply is reduced and drug absorption occurs slowly. A client may have a severe anaphylactic reaction if the medication enters the circulation too rapidly.

Skin testing requires the nurse to be able to clearly see the injection sites for changes in color and tissue integrity. ID sites should be free of lesions and relatively hairless. The inner forearm and upper back are ideal locations.

The nurse uses a tuberculin or small hypodermic syringe for skin testing. The angle of insertion is 5-15°. As the nurse injects the drug a small bleb resembling a mosquito bite should appear on the skin's surface. If a bleb does not appear or if the site bleeds after needle withdrawal, there is a good chance the medication entered SC tissues. In this case, skin test results will not be valid. Data from ID injection include a description of the precise location and time of administration. The injected site must be "read" within a prescribed time, for example 48 hours, (after the PPD injection).

Equipment

A variety of syringes and needles are available, and each is designed to deliver a certain volume of a drug to a specific type of tissue. The nurse exercises judgment when determining which syringe or needle will be the most effective.

Types of Syringes

Syringes consist of a cylindrical barrel with a tip designed to fit the hub of a hypodermic needle and a close-fitting plunger syringes in general. They are classified as being luer-lock or nonluer-lock. This nomenclature is based on the design of the syringe's tip. Luer-lock syringes require special needles, which are twisted onto the tip and lock themselves in the place. This design prevents the inadvertent removal of the needle, nonluer-lock syringes require needle that slips on to the tip. Most health care institutions use disposable single use plastic syringes that are inexpensive and easy to manipulate. The syringes are packaged separately, with or without a sterile needle in a paper wrapper or rigid, plastic container.

Needles

Needles come packaged in individual sheaths to allow flexibility in choosing the right needle. Some needles are preattached to standard-size syringes. Most are made of stainless steel and are disposable.

The needle has three parts.
1. The hub, which fits onto the tip of a syringe.
2. The shaft, which connects to the hub; and
3. The bevel or slanted tip.

Disposable Injection Units

Disposable, single dose, prefilled syringes are available for many medications. The nurse must be careful to check the medication and concentration because all prefilled syringes appear very similar.

Administering Injections

Each injection route is unique with regard to the type of tissues into which the medication is injected. The characteristics of the tissues influence the rate of drug absorption and thus the onset of drug action starts. Before injecting a drug the nurse should know the volume of the drug to be administered, the drug's characteristics, and viscosity, and location of anatomical structures underlying injection sites.

Serious consequences may occur if an injection is administered incorrectly. Failure to select an injection site in relation to anatomical landmarks can result in nerve or bone damage during needle insertion. If the nurse fails to aspirate the syringe before injecting a drug, the drug may accidentally be injected directly into an artery or vein. Injecting too large volume of medication for the site selected can cause extreme pain and may result in local tissue damage.

Many clients, particularly children, fear injections. Clients with serious or chronic illness often are given multiple injections daily. The nurse can attempt to minimize discomfort in the following ways:

1. Use a sharp, beveled needle in the smallest suitable length and gauge.
2. Position the client as comfortable as possible to reduce muscular tension.
3. Select the proper injection site, using anatomical landmarks.
4. Divert the client's attention from the injection through conversation.
5. Insert the needle smoothly and quickly to minimize tissue pulling.
6. Hold the syringes steady while the needle remains in the tissues.
7. Massage the injected area gently for several seconds unless contraindicated.

Types of Vials and Ampoules, Preparing Injectable Medicines from Vials and Ampoules

There are different types of vials such as glass plastic tubes, jar and aluminum tubes, and dispenser tubes a vial is a small container, cylindrical and made of glass, it is used of specifically for holding liquid medicine. Vials made of type I borosilicate glass are generally used for preparations that are intended for parenteral administration.

An ampoule is a small sealed vial which is used to contain and preserve a sample, usually a solid or liquid. Ampoules are commonly used to contain pharmaceuticals and chemicals that must be protected from air and contaminants.

Care of equipment: Decontamination and disposal of syringes, needles

Decontamination and disposal of syringes, needles come under biomedical waste management, with special reference to disposal of sharp.

Sharps are defined as comprising of needles, syringes, scalpels, blades, i.e., anything that cause puncture and cuts. These include both used and unused sharps.

Sharp must be collected at the point of generation in a leak proof and puncture resistant containers. Container must bear the international biohazard symbol and appropriate wording. Container should never be completely filled nor filled above the full line indicated on box.

Inhalation

The deeper passages of the respiratory tract provide a large surface area for drug absorption. Drugs can be administered through the nasal passage, oral passage or tubes that have been placed into the trachea, inhaled medication may have local effects. Drugs such as oxygen and general anesthetics create general systemic effects.

Storage and Maintenance of Drugs and Nurses Responsibilities

Storing of Medications

Care of medicine cabinet and drugs

1. To stock the medicines, each ward should be provided with a medicine cabinet.
2. It should be a large enough to accommodate all drugs to be stocked inward.
3. As far as possible, the medicine cabinet should be kept in a separate room adjacent to the nurse's room.
4. Hand washing facility should be available in that room.
5. Adequate lighting should be provided with in the cabinet or read the label clearly.
6. There should be separate compartments for different categories of drug.
7. Drugs used for external use should be kept separate from the drugs used for internal use.
8. The containers should be arranged alphabetically, so that it is easy to find them.
9. Scheduled (dangerous drug) drugs should be kept in a separate cupboard, which must have separate lock and key.
10. A senior nurse should be responsible for scheduled drugs.
11. Check the expiry date of every drug and take use of it before its expiry date is over or send it to the dispensary and get it replaced.

12. All medications should be kept closed always. The containers keeping the capsules alcoholic preparations, volatile drugs, etc., should have airtight caps. The tablets and pills tend to disintegrate if exposed to air.
13. The drugs that are unusual in color, odor, and consistency should be returned to the pharmacy and replaced with fresh ones.
14. No drug is stored without label. All the containers should have labels written neatly and legibly; the labels should contain the name of the drug, the ingredients, the strength, the dose, etc.

Therapeutic Effect, Side Effect, Toxic Effect, Allergic Reaction, Drug Tolerance, Drug Interactions, Effects of Drugs

Therapeutic Effects

The therapeutic effect is the expected or predictable physiological response a medication causes. Each medication has a desired therapeutic effect for which it is prescribed. For example, nitroglycerin is used to reduce the cardiac workload and increase myocardial oxygen supply. A single medication may have many therapeutic effects. For example, aspirin is an analgesic, antipyretic and anti-inflammatory, it reduces platelet aggregation (clumping). It is important for the nurse to know for which therapeutic effect, a medication is prescribed. This will allow the nurse to properly teach the client about the medications intended and its effect on medication.

Side Effect

Side effects are the unintended secondary effects that the medications predictably will cause. Side effects may be harmless or injurious. If the side effects are serious enough to negate the beneficial effects of medications therapeutic action the prescriber may discontinue the medication. Clients often stop taking medication because of side effects.

Adverse Effect

Adverse effects are generally considered as severe responses to medication. For example, a client may become comatose when a drug is ingested. When adverse responses to medications occur, the prescriber must discontinue the medication. Some adverse effects might be unexpected effects that were not discovered during drug testing.

Anaphylaxis

This is an immediate and severe reaction marked by increased blood pressure, local edema, prickling, feeling in the throat edema in the face and hand, cyanosis, choking, cough, dyspnea wheezing, etc. This is an emergency, unless acted quickly; death may follow, within few minutes. Sera and penicillin should be administered only after sensitivities thus were done to prevent such reaction.

Effect on Urinary System

Anuria, oliguria, hematuria, crystalluria, albuminuria, etc., might occur, where intake and output may be indicated. Frequent urine analysis and blood chemistry studies can prevent such an occurrence.

Effect on Cardiovascular System

Arrhythmia change in the rate, rhythm or volume of pulse, counting of pulse may occur for one minute will reveal such irregularities.

Blood Dispraises

A plastic anemia, thrombocytopenia, agranulocytosis, leukopenia is some of the ill effects of certain drugs. Education to the public is essential to refrain from taking drugs without physician's order and supervision.

Effects on Nervous Systems

Abnormal involuntary movements, e.g., tremor, chorea, dystonia, stimulations of the central nervous system, anxiety nervousness, insomnia, headache, double vision, convulsions, may be reposed.

Toxic Effect

Toxic effects may develop after prolonged intake of a medication or when a medication accumulates in the blood because of impaired metabolism or excretion.

Idiosyncratic Reaction

Medication may cause unpredictable effects such as an idiosyncratic reaction in which a client overreacts or underreacts to medications or has a reaction different from normal. For example, a child receiving an antihistamine (benadryl) may become extremely agitated or excited instead of drowsy. It is impossible to assess clients for idiosyncratic responses.

Allergic Reaction

Allergic reaction is another unpredictable response to a medication. They make up 5-10% of all medication reaction. A client medication allergy may be mild or severe. Allergic symptoms vary depending on the individual and the medications. The allergy to a medication may be mild or severe.

Effects on the Gastrointestinal System

Irritation of gastric mucosa, nausea, vomiting, anorexia, small bowel ulceration, abdominal pain, melena, distention and diarrhea.

Factors Influencing Drug Actions

Because of differences in the manner in which drugs act and their types of action, responses to medication vary considerably. Factors other than characteristics of the medications influence drug actions. A client may not respond in the same way to each successive dose of a medication. Likewise, the same drug dosage may cause different responses in different clients.

Genetic Differences

Genetic makeup affects the manner in which biotransformation of drugs occurs. Metabolic patterns are similar within families. Genetic factors determine whether, naturally occurring enzymes are present to assist in drug degradations. As result, members of a family may share sensitivity to the medication.

Physiological Variables

a. Hormonal differences between men and women alter the metabolism of certain drugs. Hormones and drugs compete with each other in biotransformation because they are degraded by some metabolic processes. Diurnal variations in estrogen secretions may be responsible for the cyclic fluctuations in drug reactions experienced by women.
b. Age has a direct effect on drug metabolism; infants lack many of the enzymes necessary for normal drug metabolism. A number of physiological changes accompanying the aging process influence the responses to drug therapy.

Environmental Conditions

A client's exposure to severe physical and emotional stress triggers a hormonal response that eventually interferes with drug metabolism; ionizing radiation creates a similar effect by altering the rate of enzyme activity.

Psychological Factors

A number of psychological factors influence the use of drugs and response to a medication. A person's attitude about drugs and response to a medication. A person's attitude about drugs may stem from early experiences or familial influences, seeing parent use medications frequently may cause a child to accept drugs as a normal part of life.

Diet

Drug and nutrient interaction can alter a drug's action or the effect of a nutrient. For example, vitamin K (found in green leafy vegetable) is a nutrient that antagonize the effect of warfarin sodium (coumadin), decreasing its effect on blood clotting mechanisms. Mineral oil decreases the absorption of fat-soluble vitamins. Client may be required to take nutritional supplements when taking drugs that reduce a nutrient's effects similarly withholding certain nutrients may ensure a drug's therapeutic effect.

Drug Interaction

Definition

When two or more drugs is simultaneously administered to a person, it can alter the body's reactions to any of the drugs leading to alteration of the pharmacological effect of the other drugs, then drug interaction is said to occur.

Pharmacokinetics

It is defined as the science of observing the movement of drugs through the body and the various factors that can affect this process. The principles of pharmacokinetics are applied to the passage of a pharmaceutical drug through an individual's body.

Principles of pharmacokinetics

There are four basic events that take place in the body when any drug is administered, these are:
❖ Absorption (A)
❖ Distribution (D)
❖ Metabolism (M)
❖ Excretion (E)

This is often abbreviated to the main initial as ADME.
These are concerned with the entry of the drug into the body, how it is distributed around the body, what happens to the drug molecule in the body, and finally, how it is removed from the body.

Absorption

Any drug must first enter into the body can be injected directly into the blood stream or be absorbed through the stomach, duodenum, jejunum, ileum, rectum, buccal cavity, nasal mucosa, eyes, vagina, other membranes, or skin.

In all the cases except direct injection into the blood stream, there will be a percentage of drugs, which fails to enter the body. The amount that actually enters the body is known as *bioavailability*.

Distribution

Following absorption drug must be taken in the blood plasma around the body to the site of its action. This means—it must be distributed around the body within the fluids. The measurement of which is called the: **"Volume of distribution".**

Metabolism

The body will remove all drugs over a period of time, either by exerting if unchanged, or by chemically altering it and then exerting it. The liver plays a major role in altering the other molecules and execrating it liver disease will have an effect on the rate at which a drug is metabolized.

Excretion

The kidney has the major function or excretion of a drug and its metabolites. The more water soluble the drug is the easier for the kidneys to excrete it.

Types of Medication Action

Medication varies considerably in the way they act and their types of action. Factors other than characteristics of the medication also influence medication actions. A client may not respond the same way to each successive dose of medication likewise, the same medication dosage may cause very different responses in different clients. Therefore, it is essential for the nurse to understand all the effects that medications can have when taken by or given to client.

SYSTEM OF DRUG MEASUREMENT

Medication Dose Calculation

A. Metric System

The metric system was first introduced in the early 1790s in France and accepted in most countries. The metric system is based on the decimal system, which is again based on multiples of 10, and fractions of 10. Metric system uses the same base for measuring mass, volume and length.

The basic units are

Gram: The basic unit of weights
Liter: The basic unit of fluid volume
Meter: The basic unit of length

B. Apothecary System (Customary English System)

This system was developed in the 13th century and was used in England. Canada and USA have adopted the use of this system, before they started to slowly introduce the metric system in 1975.

The basic units are:

Grain (gr.): The basic unit of weight
Minimum (Z): The basic unit of fluid volume
This system is being phased away.

C. Household System

This system is not as accurate as the metric system, because of a lack of standardization of spoons, cups and glass, but it is still in use because patients are being cared for in the home.

D. International Unit System (SI)

The SI unit is more comprehensive and incorporates much of the metric system in, 1975, WHO recommended the use of the SI unit, as an international unit of measurement.

The basic SI units used in relation to drug and fluid calculation are:

- Unit of capacity (fluid or liquid): Liter (L)
- Unit of Mass (weight): Gram (g)
- Unit of Length: Meter (m)

Example (Unit of mass)

Symbol	Unit	Meaning
Gigagram	Gm	1,000,000,000 gram
Megagram	Mg	1,000,000 gram
Kilogram	kg	1,000 gram
Hectogram	Hg	100 gram
Decagram	Dg	10 gram
Gram	g	Basic unit
Decigram	Dg	0.1 gram
Centigram	Cg	0.01 gram
Milligram	mg	0.001 gram
Microgram	µg	0.000001 gram
Nanogram	Ng	0.000000001 gram
Gigaliter	Gl	1,000,000,000 liters
Megaliter	Ml	1000,000 liters
Kiloliter	Kl	1,000 liters
Hectoliter	Hl	100 liter
Decaliter	Dl	10 liter
Liter	L	Basic unit
Deciliter	Dl	10 liter
Centiliter	Cl	0.01 liter
Milliliter	mL	0.001 liter
Microliter	µl	0.000001 liter
Nanoliter	Nl	0.000000001 liter

Other examples:

Unit of temperature: (°C) Celsius degree
Unit of pressure: (p) Pascal degree

Unit of concentration of a substance:
Mole (mol)

Converting metric units

Memorize 1 gram (g) = 1,000 milligrams (mg)
1 milligram (mg) = 1,000 microgram (µg)
1 liter (L) = 1,000 milliliters (mL)

Medication dose calculation

Formula:

$$\text{Required volume required dose} = \frac{\text{Required dose}}{\text{Stock dose}} \times \text{Stock volume}$$

OR

$$= \frac{\text{What we want}}{\text{What we have}} \times \text{Volume}$$

Required dose = Dosage ordered by the physician (What we want)

Stock dose = Dosage available (What we have)

Volume injections = The amount of solution in which the drug is available

Example

Physician ordered morphine sulfate 7.5 mg SC; drug available is 15 mg per mL. Calculate the dose you would administer to the patient.

Basic Formula

$$\text{Required volume} = \frac{\text{Required dose}}{\text{Stock dose}} \times \text{Stock volume}$$

$$= 7.5 \times 115$$
$$= 0.5 \text{ mL}$$

Calculation of IV Infusion flow rates and calculation in drops/minutes:

Formula:

$$\text{Flow rate (Drops/min)} = \frac{\text{Volume to be infused} \times \text{Drop factor}}{\text{Time of infusion in minutes}}$$

Drop factors are the number of drops per 1 mL, an IV administration set delivers. It is very important to check the drop factor mentioned on the IV administration set package, before working out the flow rate. The ordinary IV administrations deliver 15–20 drops per mL and the pediatric IV administration set delivers 60 drops per mL.

Example:
500 mL of normal saline to be given in 4 hours. IV giving set delivers 20 drops/mL. Calculate the flow rate in drops/minute.

$$\text{Drops/minute} = \frac{\text{Volume to be infused} \times \text{Drops factors}}{\text{Time of infusion in minutes}}$$

$$= \frac{500 \times 20}{4 \times 60}$$

$$= 41.6$$
$$= 42 \text{ drops/minute}$$

Example:
Physician ordered G/W 5% 80 mL hourly. Calculate the drip rate in drops/min knowing that the IV giving set drops factor is 60 drops/mL.

Formula:

$$\text{Drops/minute} = \frac{\text{Volume to be infused} \times \text{Drop factor}}{\text{Time of infusion in minute}}$$

$$= \frac{80 \times 60}{60}$$

$$= 80 \text{ drops per minute.}$$

Calculate in milliliter/hour (mL/hour)

Formula:
Flow rate (mL/hour)

Example:

$$= \frac{\text{Volume to be infused}}{\text{Time of infusion in hours}}$$

A physician orders to give 500 mL of 5% dextrose in 6 hours using an infusion pump. Calculate the flow rate in mL/hour.

$$\text{Flow rate (mL/hour)} = \frac{500}{6} = 83 \text{ mL/hour}$$

Example:
If you are ordered to administer 500 mL normal saline over 12 hours, calculate the drip rate in mL/hour.

Formula

$$\text{Flow rate (mL/hour)} = \frac{\text{Volume to be infused}}{\text{Time of infusion in hours}}$$

$$\text{Flow rate (mL/hour)} \frac{500}{12} = 41.6 \text{ mL/hour (42 mL)}$$

Broad Classification of Drugs

Medication order should include:
1. Patient name
2. Date and time the order is written

Drug	Use
Analgesics	Drug used to relieve pain
Anesthetics	Drugs, which cause loss of sensation
Anthelmintics	Drugs, which destroys and expel worms
Antipyretics	Drug, which reduces fever
Antidotes	Substances used to counteract the effects of position
Anti-infective	Drugs which act to inhibit, kill or retard the growth of microorganisms
Anti-inflammatory	The drugs, which helps to reduce the inflammation
Anticoagulants	Substances, which inhibit or decrease the blood clotting process
Antihistamines	The agents, which block the effect of histamine therefore used to prevent or relieve allergies
Antacids	Substances that react with hydrochloric acids to decrease the activity of the gastric secretions
Anticonvulsants	Those drugs used to prevent or treat convulsion and it is used in epilepsy
Antibiotic	Products that have the ability to destroy or inhibit the growth of other organisms
Broad-spectrum antibiotic	Drugs, which are effective against man strains of microorganisms
Antidiarrheal	Agents that are used to treat diarrhea
Antitussives	Drugs that inhibit the cough reflex
Antiasthmatics	Drugs which provides symptomatic relief of asthmatic attack

Contd...

Contd...

Drug	Use
Antispasmodic	An agent that relieves the spasmodic pains or spasm of the muscles.
Antifungal	An agent that relieves the spasmodic pains or spasm of the muscles.
Antiemetic	Drugs relieving or preventing nausea and vomiting.
Antitubercular	The specific drugs used in the treatment of tuberculosis.
Bronchodilator	Medicine, which relax muscles of bronchioles.
Coagulants	Those drugs that help in the clotting of blood.
Carminatives	Drugs which cause expulsion of gas from stomach and intestine.
Laxatives	Drugs used to cause intestinal evacuation.
Corticosteroids	Hormonal drugs.
Diuretics	Drugs increase the flow of urine.
Expectorants	Increase the bronchial secretions and in the expulsion of mucous.
Emmenagogs	A drug that stimulates or favors the menstrual discharge.
Galactagogues	Substances that increases the flow of milk.
Hypotensive	Any substance capable of lowering blood pressure.
Hypoglycemic	Drugs that lower the bloods sugar level.
Hematinics	An agent, which tends to increase the hemoglobin content of blood.
Sedatives	Lessen the body activity.

3. Name of the drug to be administered
4. Dosage of the drug
5. Route by which the drug is to be administered
6. Frequency of administration of the drug
7. Signature of person writing the order

Developmental Considerations

Some conditions are not recommended for medication administration such as:
1. During pregnancy: To avoid adverse effects on fetus some drugs referred as teratogenic, which will cause developmental defects in the embryo. Some drugs are contraindicated.
2. During breast feeding, infants are at risk of some drugs.
3. Children dosage should be calculated carefully, smaller than adult dose.
4. Older people are sensitive to medications.

Prevention of Needle Sticks Injuries

Steps for safe sharp removal:
1. All sharps should be disposed in a rigid puncture proof resistant container
2. Container should be three quarters full
3. All containers should have a lid, which must be tightly sealed before it goes in to disposal.

Step to prevent needle sticks injuries:
1. Avoiding recapping needles
2. Before beginning any procedure using needless plan for safe handling and proper disposal
3. Select and evaluate devices with safety features
4. Report all needle sticks and other sharp related injuries
5. Dispose of used needles in appropriate sharps disposal containers
6. Inform infection control department of hazards from needles stick injuries
7. Participate in blood-borne pathogen training
8. Follow recommended infection prevention practices, including hepatitis B vaccination.

Step to take following needle stick injuries:
If you experienced a sharp injury during your work immediately follow these steps:
1. Wash hands with soap and water
2. Flush out mouth, nose, or skin with water
3. Irrigate eyes with water, saline or sterile irrigants
4. Report to infection control department
5. Immediately seek medical treatment as per institutional policies

TOPICAL ADMINISTRATION, TYPES, PURPOSE, SITE, EQUIPMENT, PROCEDURE

Topical Administration

Drugs applied to the skin and mucous membranes principally have local effects. The topical medication is applied to the skin by maintaining or spreading it over an area, applying moist dressings, soaking body parts in a solution, or giving medicated baths. Systematic effect can occur if a client skin is thin, if the drug concentration is high, or if skin contact is prolonged. These topical medications may be applied for as little as 24 hours or up to 7 days.

Drugs can also be applied to mucous membrane. They are usually absorbed rather quickly when applied in this manner. The nurse uses the following methods for applying medications to mucous membranes:
1. Direct applications of liquid (e.g., having the client gargle, swabbing the throat).
2. Insertion of the drug into a body cavity (e.g., placing a suppository in the rectum or vagina or inserting medicated packing into the vagina).
3. Instillation (slow introduction) of fluid into a body cavity (e.g., instilling ear drops, nose drops, and bladder and rectal fluids).
4. Irrigation (washing out) of body cavity (e.g., flushing the eye, ear, vagina, bladder, or rectum with medicated fluid).
5. Spraying (e.g., instilling medication into the nose and throat).

Topical Preparations Applied to the Skin

1. Powder
2. Cream and oils
3. Ointment
4. Lotions

Application to Skin and Mucous Membranes

a. Assess the patient allergy level
b. Explain the purpose and action of medication
c. Verify area of application
d. Wear gloves
e. Remove previous application
f. Gently wash the area
g. Use the palm of your hand and press firmly
h. Perform hand washing
i. Document medication applied
j. Assess for any skin irritation

Direct Application of Liquid, Gargle, and Swabbing the Throat

Purpose:
1. To relieve pain, inflammation and congestion in the throat
2. To treat infection
3. To anesthetize the throat

Equipment:
1. Prescribed medication
2. Sterile cotton applicators
3. Small bowl
4. Tongue depressor
5. Head mirror and spotlight
6. Kidney tray
7. Paper bag
8. Towel

Procedure:
Throat paining procedure depicted in **Table 7.5**.

Table 7.5: Procedure: Throat paining.

Nursing action	Rationale
1. Identify the patient	To prevent error
2. Greet and explain the procedure to the patient	To establish rapport To gain cooperation To relieve anxiety
3. Wash hands	To prevent cross infection
4. Assemble the equipment	To save time and energy
5. Place the patient in a sitting position/upright position with head tilled backwards	To visualize the throat
6. Place the towel around the patient's neck	To protect the patient's clothing
7. Adjust the spot light behind the place	To reflect the light from head mirror
8. Pour the prescribed medication into the bowl, dip the sterile cotton applicators, and squeeze off the excess medication from the applicator	To prevent dripping of solution into the mouth
9. Instruct the patient to open his mouth and say "Aha" and depress the tongue with tongue depressor using a slight pressure	To visualize the throat. To perform the procedure. To permit an easy reach of the swab to the tonsil and posterior pharynx
10. Paint the throat gently and quickly using one swab stick to one side using half circle movements and reaching all parts of the throat	To apply medication to the throat
11. Place the patient in a comfortable position	To provide comfort
12. Clean and replace the equipment	For better organization of unit equipment
13. Wash hands	To prevent cross-infection
14. Record and report to the incharge nurse	To document the procedure. To take necessary action

Throat Gargling

Purpose:
1. To relieve congestion, swelling and pain in the throat
2. To reduce inflammation
3. To facilitate the release of secretions from the throat

Equipment:
1. Warm saline/AMC solution as prescribed
2. Kidney tray
3. Paper bag
4. Towel
5. Tissue papers

Procedure:
Gargling procedure depicted in **Table 7.6**

Insertion of Drugs into Body Cavity, Suppository/Medicated Packing in Rectum/Vagina

Insertion of Rectal Suppository

1. Identify the patient
2. Verify history of allergy
3. Explain procedure to the patient
4. Collect required suppository
5. Wear the gloves
6. Keep the patient left side in Sims position
7. Maintain privacy
8. Expose only the buttocks
9. Remove the suppository from its wrapper
10. Apply rapper
11. Apply lubricant to rounded end
12. Lubricate the index finger of your dominant hand
13. Separate the buttocks with dominant hand and instruct the patient to breath slowly and deeply through the mouth while the suppository is being inserted
14. Insert the suppository rounded end first, along the rectal wall, insert about 3–4 inches
15. Use toilet tissue to clean any stool or lubricant from around anus
16. Release the buttocks, and retain suppository for at least 5 minutes
17. Remove gloves
18. Document the procedure

Medicated Packing in Rectum/Vagina

Inserting vaginal cream:
1. Identify the patient
2. Verify history of allergy
3. Explain procedure to the patient
4. Collect required medication cream
5. Wear the gloves
6. Follow institutional policy
7. Ask the patient to void before inserting medication
8. Position the patient so that she is lying on her back with knee flexed
9. Maintain privacy with draping
10. Provide adequate light to visualize vaginal opening
11. Spread labia with fingers and clean area at vaginal orifice

Table 7.6: Procedure: Gargling.

Nursing action	Rationale
1. Identify the patient	To prevent error
2. Greet and explain the procedure to the patient	To establish rapport To gain cooperation To relieve anxiety
3. Wash hands	To prevent cross-infection
4. Assemble the equipment	To save time and energy
5. Place the patient in a sitting position with head tilled backward	For better performance of the procedure
6. Place the towel over the patient's chest	To protect the patient's clothes
7. Instruct the patient too: a. Hold the breath during gargling b. Direct the solution to all parts of the throat and gargle	To prevent aspiration of solution into the respiratory tract To promote the effect of gargle on all the parts of the throat
8. Give the patient a mouthful of gargling solution	To gargle the throat
9. Instruct the patient to spit out gargling solution into the kidney basin	To discard the gargled solution
10. Repeat the gargle following steps from 7 to 9 for 3–4 times	To get relief from pain and congestion
11. Give tissue paper to wipe the mouth	To provide comfort
12. Place the patient in a comfortable position	To provide comfort
13. Clean and replace the equipment	For better organization of unit equipment
14. Wash hands	To prevent cross-infection
15. Record and report to the charge nurse	To document the procedure To take necessary action

12. Fill a vaginal applicator with the prescribed amount of cream
13. Spread the labia and introduce the applicator gently in a rolling manner while directing it downward and backward
14. Remind the patient in supine position for 5-10 minutes after insertion
15. Remove gloves
16. Document the procedure

EAR IRRIGATION AND INSTILLATION OF EAR DROPS

Irrigation the External Auditory Canal Purposes

1. To remove discharges from the canal
2. To facilitate removal of cerumen or foreign bodies
3. To apply heat to the tissues of the ear canal

Procedure

Ear irrigation instillation procedure is shown in **Table 7.7**.

Nursing Alert

Ask the patient if he has a history of draining ears or if he had a perforation or other complications from previous ear irrigation. If the reply is affirmative, check with the physician before proceeding with the irrigation.
1. Type and amount of solution desired
2. Try containing

Protective Towels, Equipment and Solutions

a. Cotton balls and cotton applicators
b. Solution bowl and kidney basin
c. Ear syringe or irrigating container with tubing, clamp, and irrigating catheter
d. Paper bag/pedal bin for disposable cotton

Procedure

Preparatory Phase

1. After explaining procedure to the patient, place him in an appropriate position (i.e., sitting or lying with head fitted toward affected ear)
2. Position protective towel

Follow-up Phase

1. Dry external ear with cotton buds
2. Remove soiled towels, etc., and make the patient comfortable
3. Record the time of irrigation, type and amount of solution used, nature of return flow, effect of treatment

Instillation of Eardrops

Definition

Instillation of eardrops involves dropping, a prescribed solution into the external auditory canal from a dropper.

Purposes

1. To soften wax before syringing
2. To reduce inflammation and relieve discomfort
3. To combat infection

Equipment and Solutions

1. Prescribed ear drops
2. Cotton wool balls
3. Receptacle for soiled disposable

Table 7.7: Procedure: Ear irrigation and instillation of ear drops.

Nursing action	Rationale
1. Use a cotton applicator to remove any discharge on outer ear	To prevent carrying discharge deeper into canal
2. Place kidney basin close to the patient's head and under the ear	To provide a receptacle to receive irrigating solution
3. Test temperature of solution by allowing; some to run on inner aspect of wrist. Should be 35–40.6°C (95–105°F)	More comfortable for the patient; solution that are or cold are most uncomfortable and may initiate a feeling of dizziness
4. Ascertain whether implication is due to a foreign hygroscope (attracts or absorbs moisture) body before proceeding	If water contacts such a substance, it may cause it to swell and produce intense pain
5. Gently pull the outer ear upward and backward (adult) downward and backward (child)	To straighten ear canal
6. Place tip of syringe or irrigating catheter at the opening of the ear and gently stream of the fluid against the sides of canal	To permit direction for flow and outflow if stream is directed forcefully against eardrum, it is possible to rupture it
7. If an irrigating container is used, elevate not >15 cm (6 inches)	To provide safe and effective pressure of fluid if height is >6 inches, pressure will be too great and may damage tissue
8. Observe for signs of pain or dizziness	
9. If irrigating does not dislodge the wax, instill several drops of glycerin, Debrox®, or saturated solution of sodium bicarbonate, 2–3 times for 2–3 days	

Table 7.8: Procedure: Instillation of eardrops.

Nursing action	Rationale
1. Explain the procedure to the patient	To gain his consent and cooperation
2. Collect and prepare the equipment	
3. Assist the patient to sit in an upright position with his head tithed slightly from the affected ear	
4. Check the drug prescription with the ear drops label and expiry date	To avoid getting wrong mediation
5. Wash and dry hands	
6. Pull the pinna of the ear gently in an upward and backward direction	To straighten the ear canal
7. Insert the prescribed number of ear drops into the canal	
8. Position a piece of cotton wool at the entrance of the canal	To avoid tickling of medicine from the canal
9. Dispose of the equipment	
10. Wash and dry hands	
11. Documents the procedure	

Procedure

Ear drops instillation procedure is shown in **Table 7.8**.

APPLICATION OF DRUGS IN OTHER FORMS (TROPICAL DRUGS) (TABLE 7.9)

Equipment

1. Flat wooden spatula
2. Sterile topical swabs
3. Applicators

Procedure

Application of tropical drugs is depicted in **Table 7.9**.

Table 7.9: Procedure: Application of drugs in other forms (tropical drugs).

Nursing action	Rationale
1. Explain the procedure to the patient	To obtain the patient's consent and cooperation
2. Use aseptic technique if the skin is broken	To prevent local or systemic infection
3. Remove semisolid or stiff preparations from their containers with a flat wooden spatula. Use a different spatula each time if more of the preparation is required	To prevent cross infection
4. If the medication is to be rubbed into the skin, then the preparation should be placed on a sterile topical swab, wearing of gloves may be necessary	To avoid cross infection. To protect the nurse
5. If the preparation causes staining, advise the patient of this	To ensure that adequate precautions are taken

INHALATION

Inhalation of medication are aerosol administered in small dosage and breathed in by the patient, which helps drugs to be absorbed easily from lower respiratory tract. Bronchodilator helps relaxed passage provide an opened respiratory passageway. Inhalation drugs administered by inhaler, the hand held metered dose inhaler is often used.

Guidelines for Using Inhaler

1. Assess the patient—which inhaler is using
2. Demonstrate how to use nebulizer
3. Verify allergy
4. Explain action of medication

Steps of Administrating Meter Dose Inhaler

1. Remove the mouthpiece cover and shake inhaler well
2. Remove the cover
3. Have the patient place the mouthpiece into mouth, grasping securely with teeth and lips
4. Ask the patient to take deep breath, exhales hold the inhaler 1–2 inches away from the mouth
5. Inhale slowly and deeply and continues to inhale for a full breath
6. Instruct patient to hold breath for 5–10 seconds and then exhale slowly through pursed lips
7. Have the patient gargle and rinse with tap water after using inhaler

Steps of Administrating Small Volume Nebulizer

1. Perform all preparation steps as above
2. Remove the nebulizer cup from the device
3. Place premeasured unit dose medication in the bottom
4. Screw the top portion of the nebulizer cup back and attach the cup to the nebulizer

5. Attach one end of tubing to the stem and other end to the air compressor or oxygen source
6. Turn on air compressor or oxygen
7. Have the patient place the mouth piece into mouth and grapes securely with teeth and lips
8. Have patient inhale slowly and deeply through the mouth and hold each breath slight pause before exhaling
9. Have patient continue till all medication in nebulizer is aerosolized
10. Have the patient gargle the mouth after using the nebulizer

Insulin Administration

Procedure for insulin administration is depicted in **Table 7.10**.

Purpose

To control the blood glucose level in a diabetic patient.

Table 7.10: Procedure: Insulin administration.

Nursing action	Rationale
1. Check the physician's written order	To obtain specific instructions and information
2. Identify the patient (refer to identification protocol)	To fulfill legal requirement and hospital policy
3. Explain procedure to the patient. Encourage the patient to participate in the procedure	To allay patient's fears and gain confidence and cooperation. To promote patient's education
4. Ensure privacy	To avoid unnecessary embarrassment to the patient during the procedure
5. Wash and dry hands	To prevent cross infection
6. Prior to withdraw insulin, roll the vial between hands (long acting only)	To ensure proper mixing
7. Clean the top of the insulin vial with spirit swab and leave to dry	
8. Draw air into the syringe corresponding to the prescribed amount	To facilitate easy withdrawal
9. Stand insulin vial upright, insert needle and inject air into the vial	
10. Turn the vial upside down with the needle still inserted. Make sure that the needle, level is below the surface level of insulin. Pull back the plunger and extract the required amount of insulin	
11. Tap the syringe barrel and push in the plunger to correct level. Withdraw needle and syringe from vial by pulling on barrel	To expel any air bubbles. To prevent accidental pulling of plunger

Equipment

1. Clinically clean tray
2. Sterile and disposable insulin syringe and needle
3. Spirit swab
4. Prescribed type of insulin and physician's prescription

Types of Insulin

1. Short-acting insulin
2. Intermediate acting insulin
3. Long-acting insulin

Mixing Medication from Two Vials

Definition

Occasionally, the nurse must mix medications from two vials or from a vial and an ampoule **(Table 7.11)**. Mixing medications from a vial and ampoule is simple, by adding air to the ampoule

Table 7.11: Procedure: Mixing parenteral medication from two vials.

Medications from vials	
Nursing action	Rationale
1. Check the physician's medication order	To obtain specific instructions/information
2. Determine medications to be mixed and sterility of vials/ampoules. Determine correct dose and amount	To prevent the risk of error and ensure that correct dosage is prepared
3. Wash and dry hands.	To prevent cross infection.
4. Assemble supplies at clean work area/or treatment room	To perform the procedure in an appropriate area
5. Take syringe and aspirate volume of air equipment to first medication's dosage (vial A)	Air must be introduced into vial to create positive pressure needed to withdraw solution
6. Stand vial A upright-insert needle. Inject air into vial A, making sure needle does not touch solution	To prevent cross contamination
7. Withdraw needle anal syringe and then aspirate air equivalent to second medication's dose (vial B)	Air injected into vial to withdraw desired dose
8. Stand vial B upright-insert needle into vial B, inject air. Invert vial then fill syringe with prescribed volume of medication from vial B	
9. Withdraw needle and syringe from vial by pulling on barrel. Check the dose	To prevent accidental pulling of plunger, which may cause loss of medication. To ensure correct dose is prepared

Contd...

Contd...

Nursing Action	**Rationale**
10. Determine, at which point on the syringe scale, the combined volume of medication measures	To prevent accidental withdrawal of too much medication from second vial
11. Insert needle into vial A, being careful not to push plunger and expel medication into vial. Invert vial and carefully withdraw desired amount of medication into syringe	Positive pressure within vial A allows fluid to fill syringe without the need to aspirate
12. Withdraw needle and expel any excess air from syringe	Air bubbles should not be injected into tissues
13. Change needle on syringe. Do not remove cap or sheath from needle	New needles prevent tracking of medication into tissues
14. Dispose of soiled needle and supplies in proper receptacles	To control spread of infection and prevent accidents
15. Wash and dry hands	

then withdraw the medication. The nurse first prepares medications from the vial first and then, using the same syringe and needle withdraws medication from the ampoule.

Purposes

To avoid having to give the patient more than one injection at a time.

Nursing Alert

1. It is essential that any medications mixed must be compatible.
2. When mixing medications, the nurse must simply remember the differences in how to correctly aspirate fluid from each type of container.
3. When using multidose vials, the nurse must not contaminate the vial's contents with medication from one ampoule or vial to another.
4. If excess medication is accidentally withdrawn from vial B, the procedure of reconstitution must be recommenced.

Equipment

1. Single-dose or multidose vials and ampoules containing medications
2. Syringe with needle
3. Extra sterile disposable needles
4. Alcohol swabs
5. Containers for disposing of syringes, needles, and vial'ampoules
6. Medication prescription sheet

Mixing Insulin

Insulin is a hormone used in the treatment of diabetes, a combination of different types of insulin to control blood sugar levels could be required. Regular insulin is a clear solution that can be given subcutaneously or intravenously. Modified types of insulin are cloudy solutions because of the addition of a protein, which slows absorption **(Table 7.12)**.

Table 7.12: Procedure for mixing insulin.

Nursing action	**Rationale**
1. Check the physician's medication sheet	To obtain specific instructions/information
2. Determine insulins to be mixed and sterility of vials	To prevent the risk of error and ensure that correct dosage is prepared
3. Wash and dry hands	To prevent cross contamination
4. Assemble supplies at clean work area/or treatment room	To perform the procedure in an appropriate area
5. Take insulin syringe and aspirate volume of air equivalent to dosage to be withdrawn from modified insulin	Air must be introduced into vial to create pressure needed to withdraw solution
6. Stand vial upright, insert needle. Inject air into vial of modified insulin. Make sure that the needle does not touch the solution	To prevent cross contamination
7. Withdraw needle and syringe from vial and aspirate air equivalent to be withdrawn from unmodified regular insulin	Air is injected into vial to withdraw desired dose
8. Insert needle into vial of unmodified regular insulin, inject air, and then fill syringe with proper regular insulin dose	Always fill syringe with unmodified regular insulin first to prevent contamination of the regular insulin bottle with NPH or lente insulin. The immediate effect required from short-acting regular insulin can be modified, if contaminated by longer acting insulin
9. Withdraw needle and syringe from vial by pulling on barrel. Check the dose	To prevent accidental pulling of plunger, which may cause loss of medication? To ensure correct dose prepared
10. Determine at which point onto syringe scale combined units of insulin measures	To prevent accidental withdrawal of too much insulin from second vial
11. Insert needle into vial of modified insulin. Be careful not to push plunger and expel medication into vial. Invert vial and carefully withdraw desired amount of insulin into syringe	Positive pressure within vial of modified insulin allows fluid to fill syringe without the need to aspirate

Contd...

Contd...

Nursing action	Rationale
12. Withdraw needle and check insulin level in syringe. Check dosage. Change needle on syringe	To ensure an accurate dose. Insulin overdose can cause serious hypoglycemia. Accurate dose ensures safe medication administration
13. Dispose of soiled supplies in proper receptacle	To control spread of infection
14. Wash and dry hands (refer to hand wash procedure)	

Nursing Alert

1. Regular insulin can be mixed with any other type of insulin.
2. Lente insulins can be mixed with regular insulin, but should not be mixed with any other types of insulin.
3. Mixtures of insulins should be administered within 5 minutes of preparation, at the regular insulin binds neutral protamine Hagedorn (NPH) and the action of regular insulin is reduced.
4. First withdraw unmodified regular insulin to prevent contamination of the regular insulin bottle with NPH or lente insulin. Second, the immediate effect required from short acting regular insulin can be modified further if contaminated by longer-acting insulins.
5. Always refer to guidelines of the manufacturer.

Heparin Lock

Definition

Heparin lock is an intermittent infusion that permits administration of periodic intravenous medications/solutions without continuous fluid administration and aspiration of blood samples for laboratory analysis the procedure is explain below in **Table 7.13 to 7.15**.

Equipment

1. #21-gauge intermittent infusion reservoir, cannula or catheter infusion device with latex port adapter attached
2. Foil-wrapped alcohol sponge so iodine-based antiseptic
3. Rubber tourniquet
4. 2 × 2 inch gauze squares
5. ½ inch tape
6. Tuberculin syringe containing prescribed 0.5 mL heparin solution (100 U/mL) or other prescribed amount of heparin
7. One 5–10 mL syringe containing normal saline solution with # 25-gauge needle

Table 7.13: Procedure: Administration of heparin lock.

Nursing action	Rationale
1. Check the physician's order, progress notes, and care plan	To obtain specific instructions and/or information
2. Identify the patient	To perform the right procedure on the right patient
3. Explain nature and purpose of heparin lock to the patient	His understanding will facilitate proper functioning of the lock
4. Wash and dry hands (refer to handwashing procedure)	To prevent cross contamination
5. Ensure patient's privacy	To avoid unnecessary embarrassment to the patient during the procedure
6. Prepare selected site for infusion reservoir as described in vein puncture	
7. Cleanse rubber injection port of heparin lock	Firmly rub, using alcohol sponge
8. Insert #25-gauge needle a syringe containing normal saline solution into injection port	Small gauge needle will prevent large puncture openings
9. Flush cannula-reservoir system with solution (usual volume is 1–2 mL)	This will release air bubble from reservoir
10. After confirming the position of the needle in the vein, secure wings with adhesive	Carefully aspirate blood to verify needle position
11. Inject 2 mL of normal saline solution	Observe site for evidence of infiltration
12. Remove saline syringe with needle from injection port	Continue to observe site for evidence of infiltration
13. Cover with 2 × 2 inch gauze square; secure with ½ inch tape	To reduce possibility of infection
14. Replace with needle and syringe containing heparin holding solution	Strict asepsis is observed in making this switch
15. Inject 0.5 mL heparinized saline solution (or other prescribed dose)	Heparinized saline solution will keep the line open for the next injection
16. Remove needle and syringe from injection port	

Table 7.14: Administration of heparin medication.

Nursing action	Rationale
1. Prepare the medication to be administered by drawing it into the appropriate syringe	
2. Draw 2 mL of normal saline solution into each of 2 syringes	Heparin is incompatible with many antibiotics; saline solution is used before and after administration to prevent mixing of 2 incompatible drugs
3. Draw heparinized saline solution into a syringe if prescribed	
4. Explain to the patient what you are about to do	
5. Cleanse injection site of the heparin lock with methylated spirit. Insert normal saline syringe needle into port and aspirate slightly	When positive blood return is not obtained, monitor site carefully to detect infiltration
6. Inject normal saline to flush reservoir of heparinized saline and remove syringe	Note any signs of inflammation or infiltration, also observe the patient for signs of discomfort. If such signs are present, discontinue injection
7. Insert medication syringe, administer drug, and remove syringe	Maintain stability of system by inserting sterile equipment
8. Insert saline syringe, and flush reservoir slowly, then remove syringe	Saline solution will clear the reservoir of medication and prepare the way for heparinized saline solution
9. Inject Heparinized saline solution into reservoir if prescribed	The usual heparin is 10–100 units in 1–2 mL
10. Remove heparin syringe and needle from injection port	Treatment is completed

Table 7.15: Follow-up activities.

Nursing action	Rationale
1. Maintain patency of heparin lock by flushing it every 8 hours	If resistance is met, device should not be flushed. Attempt to remove occlusion via aspiration. If unable to restore patency, remove IV device
2. Record all actions and medications	

Contd...

Contd...

Nursing action	Rationale
3. Heparin lock should not be left in place longer than 48–72 hours	NITA standards; communicable disease center guidelines
4. IV administration sets for intermittent therapy should be changed every 24 hours or immediately upon contamination. A new sterile needle should be used for each entry into the intermittent cannula device	Since the tubing is not maintained as a closed system, it is at higher risk for infection

Wing Tipped Cannula Insertion

Equipment

Same as cannulation guidelines:
1. Tape—½" × 2" strip × 2
2. Tape—1" × 3" strip × 2

Substitute for cannula: One wing-tip cannula (gauge and length depending on reason for insertion and condition of veins). Procedure is explained in **Table 7.16**.

Table 7.16: Procedure: Wing tipped cannula insertion.

Nursing action	Rationale
1. Follow steps 1 to 7 in cannulation guideline	
2. While site is drying, prepare equipment. Draw up 5 mL sterile saline from ampoule using needle. Attach syringe to winged-tip cannula tubing and flush with saline. Using device only for blood sampling, attach empty sterile syringe to end of tubing	Needles must be discarded after one use
3. Prepare tape as instructed	
4. Reapply tourniquet	
5. Pinch wings firmly together between thumb and index finger of one hand	Bevel up
6. Apply skin traction	Same as cannula insertion Step 13
7. Hold tip of cannula with bevel up in direction of venous flow	

Contd...

Contd...

Nursing action	Rationale
8. Place tip of needle on skin directly over the vein. Pierce through skin and tissue and into the vein with one motion (approximately 30° angle)	If not successful, pull needle back to where bevel entered beneath the skin surface, locate vein and attempt again
9. Verify entry into vein by flashback of blood	
10. Decrease angle of cannula until it is parallel to the skin and simultaneously lift entire needle up	To avoid piercing through the vein's bottom wall
11. Advance cannula cautiously into the lumen of the vein	Remember to keep the needle lifted up
12. Release traction	
13. Position wings flat on skin surface	
14. Stabilize the needle in place with your thumb	
15. Release tourniquet	
16. Draw back on syringe to ensure blood return	
17. Connect IV infusion tubing	See cannula procedure
18. Place ½" × 2" tape one strip over each wing "H" parallel to the cannula	"H" taping—anchoring tape should not touch the insertion site
19. Place 1" × 3" tape across the plastic wings	"H" taping—anchoring tape should not touch the insertion site
20. Cover site with dressing (date and time should be on tape)	
21. Coil excessive tubing up and tape in convenient place on patient's skin	
22. Follow down procedure	

MEANING OF PARENTERAL ROUTE OF EPIDURAL, INTRATHECAL, INTRAOSSEOUS, INTRAPERITONEAL, INTRAPLEURAL, INTRA-ARTERIAL

Epidural Injection

An epidural involves injecting medication around spinal cord to epidural space. The epidural space is surrounded by spinal cord.

Epidural analgesia can be used to provide pain relief during the immediate postoperative phase after thoracic, abdominal, orthopedics and vascular surgery and chronic pain situation.

Intrathecal Injection

Intrathecal so-called subarachnoid space, the intrathecal space is the fluid filled area located between the innermost layer of covering the pia matter of the spinal cord and middle layer of covering the arachnoids matter.

An intrathecal injection can help control pain after surgery. An anesthesiologist gives injection around the spinal cord. An intrathecal injection can reduce the amount of other medicines needed to control pain.

Intraosseous Injection

Intraosseous injection is the process of injecting medication, fluids or blood products directly into the marrow of bone. This a non-collapsible entry point into the venous system.

Intraosseous location such as sternum, clavicle, humeral head, iliac crest, distal femur, proximal tibia, distal tibia site and calcaneus are potential site for intraosseous space.

Intraperitoneal Injection

Intraperitoneal (IP) injection is the injection of a substance into the peritoneum, within the peritoneal cavity. The injection site will be in the lower left or right quadrant of the abdomen. There is a fast uptake of the drug from the peritoneal cavity.

Intrapleural Injection

An intrapleural drug in injected through the chest wall into the pleural space or instilled through a chest tube placed intrapleural for drainage. Intrapleural administered drugs diffuse across the parietal pleura and innermost intercostals nerves. During intrapleural injection of a drug, the needle passes through the intercostals muscle and parietal pleura on its way to the pleural space.

Drugs commonly given by intrapleural injection include tetracycline, streptokinase, anesthetics, and chemotherapeutic agents.

Intra-arterial Injection

Intra-arterial medication is administered directly into the arteries. Intra-arterial infusions are common in clients who have arterial clots.

IMPORTANT DATES IN NURSING (OUTLINES OF WORLD NURSING HISTORY)

1. **5000 to 4000 BC.** Egyptian medicine
2. **3000 BC.** Beginning of Chinese medicine
3. **2000 BC.** Babylonian medicine
4. **1200 BC.** Vedas written in India
5. **400 BC.** Hippocrates the Greek, father of medicine
6. **250 BC.** King Asoka, the best era of medicine in India
7. **936.** First hospital in England, at York

UNIT 7: Introduction to Clinical Pharmacology

8. **1123.** St. Bartholomew's Hospital, London founded
9. **1213.** St. Thomas' Hospital, London, founded
10. **1517.** The reformation began
11. **1600 to about 1850.** The dark period of nursing
12. **1633.** Sisters of charity organized
13. **1640.** First hospital built by the Ursuline Sisters, at Quebec
14. **1664.** Hotel Dieu of Montreal built
15. **1836.** Flinders Deaconess Hospital at Kaiserswerth opened
16. **1859.** The school of La Source founded
17. **1820.** Florence Nightingale was born
18. **1851.** Took training at Kaiserswerth
19. **1854-56** In Crimean War.
20. **1856.** The Nightingale Fund
21. **1860.** Founded the Nightingale school at St. Thomas
22. **1874.** First school of nursing established, at St. Catherine's Ont
23. **1910.** Florence Nightingale died.
24. **1858.** William Rathbone organized visiting nursing in Liverpool
25. **1881.** Army Nurse Crops established
26. **1885.** The Lady Dufferin fund established
27. **1893.** The British Journal of Nursing established
28. **1900.** The International Council of Nurses founded
29. **1919.** Registration bill passed by British parliament
30. **1922.** International course in public health nursing established at Bedford college, London
31. **1730.** Blockley Hospital, Philadelphia
32. **1770.** The New York hospital founded
33. **1800.** Valentine Seaman of the New York hospital began to teach nurses systematically
34. **1809.** American branch of sisters of charity founded
35. **1839.** The Nurse Society of Philadelphia began training of midwives
36. **1861.** The Woman's Hospital of Philadelphia planned a course in nursing, it was reorganized in 1872
37. **1872.** New England Hospital for Women began its School of Nursing
38. **1873.** Bellevue Hospital, New York. New Haven Hospital, Conn. Massachusetts General Hospital Boston
39. **1877.** First organized visiting nurse society (New York)
40. **1881-1890.** Period of organization of many protestant religious hospitals and schools of nursing
41. **1882.** First school of nursing in a mental hospital, McLean at Waverly, Massachusetts
42. **1882.** Period of organization of many catholic school of nursing
43. **1866.** Founding of the Red Cross Society
44. **1882.** United States entered the Red Cross Society
45. **1885.** First school of nursing in Australia
46. **1888.** First school of nursing established in New Zeeland
47. **1888.** Organization of Mills School for Men Nurses, Bellevue Hospital, NY.
48. **1895.** Nurse appointed as assistant inspector of hospitals in New Zeeland
49. **1912.** Florence Nightingale medal established by the International Red Cross Society
50. **1920.** Division of nursing of the league of Red Cross Societies established
51. **1920.** Military rank given to American Nurses
52. **1902.** Establishment of school nursing, New York City
53. **1919.** First University School of Nursing at University of British Columbia
54. **1931.** The League of Nations appointed a nurse as health secretary. She was an American, Miss Hazel Goff, who had worked under the American Red Cross Society and the Rockefeller Foundation in Eastern Europe
55. **1922.** The ICN appointed a committee on international standards in nursing education
56. **1936.** Standard curriculum published

WORLD NURSING ORGANIZATION HISTORY

1. **England**
   - The national council of nurses for Great Britain and Ireland, a union of alumni societies, was formed in 1908.
   - The British College of Nurses, was founded in 1926 by Mrs Bedford Fenwick, it has over 20,000 members, with headquarters in London.
   - The General Nursing Council for England and Wales is the national board for approval of schools of nursing, planning curricula, holding examination and registering nurses. It is a statutory body, established in 1919.

2. **Canada**
   - The Canadian Society of Superintendent of training schools for Nurses was organized in 1908. In 1917, its name was changed to the Canadian Association of Nurse Education, and its membership opened to all engaged in training nurses.
   - The Canadian National Association for Trained Nurses was organized in 1908. It is now the Canadian Nurses Association.

3. **Scotland**
   - The Matrons' Council of Scotland
   - The Scottish Nurses Association

4. **Ireland**
   - The Irish Nurses Association was formed first in 1900, as the Dublin Nurses Club. It becomes the national association in 1904. It is now the National Council of Trained Nurses of the Irish Free State.

5. **France**
   - A National Association of Trained Nurses of France was organized in 1924.

6. **Germany**
   - The German Nurses Association was organized in 1903. It is now Nurses Association of Germany. It has headquarters in Berlin.

7. **Belgium**
   - There is a National Federation of Belgian Nurses and a General Nursing Council attached to the ministry of health.
8. **Holland**
   - Nosokomos, the Dutch Nurses Association was organized in 1900.
   - The Male Nurses of Holland have a national association.
9. **Sweden**
   - The General Council of Swedish nurses was organized in 1910. It is now the Swedish association.
10. **Norway**
    - The National Council of Nurses, now the Norwegian Nurses Association was formed in 1912.
11. **Denmark**
    - The Danish Council of Nurses was formed in 1899.
12. **Iceland**
    - The Icelandic Nurses Association has its headquarters at Reykjavik, the capital.
13. **Switzerland**
    - There is a Swiss Nurses Association
14. **Italy**
    - The National Organization is the Fascist syndicate for professional nurses.
15. **Greece**
    - The Graduate Nurses Association of Greece was founded in 1924.
16. **Yugoslavia**
    - The Yugoslavian Graduate Nurses Association has its headquarters in Belgrade.
17. **Bulgaria**
    - The Bulgarian Nurses Association was organized in 1924.
18. **Poland**
    - The National Council of Polish Professional Nurses was organized in 1925.
19. **Czechoslovakia**
    - The Graduate Nurses Association of Czechoslovakia has its headquarters in Prague.
20. **Estonia**
    - There is an Estonian Nurses Association founded in 1923 and a Latvian Red Cross Nurses Association founded in 1922.
21. **Finland**
    - The Association of Nurses in Finland, now the National Council of Nurses of Finland, was organized in 1898.
22. **Australia**
    - The Australasian Trained Nurses Association was organized in 1899. The Royal Victorian Trained Nurses Association was organized in 1901, with a doctor as president. In 1911, it elected a nurse as the president. There is a branch of the British Nurses Association in South Australia.
23. **New Zealand**
    - The New Zealand Trained Nurses Association was formed by uniting four local associations, those of Wellington, Dunedin, Auckland, and Christchurch. A central council was elected in 1909.
24. **South Africa**
    - The South African Trained Nurses Association was founded in 1914. It has nine branches.
25. **India**
    - The Association of Nursing Superintendents of India was organized in 1905.
    - The Trained Nurses Association of India, organized in 1910 the Bombay Presidency Nurses Association held its first examination for nurses, a beginning of registration.
26. **China**
    - The Nurses' Association of China was organized in 1909. At the request of the government its name was in 1936 changed to the Nurses Educational Association of China. It has both Chinese and foreign members, the president being Chinese. It has a central examining and registration board.
27. **Japan**
    - The Nurses Association of Japan founded in 1929, it has headquarters at Tokyo.
28. **The Philippines**
    - The Filipino Nurses Association has headquarters at Manila.
29. **Korea**
    - The Nurses Association of Korea was formed in 1923.
30. **Cuba**
    - The National Association of Nurses of Cuba was formed in 1909.
31. **Brazil**
    - The Brazilian Graduate Nurses Association has its headquarters at Rio de Janeiro.
    - The International Catholic Federation of Nurses, started in United States, has branches in Canada, Germany, France, and Holland.

World Nursing Organization history at that time of beginning, present status changed in countries.

WORLD HISTORY OF NURSING JOURNAL

In 1935, there were 56 national nursing journals, published in 17 languages.
1. **United States:** The American Journal of Nursing was established in 1900 as a stock company of nurses. It is the property and official organ of the American Nurses' Association, the official organ of the national league of nursing education and of nearly all of the state societies. Miss Sophia Palmer of Rochester, NY, was its editor until her death.
   - **The trained nurses and hospital review** was established in 1888. It was the first nursing and

hospital journal and did a valuable pioneer work. In 1989, it combined with the journal of practical nursing, and later absorbed, one at a time. The nightingale, the nurse, the nursing world, and the nursing record. It was for 10 years the only nursing and hospital journal of America.

- The pacific coast Journal of Nursing was established in 1909 by the Visiting Nurse Association of Cleveland, Ohio, it is the official organ of the national organization for public health nursing. It is now named public health nursing.

2. **Canada:** The Canadian nurse began in 1905 as an alumnae quarterly of Toronto General Hospital.
3. **England:** The British Journal of Nursing was established in 1839 as an outgrowth of the nursing record of 1888.
    a. Nursing notes and Midwives Chronicle: a weekly is the official organ of the midwives institute.
    b. Nursing mirror was originally included in the hospital the hospital the organ of the hospitals association of Great Britain.
    c. The nursing times is a weekly.
4. **Ireland:** The Irish Nursing and Hospital World is the official organ of the national society.
5. **Scotland:** The Scottish Nurse is published in Glasgow.
6. **France:** An official magazine, The French Nurse was started in 1924.
7. **Germany:** Unterm Lazarus Kreuz was established in Berlin in 1906, it is the official organ of the German Nurses Association.
8. **Holland:** Nosokomos, the (nursing) was established in Amsterdam near 1905. The Journal of Nursing was a bimonthly published by the Bond established in 1890.
9. **Sweden:** Svensk Sjukskoterskelidning is the official publication of the national association. The Swedish Nurses Journal "Humanitet" was established at Stockholm in 1909.
10. **Norway:** The Nursing Journal was established in 1912. It is the official journal.
11. **Denmark:** The Journal of Nursing was established at Copenhagen in 1901, it is the official organ of the national society.
12. **Belgium:** De Vlaamsche Verpleging was published at Antwerp before the war, is the Official Nursing Journal of Belgium.
13. **Finland:** Epione, established in 1907, is the official organ of the National Nursing Association, it is published at Helsinki.
14. **Bulgaria:** An Official Nursing Journal, Sestra, was begun in 1924.
15. **Czechoslovakia:** A nursing journal called, News, was first published in 1925 and is continued.
16. **Yugoslavia:** Yugoslavia has nursing journal.
17. **Poland:** The Polish Nurse was published first in 1929. It is the official magazine.
18. **Greece:** The Greek Red Cross publishes the nursing journal of the country.
19. **Switzerland:** The Swiss nursing magazine, a publication of years, standing is managed by doctors.
20. **Latvia:** Latvia began in 1929 to publish a quarterly nursing journal. It is called the nurse (zelsirdiga Masa).
21. **Australia:** The Australian Nurse's Journal published at Sydney, NSW, is the official, organ of the Australian Trained Nurses Association. Una, published at Melbourne, is the official organ of the Royal Victorian Trained Nurses Association.
22. **New Zealand:** Kaitiaki, a quarterly established in 1908, was until 1923 the private property of Miss Hester Maclean, its editor. At that time it was taken over by the National Nurses Association and made an official magazine.
23. **South Africa:** The South African Nursing record was founded in 1913 by Dr Tremble, who was its editor. It is the official organ of the South African Trained Nurses Association.
24. **India:** The Nursing Journal of India was established in 1910. It is the official organ of the two nursing societies.
25. **China:** The quarterly Journal of Chinese Nurses was established in 1919. It is owned and published by the Nurses Association of China. It is printed in both English and Chinese.
26. **Korea:** The Nursing Journal of Korea is published in two languages.
27. **Japan:** A nursing magazine "Doho" (the nurse), was established in 1997.
28. **The Philippines:** The quarterly journal, the Filipino Nurse, was begun in 1925. It is published by the Filipino Nurses Association and is in English.
29. **Cuba:** The Official Nursing Journal of Cuba is La Enfermera Nacional. It is published from Havana.

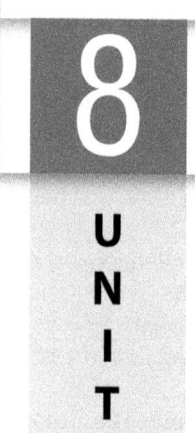

First Aid

LEARNING OBJECTIVES

After completing this unit, learner will be able to:
- Definition, aims of first aid
- Describe general principles of first aid
- Explain concept of emergency
- Describe procedures and techniques in first aid
- Describe preparation of first aid kit
- Explain dressing, bandaging, splinting (spiral, reverse spiral, figure of eight, breast, jaw, spica, shoulder, hip, ankle, thumb, finger, stump, single and double eyes, single and double ears, breast, jaw, capeline), triangle bandage uses, abdominal binder and bandage, breast binder, T and many tail bandage, knots reef, clove
- State transportation of injured
- Describe CPR: External cardiac massage
- Discuss first aid in emergencies
  - Asphyxia, drowning, shock
  - Wounds and bleeding
  - Injuries to the bones, joints, strains hanging, falls
  - Burns and scalds
  - Poisoning—ingestion, inhalation, bites and stings
  - Foreign body in eye, ear, nose and throat
- Explain community emergencies and community resources
  - Fire, explosion, floods, earthquakes, famines, etc.
  - Role of nurses in disaster management
  - Rehabilitation
  - Community resources
    ◊ Police, ambulance services
    ◊ Voluntary agencies-local state national and international

INTRODUCTION

First aid has been practised ever since the beginning of humanity. Learning *first aid* is the civic responsibility of every citizen. All of us should be able to perform first aid because we will eventually find ourselves in a situation requiring it, either for another or for ourselves. The risk of injury while traveling, working or playing is so great, that most people sustain a significant injury at sometime during their lives.

An organized worldwide effort at recognizing the importance of first aid came only in the year 1877 with the formation of the St. John Ambulance Association of England named after the great Apostle St. John. Mahatma Gandhi also was a great supporter of the cause of first aid, and led a band of dedicated Ambulance Corps volunteers during the time of the Boer war (1899) and during the time of Zulu Rebellion (1906).

DEFINITION OF FIRST AID

First aid is the first and immediate assistance given to any person suffering from either a minor or serious illness or injury, with care provided to preserve life, prevent the condition from worsening or to promote recovery.

What is First Aid?

First aid is the immediate treatment given to the victim of an accident or sudden illness, before medical help is obtained. First aid does not take the place of proper medical treatment. It consists only of giving temporary assistance until competent medical care is obtained if needed, or until the chance for recovery without medical care is ensured. Most injuries and illnesses require only first aid care. Properly applied, first aid may mean the difference between life and death, rapid recovery and long hospitalization, or temporary disability and permanent injury.

AIMS OF FIRST AID

The main aims of first aid are:
- To preserve life
- To promote recovery
- To prevent the worsening of the victim's condition
- To transport the victim safely to the healthcare facility, if needed

GENERAL PRINCIPLES OF FIRST AID

Keep Calm

The most basic principle of first aid is to keep calm at the accident scene. Doing so will help to decrease the victim's fears and anxieties, and will help to ensure that the best first-aid care is provided during stabilization and treatment. Remember, excitement is contagious–keep yourself calm.

Identify Yourself

Accident victims may be very upset and reluctant to accept assistance from a stranger. If you force the victim to accept assistance, your offer might be rejected. You should earn his/her confidence by conducting yourself in a professional manner.

Evaluate the Situation

When you approach the accident scene, make a quick and thorough assessment of what may have happened. Be alert. Use all your senses for complete observation and anticipate the types of injuries, if any, that may have resulted. Your ability to complete on objective evaluation of what happened will help to determine the immediate corrective action required and will help to ensure that adequate first aid is provided.

Protect the Accident Scene

To ensure the safety of the victim(s) and yourself, you must control or eliminate any immediate danger or potential for additional injuries. When this is not possible, the victim(s) should be moved to a place where first-aid core and assistance can be safely provided. Anticipate danger or you may become the next accident victim.

Keep by Standers Away

An accident scene tends to attract spectators. In many cases, these onlookers have an adverse effect on the victim by creating confusion and/or causing unnecessary alarm which may increase the likelihood that the victim will go into shock. Whenever possible, disperse spectators as soon as possible and protect the victim's privacy.

Be Aware of Common Responses at an Accident Scene

An accident scene can create confusion that may cause the individuals involved to make irrational decisions. Be aware of the following normal responses:
a. **First-aid administrant:** The first-aid administrant may do nothing for fear of making the situation worse. She may move the victim and/or administer liquids for no reason other than "to do something," or may interfere with others who are providing assistance thinking, "I can do it better".
b. **Accident victim:** The accident victim may cry, shout or exhibit extreme behavior. He/she may get up, walk around, leave the scene or refuse medical assistance for fear it might make the situation worse. The victim may also become depressed, uncooperative or irrational.

Make the Victim Comfortable

Talk calmly and with authority. Advise the victim that you will provide assistance. Place the victim in a comfortable position. Be reassuring and responsive to the victim's concerns. Encourage him/her to relax. Let the victim tell you when he/she feel comfortable.

Keep the Victim Lying Down (If Possible)

It is easier to provide care while the victim is lying down. You should never move or force the victim to lie down until all major injuries (real or suspected) are stabilized. Move slowly while providing first aid. Do not force the victim to do anything that causes discomfort or create additional stress.

Check the Victim for ID

Essential first aid does not include identifying the victim; however, checking the victim's personal belongings may provide important information such as medical conditions, allergies, blood type or medications. It may also be necessary to notify the victim's relatives if the injuries are serious or fatal. Always be certain that you have sufficient witnesses if you look through the victim's personal belongings.

Examine the Victim

A quick but thorough examination is necessary to determine the extent of injury. Talk to the victim and keep his/her attention while you conduct the examination. Be sure you check all parts of the body. Always respect the victim's right to privacy. Solicit the help and witnesses if needed.

Never Permit the Victim to Know the Extent of Injury

The victim knows he/she is injured and in pain. Do not arouse additional concern with facial reactions or remarks about the seriousness of the injuries. These actions can adversely affect the victim's mental attitude, can cause shock or may influence the victim's recovery rate.

Prepare for the Worst

It is not always possible to accurately determine the extent of injury. The care you give should be guided by the victim's complaints and your assessment of what might have occurred. There is no harm in providing too much first aid. A victim will not typically complain if too much first aid is provided (e.g., applying splint when the arm or leg is not broken). Conversely, providing insufficient first aid may cause serious problems in the future. Aim to provide the best care possible. Know first-aid priorities.

The four major injury types that require first aid in order of importance include:
1. Serious bleeding (arterial)
2. Cardiac arrest/stoppage of breathing
3. Internal poisoning
4. Shock

After providing care for the above conditions, then consider addressing the following injuries:
1. Fractures
2. Burns
3. Concussions
4. Lacerations
5. Animal bites
6. Other injuries

These types of injuries are not generally life-threatening; however, they can be serious and may lead to shock or even death.

1. **Be familiar with first-aid equipment and materials:** Adequate first-aid equipment and materials are not always readily available at an accident scene. Do not excite the victim by expressing your concern. Attempt to improvise. If you cannot provide adequate assistance, make the victim as comfortable as possible and call for help.

2. **Keep the victim warm:** Cover the victim to protect from the elements and to maintain normal body temperature. Do not overheat the victim. In hot weather, provide shade for the victim. In cold weather, if hot packs are used, make certain that you do not burn the victim. Do not give liquids to an unconscious victim. An unconscious victim may have serious internal injuries and/or may require surgery following transport to a hospital. Moistening the lips will usually provide relief from thirst and satisfy the victim's need for something cool until medical specialists can evaluate his/her condition. Do not permit injured victims to drink large amounts of fluid.

3. **Obtain emergency transportation:** Moving the victim and/or providing emergency transportation is usually necessary for two reasons:
   a. To move the victim to a place where first aid can be safely administered. Do not care for a victim in the middle of a highway or in a burning building-you may be the next victim.
   b. To move the victim to a hospital or physician's office so that additional medical treatment can be provided.

   Whenever possible, obtain professional assistance when transporting an injured victim. Never transport an injured victim in your own automobile unless there is no other alternative.

4. **Provide complete information to emergency personnel:** Excitement at the accident scene is contagious and this causes individuals to forget the facts and become emotional. Remember, help cannot arrive if it does not know where to go. Provide the following information to emergency personnel:
   - Location of emergency
     a. On highways, use route numbers, direction of travel and mile markers
     b. On city streets, use street name, nearest address or street intersection
     c. In other areas, use easily recognizable land marks
   - An account of the incident; number and severity of injuries.
   - Total time elapsed since injuries occurred.
   - Assistance currently being provided.

5. **Appoint someone to watch for emergency vehicles:** Make certain that someone is always available to watch for and to direct emergency vehicles. Nothing is more frustrating for emergency medical crews than to arrive at an accident scene with rescue equipment and be unable to locate the victim(s). Always watch for emergency vehicles. Be ready to provide directions when help arrives.

6. **Cooperate at the accident scene:** Any method or procedure that gets the job done without causing additional injury to the victim is okay. If you see that a procedure is not meeting this objective, suggest a better method and provide an explanation. Do not create confusion at the accident scene. Assist-do not hinder-the administration of first aid.
7. **Do not allow the victim to overhear your conversation:** When an accident victim overhears discussions about the seriousness of injuries, first-aid care requirements, methods of improvising, need for transportation and other issues, the immediate result is an increased concern. Furthermore, when disagreements are overheard at an accident scene, the victim(s) and the observers quickly lose confidence in the quality of the care being provided. Discuss treatment procedure and differences of opinion where you will not be overheard.
8. **Do not leave a seriously injured victim unattended:** Most accident victims have a major concern about the extent of their injuries. If left alone, they may begin to investigate. Awareness of their condition may increase anxiety and cause shock or they may simply getup and begin wandering. By staying with the victim you can continue to be reassuring and the victim will usually remain at rest until additional emergency help arrives.
9. **Administer all necessary first aid before the victim transported**
    - Control serious bleeding
    - Begin resuscitation
    - Immobilize fractures
    - Treat for shock
    - Reassure victim
    - Alert the hospital.
10. **First aid is immediate and temporary care:** First aid is the immediate and temporary care given to the victim of an accident or sudden illness until the services of a physician can be obtained.
11. **Remember, you are not a physician:** You are not certified to make a medical decision or determination. You are providing emergency care for victim of an accident until professional medical assistance can be obtained. You should be reassuring without representing yourself as a physician.
12. **First aid is more than a bandage:** Have a definite reason for what you do. Most importantly, keep yourself calm-excitement is contagious. Learn more about first aid and update your knowledge on first aid.

Rules of First Aid

- Do not delay in reaching the accident spot.
- Be calm, methodical and quick.
- Look for breathing, bleeding and signs of shock.

The first priority is to assess a person's **airway, breathing** and **circulation** (*ABC*). Problem in any of these areas is always fatal if not corrected. The airway (A) the passage through which air travels to the lungs-can become blocked. Various illnesses and injuries can cause breathing (B) to cease. Cardiac arrest-cessation of the heart beat-stops blood from circulating (C) through the body.

CONCEPT OF EMERGENCY

First aid sometime referred to as *emergency aid,* and is the first skilled assistance given to a victim (sick or injured). On the occurrence of accident or sudden illness in order to preserve life, prevent further injury and relive suffering until qualified medical care is available.

PROCEDURES AND TECHNIQUES IN FIRST AID

PREPARATION OF FIRST AID KIT

What is First Aid Kit?

A first aid kit is a collection of supplies and equipment used to give immediate medical treatment. There is wide variation in the contents of first aid kits based on the type of emergency occurs and place at which emergency occurs.

Basic first aid kit should contain:
1. Plasters in a variety of different sizes and shapes
2. Small, medium and large sterile gauze and dressings
3. Sterile eye dressings
4. Triangular bandages
5. Crepe bandages
6. Safety pins
7. Disposable sterile gloves
8. Tourniquet
9. Adhesive tape
10. Band-aid in several size
11. Antibiotic ointment

DRESSING, BANDAGING AND SPLINTING

Wound Dressing: Care of Wounds (Table 8.1)

Definition

A wound is a break in the continuity of the soft parts of body structures, resulting from surgical intervention or injury, causing disruption to the normal tissue pattern.

Table 8.1: Dressing of wound: Procedure.

Nursing action	Rationale
Check the physician's order, progress notes and nursing care plan. It is best to schedule the procedure at the least disruptive time and at least 30 minutes following any cleaning and bed making activity. If the wound is painful, it is wise to perform the procedure 20–30 minutes after analgesic has been administered.	To obtain specific instructions and/or information.
Identify the patient Check identification against the physician's order.	To perform the right procedure on the right patient.
Explain the procedure to the patient Allow him to ask questions.	To allay fears and gain patient's confidence and cooperation. To promote patient's education.
Ensure privacy.	To prevent undue exposure and avoid unnecessary embarrassment to the patient during the procedure.
Assist the patient to get into a comfortable position. Adjust the bed to your waist level if possible.	To maintain body alignment and promote comfort.
Place absorbent pad.	To protect the patient from wetness and keep the bed clean and dry.
Assemble equipment at the patient's bedside and within easy reach.	To gain time and easy handling of equipment.
Wash and dry hands. Asepsis must be maintained throughout the procedure.	To prevent cross-infection. To prepare the sterile package. To prevent local and systemic infection.
Prepare equipment using aseptic technique.	
Get a forceps from the sterile package if not using clean sterile glove. Keep the sterile package covered.	To handle the soiled dressing when removed. This forceps is considered contaminated and should not be used later.
Remove tape along longitudinal axis, slowly and gently. • Peel back edges by holding skin tact and pushing away from tape. • Remove tape near a wound by pulling toward the wound. • Use a suitable solution, e.g., normal saline, if the tape does not pull away easily.	Removing tape in the same plane is less injurious and less painful. It is less traumatic to push skin away from tape than to pull tape from the skin. Pulling away from a wound may tear some of delicate newly formed tissues.
Using forceps or clean gloves, remove the soiled dressing by grasping its outer part.	
Inspect the soiled dressing and packing for drainage.	
Examine the wound, inspect for size, color, edema, drainage, odor, and amount of granulation tissue. Report abnormalities.	
Dispose of the soiled dressing.	
Obtain a wound culture if needed.	
Wash and dry hands.	
Pour solution(s) into sterile container(s).	
Wear sterile gloves if required.	
Perform dressing using aseptic technique.	
Clean and rinse the wound with the prescribed disinfectant solutions.	In case of surgical wound, the suture line is the least contaminated area and should be cleansed first. The dominant hand is considered sterile and is used to obtain supplies from the sterile field. Always work from areas of less contamination (clean to dirty).
Blot the surrounding area dry with sterile gauze pods.	
Cover the wound with sterile dressing.	The dressing should be loosened enough to allow circulation.
Anchor the dressing securely in place. Apply minimum taping necessary to keep dressing in place.	Nonallergic tape is most desirable since it reduces the risk of skin breakdown, is more porous than adhesive tape, and allows air to penetrate it.

Contd...

Contd...

Nursing action	Rationale
Replace the patient's gown or clothing and place the patient in a comfortable position.	
Reposition the bed and raise bed-rails back if required.	
Clean and dispose of equipment as appropriate.	
Clean non-disposable equipment and send to CSSD for sterilization.	
Wash and dry hands.	
Document the procedure in the appropriate charts. Note: Condition of the wound, color, amount and odor of the drainage if present, appearance of the wound, and patient's tolerance and response to treatment.	
Report any abnormal findings.	

Purposes

1. To remove bacteria and foreign bodies from the wound.
2. To debride tissue, or foreign objects that interfere with healing process.
3. To prevent and reduce contamination.
4. To help absorbed drainage and fluid wastes.
5. To control bleeding.
6. To immobilize the injured tissues that healing can occur.
7. To prevent additional trauma.
8. To reduce pain and discomfort.
9. To assess the healing process.

Equipment

1. Clean dressing trolley with sterile instrument dressing set—sterile dressing package 4 × 4 gauze, absorbent pads, cotton swabs, solution cups (2)
2. Cleansing/disinfectant solution and topical medication as per physician's order
3. Clean gloves if required
4. Sterile gloves if required
5. Adhesive tape
6. Bandages
7. Plastic bag for discarded dressing

For wound irrigation add—

8. Disposable apron
9. Sterile wound drain if required
10. Sterile irrigation package
11. Sterile safety pin if required
12. Clean gloves
13. Sterile gloves
14. Sterile syringes and needles
15. Irrigation solution as ordered
16. Receptacle(s)

Bandages

A bandage is a strip of cloth, gauze or elasticized material used to wrap a body part. Bandages are available in various widths, most commonly from 1–6 inches and are usually supplied in rolls for easy application.

Types of Bandages

According to material used:

- **Gauze bandage:** It is lightweight, porous, inexpensive, molds easily to the body and permits air circulation to prevent skin maceration.
- **Elastic bandage:** It is used to exert pressure over a body part, support and improve the venous circulation in the legs.
- **Flannel and muslin bandage:** It is thicker than gauze and thus stronger for supporting or applying pressure. It also provides warmth.
- **Plastic adhesive bandage:** It is waterproof and thus retains wound drainage or keep the body area dry. It also provides some pressure because of elastic property.

According to shape:

- Roller bandages
- Triangular bandages
- T-binder.

General Purposes of Bandages

- To maintain direct pressure over a dressing in order to control bleeding
- To hold dressings or splints in position
- To prevent swelling
- To provide support for a limb or joint
- To restrict movement
- To assist in lifting or carrying casualties (occasionally)
- To absorb the discharge from wounds
- To protect from the invasion of prior organisms.

The width of the bandage used depends upon the size of the body part to be bandaged. The larger the circumference of the part, the wider the bandage. Padding with pads or gauze squares is frequently used to cover bony prominences such as the elbow, or to separate skin surfaces such as fingers.

Width of the bandage	Body part
1 inch	Finger
2 inches	Arm
3–4 inches	Leg
4–6 inches	Thigh

Basic Terms for Roller Bandages

Circular turn
Circular turns are used to cover small body parts such as digit or wrist and are used mainly to anchor and terminate bandages.

Steps
- Unroll 3-4 inches of bandages.
- Place the tail of the bandage on the anterior surface of portion of body to be covered and hold with thumb of nondominant hand.
- Encircle the body part a few times or as often as needed each turn directly covering the previous turn.
- Secure end of bandage with a safety pin or clip. If end of bandage has raw edge, fold 12-1 inch underneath before securing bandage. Gauze bandage may be secured with a strip of adhesive tape.

Spiral turn
Spiral turns are used to bandage parts of the body that have uniform width, e.g., upper arm or upper leg.

Steps
- Anchor bandage at distal end of body part with two circular turn.
- Make a series of spiral turns at about a 30° angle, each turn overlapping the previous one by two-thirds the width of the bandage.
- Terminate the bandage with two circular turns and secure end of bandage.

Spiral reverse turn
Spiral reverse turns are used to bandage inverted cone-shaped body parts such as forearm, or calf.

Steps
- Anchor bandage at distal end with two circular turns.
- Bring the bandage upward at about a 30° angle.
- Place the thumb of the free hand on the upper edge of the bandage.
- Unroll the bandage about 6 inches, and then turn the hand so that bandage falls over itself.
- Continue advancing bandage until desired proximal pint is reached. Make each bandage turn at the same position so that the turns of the bandage will be aligned.
- Terminate the bandage with two circular turns and secure the bandage.

Figure of eight turns
Figure of eight turns often used for immobilization. It is effective for use around joints such as knee, elbows, ankle and wrist.

Steps
- Anchor bandage at center of joint.
- Ascend obliquely around upper half of circular turn above joint followed by turn that descends obliquely joint.

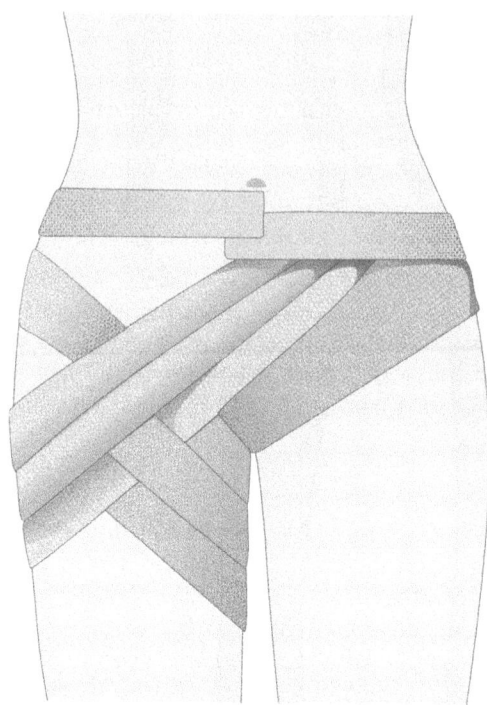

Fig. 8.1: Spica for groin.

- Continue in same manner, overlapping half of previous turn until desired immobilization is attained.
- Terminate the bandage above the joint and secure the end.

Spica bandage
It is a variation of figure of eight bandage. It is commonly used to bandage hip, groin, shoulder, breast or thumb (**Fig. 8.1**).

Steps for thumb spica
- Anchor the bandage around the wrist.
- Bring the bandage down to the distal aspect of the thumb, encircle the thumb, bring back up and around the wrist, then back down and around the thumb, overlapping the previous turn by two-thirds the width of the bandage leaving the tip of the thumb exposed for enabling to check blood circulation to the thumb.
- Repeat the above step until the thumb is covered.
- Terminate the bandage around the wrist and secure the end (**Fig. 8.2**).
- **Recurrent turns:** It is also called as stump bandage or capeline bandage. It is used for fingers or for the stump of an amputated limb and the skull.

Steps
- Anchor the bandage at proximal end of body part to be covered.
- Make reverse turn at center front, advance over distal end of the body part to center back, forming covering perpendicular to circular turns.

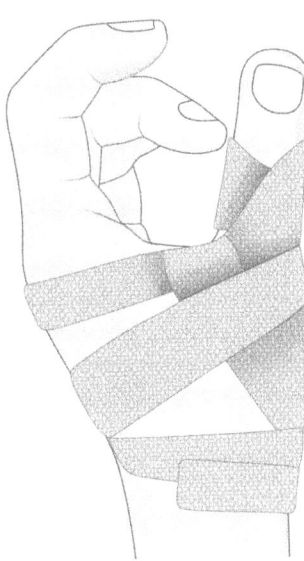

Fig. 8.2: Thumb spica.

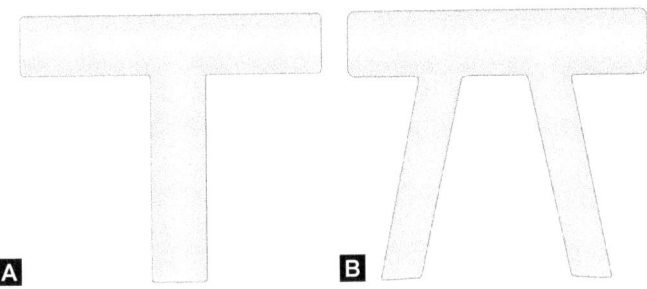

Figs. 8.3A and B: T-binders: (A) This may be used to hold the dressing in place on the perineum and groin. A single T-binder is used for females to provide support for external genitalia. The top of the T is placed around the waist, and the stem is passed between the legs and pinned to the belt created at the waist; (B) The double T-binder is used for males to provide support for the eternal genitalia.

- Holding with the other hand make a reverse turn at the back, bring bandage forward, overlapping of perpendicular bandage.
- Make reverse turn at front and overlap opposite side of center, continuing on to back.
- Repeat the above steps until entire area is covered.
- Terminate the bandage and secure the end.

Removing the Roller Bandage

It is best to cut a roller bandage with a bandage scissors to prevent manipulation of the part. Cutting should be done on the opposite side of the injury or the wound from one end to the other. If the bandage is to be reused it may be unwound by keeping the loose end together and passing it as a ball from one hand to the other while unwinding it.

Applying Binders

Binders are bandages made of large piece of material specially designed to fit a specific body part. Most binders are made of elastic, cotton, muslin or flannel. Binders are used to support large areas of the body such as the abdomen, arm or chest.

T-binders (Figs. 8.3A and B)

It looks like the letter T and is used to secure rectal or perineal dressings. The single T-binder is used for females and the double T-binder is used for males. The belt is secured around the client's waist with single tail or double tails are passed between the legs from back to front and pinned to the belt making sure that the tail fits smoothly and against the dressing.

Breast binders

It looks like a tight fitting sleeveless vest. It provides support after breast surgery or exerts pressure to reduce location in a woman after childbirth **(Fig. 8.4)**.

Abdominal binders
a. Straight abdominal binders
b. Scultetus or many tailed binders **(Figs. 8.5A to C)**.

A straight binder is a straight piece of material about 15–20 cm wide and long enough to more than circle the torso. It supports the large abdominal incisions that are vulnerable to tension or stress as the client moves or coughs.

A many tailed binder or Scultetus binder consists of rectangular pieces of material with tails that are about 5 cm wide attached to its sides. The binder supports the abdomen or holds dressings on it or on the chest.

Method
- With the client in a supine position, place the abdominal binder smoothly under the client with the upper border of the binder at the waist and the lower border at the level of the gluteal fold to prevent interference with respiration if placed above the waist or interference with walking and elimination if placed too low.

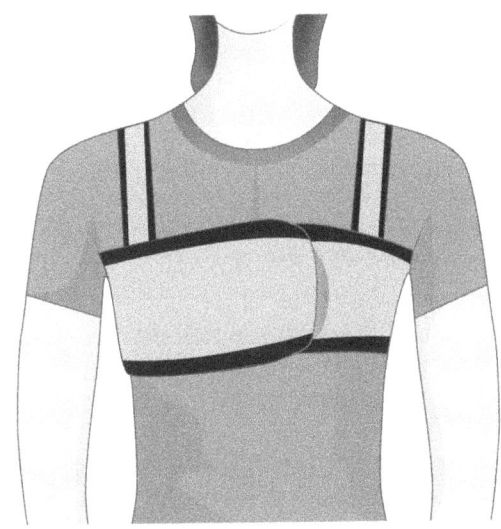

Fig. 8.4: Breast binder.

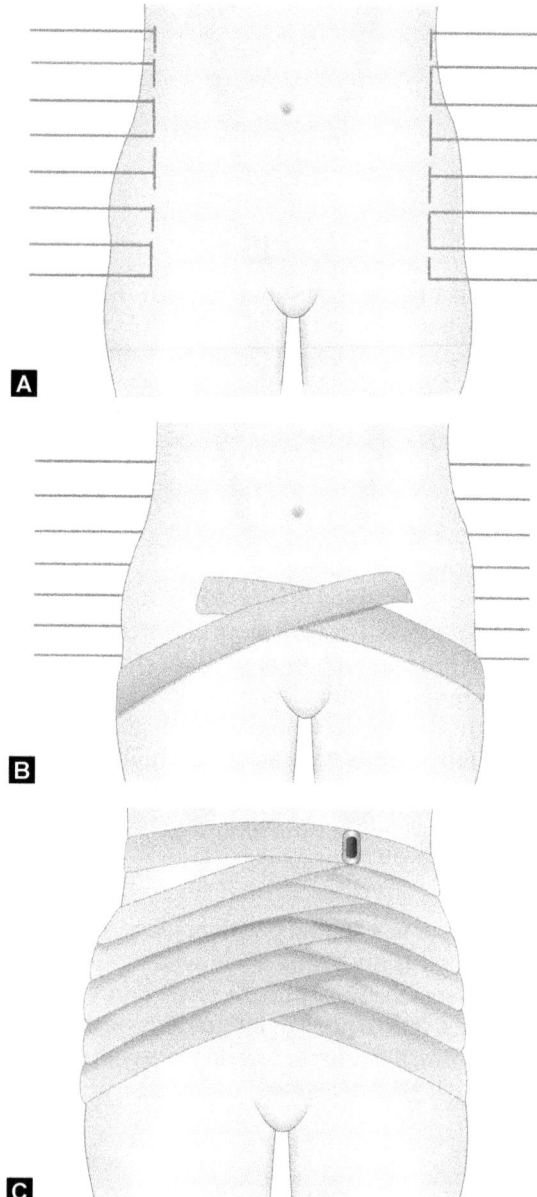

Figs. 8.5A to C: Scultetus binder: (A) It consists of a bandage with two sets of strips on either side; (B) Starting at the bottom of the binder, the tails are brought up and across the abdomen or chest, alternating with each side in an overlapping manner in a slightly upward angle; (C) The tails are pulled taut so that the binder fits snugly. The last two tails are crossed and pinned to the first tails, if possible, and fastened with safety pins.

- Apply padding over the iliac outs if the client is thin.
- The tails are brought out to the sides of the client's body with the bottom tail in position to wrap around the lower part of the abdomen first.
- A tail from each side is brought up and placed obliquely over the abdomen until all tails are in place. The last tails are fastened with safety pins.

Triangular arm slings

It supports the arms, with muscular sprains or fracture to reduce or prevent swelling of hand.

Method

- Place one end of the unfolded triangular binder over the shoulder of the uninjured side so that the binder falls down the front of the chest or the client with the pint of the triangle (apex) under the elbow of the injured side.
- Take the upper corner and carry it around the neck until it hangs over the shoulder on the injured side.
- Bring the lower corner of the binder up over the arm to the shoulder of the injured side.
- Using the reef knot and secure the bandage at the side of the neck on the injured side.
- Fold the sling neatly at the elbow and secure it with safety pins or tape.

Reef knot

Always secure the ends of a bandage with a reef knot because it will not slip, it lies flat and it is easy to untie. Make sure that the knot does not press on or a bone or into the skin. If the knot is uncomfortable, place some soft padding under it.

Method

- Hold one end of the bandage in each hand; take the left end over the right and under.
- Bring the ends up again. Take the right end over the left and under. Pull the knot firm.

Application of Elasticated Tubular Bandage (Tubigrip) (Table 8.2)

Definition

Tubigrip is an elasticated tubular bandage.

Purposes

- It provides support to tissues in case of strains, sprains, joint effusion and muscle injury.
- It aids in venous and lymphatic return in case of venous disorders of the legs and arms.
- It helps in relieving pain.
- It is used as an alternative to compression bandage.

Equipment

- Tubigrip - appropriate - see manufacturer recommendation
- Tubigrip applicator (if available)
- Scissors

Splinting

The device of this invention lies in the field of splints or braces for application to traumatized portions of a human body and is directed more particularly to a device of this class which is useful in maintaining during the healing period a traumatized nose resulting from injury or surgery in the desired size and shape after squeezing out all of the edema fluid from the tissues.

Table 8.2: Procedure: Application of elasticated tubular bandage (Tubigrip).

S. No.	Nursing action	Rationale
1.	Explain the procedure to the patient and cheek the physician's written order	To obtain the patient's cooperation and consent
2.	Keep the patient in a comfortable position and ensure privacy	To ensure the comfort and dignity of the patient
3.	Ensure the area is clean and dry	To avoid irritation and discomfort
4.	If the skin is torn, apply appropriate drug as per physician instruction	
5.	Cut Tubigrip to twice length required for the limb allowing an extra 2–3 cm for overlap	Allow maximum support
6.	Load Tubigrip into the applicator if available	Applicator makes application easier over the painful limb
7.	Insert the limb into the applicator at the end of the Tubigrip is held in position while the applicator is gently removed leaving the Tubigrip in place	Form a double layer by doubling back the Tubigrip. Note: If applicator is not available, pull Tubigrip onto limb, like a stocking and double Tubigrip back over limb
8.	Advice the patient not to roll the Tubigrip	By rolling Tubigrip to form a tight hand blood supply to the distal end of the limb may be compromised
9.	Clean and disposal of equipment	
10.	Wash and dry hands	Document the procedure in appropriate chart/form

For many years, it has been common practice to form splints from plaster of Paris for use in maintaining immobility of bony segments after surgery. They are difficult to make and difficult to retain in place, requiring excessive taping or bandaging, in addition to being uncomfortable and unsightly. Various other approaches have been tried with indifferent success.

Indications

Temporary immobilization to improve pain and discomfort, decrease blood loss, reduce the risk for fat emboli and minimize the potential for further neurovascular injury associated with:
- Fractures
- Sprains
- Reduced dislocations
- Tendon lacerations
- Deep lacerations across joints
- Painful joints associated with inflammatory disorders.

Contraindication

- Fixed contractures
- Large draining wounds
- Excessive swelling or edema
- Continuous spasticity
- Excessive pain

Materials

- Plaster rolls or sheets
  - Strips or rolls of various widths made from crinoline-type material impregnated with plaster which crystallizes or "sets" when water is added.
- Prefabricated splint rolls (Ortho-Glass)
  - Layers of fiber glass between polypropylene padding.
- Stockinet
- Cast padding
- Elastic bandages
- Adhesive tape
- Heavy scissors
- Bucket
- Protective sheets or pads to protect patient clothing
- Gloves

Patient Education

- Instructions should be both verbal and written.
- Explain and demonstrate the importance of "elevation" to minimize swelling and decrease pain.
- Apply ice bags or cold packs (bags of frozen vegetables also work well) for at least 30 minutes at a time during the first 24–48 hours after injury to decrease swelling and pain.
- Avoid getting the splint wet—same splints may be removable for bathing purposed, otherwise plastic bags may be placed over the splint to keep it dry while bathing.
- Explain signs of infection and vascular compromise, instruct patient to seek help for any concerns.
- Instruct patient to return for evaluation of damaged/broken or wet splint.
- Discuss follow-up guidelines.

Procedure/Technique

- **Prepare the patient:**
  - Cover patient with sheet or gown to protect clothing
  - Inspect skin for wounds and soft tissue injuries
  - Clean, repair and dress wounds as usual prior to splint application
- **Padding:**
  - Apply stockinet to extremity to extend several centimeters beyond edges of plaster, so that it may be folded

back over the edges of the splint after plasters is applied to create a smooth edge.
- Roll on 2-3 layers of cast padding evenly and smoothly (but not too tight) over the area to be splinted.
- Extend the padding out beyond the planned area to be splinted so that it can be folded back with the stockinet over the edges of plaster to create smooth edges.
- Each turn of the cast padding should overlap the precious by 25-50% of its width.

An alternative to circumferential stockinet and cast padding is to place 2-3 layers of padding directly over wet plaster, and then apply this lined splint over the area to be immobilized and secure it with an elastic bandage.

❖ **Prepare the plaster splint material:**
  - Ideal length and width of plaster depends on body part to be immobilized in the splint.
  - Estimate the length by laying the dry splint next to the area to be splinted.
  - Be generous in estimation length, the ends can always be trimmed or folded back.
  - Width should be slightly greater than the diameter of the limb to be immobilized.

❖ **Cut or tear the splint material to the desired length:**
  - Choose thickness based on body part to be immobilized, patient body habitus, and desired strength of splint.
    - Average of 8-12 layers
    - Less layers (8-10) for upper extremities
    - More layers (12-15) for lower extremities
    - More layers may be needed for large patients.
  - Fill a bucket with cool water, deep enough to immerse the splint material into:
    - Using cool water decreases the chances of thermal burns, but takes longer for the splint to dry.

❖ **Application of the splint:**
  - Submerge the dry splint material in the bucket of water until bubbling stops.
  - Remove splint material and gently squeeze out the excess water until plaster is wet and sloppy.
  - Smooth out the splint to remove any wrinkles and laminate all layers.
  - Place the splint over the cast padding and smooth it onto the extremity.
  - An assistant (or a cooperative and willing patient) may be required to hold the splint in place while you adjust the splint.
  - Fold back the edges of the stockinet and cast padding over the ends of the splint.
  - Secure the splint with on elastic bandage.
  - Place the extremity in the desired position and mold the splint to the contour of the extremity using the palms of your hand (avoid using your fingers to mold in order to decrease indentations in the plaster which can lead to pressure sores).
  - Hold the splint in the desired position until it hardens.

❖ **Check and finish the splint:**
  - Check for vascular compromise.
  - Check for discomfort or pressure pints.
  - Apply tape along the sides of the splint to prevent elastic bandages from rolling or slipping (avoid circumferential tape to allow for swelling).
  - Provide sling or crutches as needed.

Complications

Compartment syndrome
❖ Usually less common in splints than with circumferential casts.
❖ It may occur associated with splints from constricting Webril™ (cast padding) or elastic bandages that cause increased pressure within a closed space on an extremity.
❖ Increased pressure leads to inadequate tissue perfusion and loss of tissue (muscle, vascular and nerve) function within the compartment.

Presenting signs and symptoms: Pain, pallor, paresthesia, paralysis, and pulselessness, but seldom all occur simultaneously, and when they do—indicate a late finding associated with poor prognosis.
❖ Pain in the extremity
❖ Significant pain with passive stretching of ischemic muscle tissue
  - Diminished distal pulses and sensation
  - Delayed capillary refill, and pale cool skin

Prevention
❖ Avoid wrapping bandages too tightly or making circumferential splints
❖ Elevate the extremity to decrease swelling
❖ Apply topical cold packs
❖ No weight bearing
❖ Early (24-48 hour) follow-up for high-risk injuries.

Management
❖ Remove all constricting bandages and splint materials
❖ Consider compartment pressure monitoring
❖ Early consultation with orthopedist and/or vascular surgeon for possible fasciotomy.

Pressure Sores
❖ It is uncommon with short-term splinting.
❖ It can result from stockinette wrinkles, irregular wadding of padding, insufficient padding over bony prominences or indentations in plaster form using fingers to mold splint.
❖ If suspected, remove the splint materials and check the skin carefully, care for wounds and revise the splint if necessary.

Heat Injury
❖ It can result from drying plaster which produces heat and may cause burns to underlying skin.
❖ To reduce risk for thermal injury, use cool water to wet the splint material and keep splint thickness <12 sheets of plaster.

Infection

- More common with open wounds, but may occur with intact skin
- Clean and debride wounds well prior to splint application
- Consider using a removable splint for periodic wound checks.

Joint Stiffness

- Expected to some extent after any immobilization of a joint
- Avoid prolonged immobilization if possible.

Documentation

- Note the indication for the splint
- Describe any wounds and their location under the splint
- Document the neurovascular examination findings
- Describe the type of splint applied, area immobilized, and materials used to make the splint
- Indicate what follow-up is planned for reassessment of injury.

Bandaging

- *Spiral bandaging* is described in **Figures 8.6A to C.**
- *Figure of eight bandaging* is described in **Figures 8.7A to C.**
- *Recurrent bandaging* is described in **Figures 8.8A to D**.

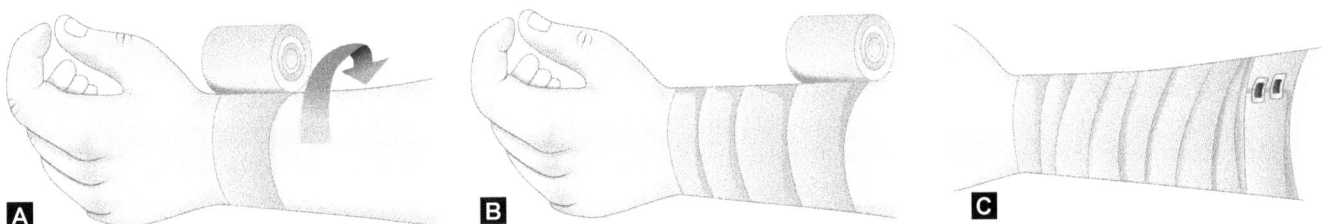

Figs. 8.6A to C: Spiral bandaging: (A) Overlap the bandage to secure it in position; (B) Each subsequent wrap slightly overlap the previous wrap; (C) At the end, wrap the bandage twice to anchor it.

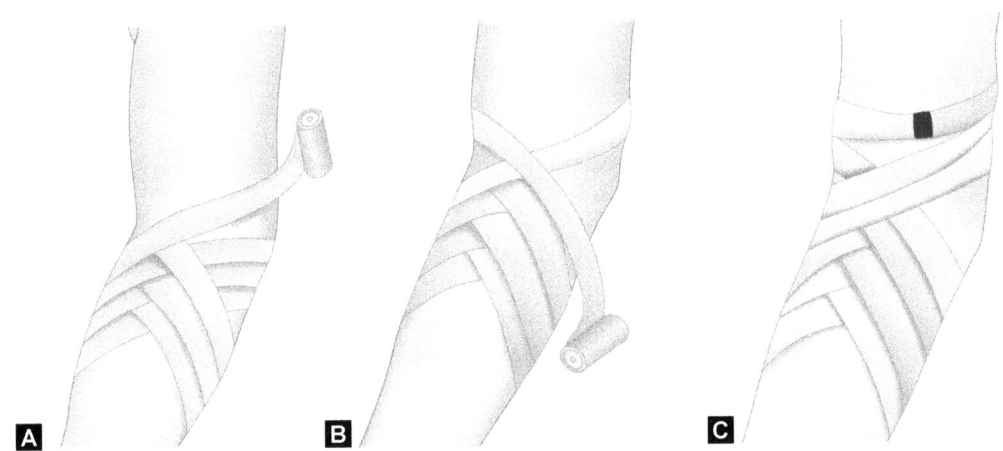

Figs. 8.7A to C: Figure of eight bandaging: (A) Make oblique overlapping turns, ascending and descending alternately; (B) Continue in a figure of eight pattern; (C) Wrap the bandage twice at the end to anchor it.

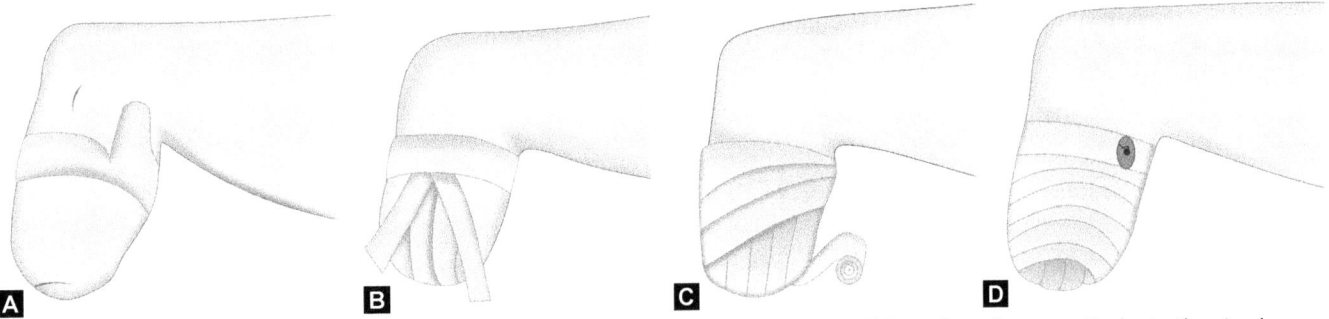

Figs. 8.8A to D: Recurrent bandaging: (A) Anchor the bandage with two circular wraps; (B) Turn the roll perpendicular to the circular wrap and pass it up and over the end of the appendage; (C) Anchor the loose ends of the perpendicular wraps with circular oblique wraps; (D) Anchor the final bandage with tape strips.

CARDIOPULMONARY RESUSCITATION: EXTERNAL CARDIAC MASSAGE

Heart Attack

A heart attack or myocardial infarction is due to an obstruction in one of the coronary arteries. Although the heart attack itself is sudden, it is the result of a slowly developing disease (arteriosclerosis) of the coronary arteries, because the heart muscle requires a continuous supply of oxygen, a portion of the muscle ceases to function.

Healthy heart has controllable and uncontrollable or modifiable or nonmodifiable risk factors.

Cholesterol

Why Cholesterol is Important?

Coronary heart disease causes millions of deaths in the world, coronary heart disease occur when cholesterol clots the coronary arteries. These small blood vessels surround the heart and carry oxygen and nutrients to the heart muscle. Coronary heart disease may not cause symptoms.

High blood cholesterol, high blood pressure, and smoking can increase the risk of coronary heart disease. Reducing this factors make it less likely that patient will develop the disease.

What is Cholesterol?

Cholesterol is a complex fat-like substance. Most of the cholesterol in our bodies is produced naturally in the liver, while too much cholesterol can be harmful. A little is needed for many body functions. It is found in all cells and the body uses it, to help make many important substances, including some hormones and vitamin D. Cholesterol can become a risk to health when there is more in blood than individual body needs. The extra cholesterol may build up in the walls of the arteries.

Why Does High Cholesterol Occur?

Many factors, including obesity, certain inherited tendencies, and lack of exercise, can raise cholesterol. However, one of the most common and controllable factors is diet. When we eat large amount of animal foods, oils, whole milk, and eggs, these may cause extra cholesterol and fats to build up. Fats particularly saturated fats add to the problem of high cholesterol. Saturated fats occur mainly in foods that come from animals, while unsaturated fats occur mainly in plant foods. Most fish and poultry are low in saturated fats.

Saturated fats: These come mainly from animals and tend to be solid at room temperature. An example is the marbling seen in red meat. Certain vegetable fats include tropical oil, such as palm and coconut oils and hydrogenated oils, such as those found in solid margarine.

Unsaturated fats: These come primarily from vegetables. Most of them are liquid at room temperature such as corn and sunflower oil, there are two basic types of polyunsaturated and monounsaturated. Switching to unsaturated fats may help to lower blood cholesterol.

Lipoproteins

Lipoproteins are natural body substances that help to control blood cholesterol levels. They are the carriers of cholesterol in the blood. LDL is the bad lipoprotein because it tends to keep cholesterol in the blood vessels, forming fatty build up.

What Can I Do If I Need Treatment?

The first step in reducing blood cholesterol to healthy levels is to follow a low fat, low cholesterol diet, in general a low fat diet requires that eat less high saturated fat and high cholesterol foods, eggs, and dairy products, and more fruits, grains and vegetables. A low fat diet can contain small portions of meat, such as turkey, and chicken without the skin, fish, boiled or baked without butter is another protein source.

Emergency Cardiac Care

Definition

Cardiac arrest

Cardiac arrest is the abrupt cessation of effective cardiac pumping activity resulting in cessation of blood circulation.

Resuscitation

It is the restoration of vital functions.

Clinical death

It is the absence of vital signs, heart beats and breathing have stopped. This process is reversible.

Biological death

It is the irreversible cellular damage, permanent cellular damage due to lack of oxygen. This is irreversible.

Basic cardiac life support

It is the particular phase of emergency cardiac care that either:
- Prevents circulatory or respiratory arrest, or insufficiency through prompt recognition and intervention.
- Externally supports the circulation and ventilation of a victim of cardiac or circulatory arrest through cardiopulmonary resuscitation (CPR).

What is CPR?

It is the phases of emergency cardiac care (ECC), which includes a series of assessment, and interventions that support cardiac and respiratory function proper and prompt CPR serves to:
- Maintain cardiopulmonary function, by providing oxygen to brain and heart during respiratory and or cardiac arrest until advanced life support can be provided.
- Prevent cardiac arrest.
- Restore cardiopulmonary function.

Why CPR Training is Needed?

Because cardiac arrest is responsible for many deaths, and CPR can help to save the lives of people. The basic rescue in CPR is to recognize and treat and react to emergency situations.

CPR is an emergency procedure used when a person is not breathing and his heart stops beating. CPR alone does not save lives. The purpose of CPR is to keep the victim's brain and heart supplied with blood and oxygen until medical help arrives.

Basic rescue techniques are to keep blood and oxygen flowing when the heart stops beating or there is an airway obstruction (a blockage of air passages caused by food or small objects).

Chain of Survival

These are the steps or links that give the victim of a medical emergency the best chance of living:
- Early access to medical treatment
- Early CPR
- Early defibrillation
- Early advanced life support.

If any link is weak or missing, the chances of survival are lessened.

Cardiopulmonary resuscitation alone is not the only answer to saving lives. If you reduce risk factors and respond to early warning signs will help to reduce the need for CPR and improve the quality of life. Knowing some basics of how human body works is the first step to understanding CPR, cardiovascular disease, warning signs and risk factors.

Circulatory System

Every part of body needs oxygen to survive. When there is not enough oxygen, cells in the body may be damaged.

Heart is a hollow muscle about the size of your fist. It is in the chest behind the lower part breast bone. The heart is a two-sided pump. The right side of the heart receives blood from the body and sends it through the lungs, where waste (carbon dioxide) is removed and fresh oxygen is added. The left side of the heart receives the oxygenated blood from the lungs and sends it through large vessels (arteries) to the rest of body. With each beat of the heart, blood rushing through the arteries creates a pulse that we can feel. The pulse varies according to age, fitness and level of activity.

Each time you breathe in, your lungs fill with fresh air containing oxygen. When you breathe out, you remove waste like carbon dioxide. The air that enters your lungs contains about 21% oxygen. Air that you breathe out contains about 16% oxygen and about 5% carbon dioxide, so the air you breathe out still has enough oxygen to help a person who has stopped breathing.

The average adult's heart beats about 70 times a minute, and it never rests. Each hour the heart pumps about 4,200 times, that means each day the heart beats 100,800 beats, totaling 36,792,000 every year. If man live to be 75 years old, heart will beat 2,759,400,000 times almost 3 billion beats.
- 0-minute breathing stops heart will soon stop beating
- 1–4 to 6 minute brain damage possible
- 2–6 to 10 minutes brain damage likely
- 3 to over 10 minutes irreversible brain damage is certain.

The brain cells stop functioning very quickly when oxygen is not available. A person may lose consciousness and stop breathing if brain goes without oxygen for 4–6 minutes some parts may be permanently damaged.

Airway obstruction is a blockage of the air passage, preventing air from reaching the lungs. In a conscious person, the most common cause of airway obstruction may be a small object or piece of food blocking the airway. The airway may be partially or entirely blocked. The person with partially blocked the airway the person will still get air to move in and out and can cough or speak (do not interfere while the person continues efforts to clear a partially blocked airway). Encourage the person to continue coughing to expel the object if the person cannot speak or cough and skin color turns bluish gray, there is a complete airway obstruction and the person needs immediate help. In an unconscious person, the base of the tongue is the most common cause of airway obstruction.

Indications for Basic Cardiac Life Support

Coming upon a collapsed person can be a frightening experience. You want to ensure that the rescue attempts a safe and effective as possible. You should take charge, assess hazards for yourself and others, and make sure that area is safe. Initial caution may prevent further injuries, hazards which may include electrical wires, fire or gas leakage.

Respiratory Arrest

When there is a primary respiratory arrest, the heart can continue pump blood for several minutes. Existing stores of oxygen in the lungs and blood will continue to circulate to the brain and other vital organs.

Causes of respiratory arrest
- Drowning
- Cerebrovascular accidents
- Foreign body obstruction
- Smoke inhalation
- Drug overdose
- Suffocation
- Electric shock
- Cardiac arrest

Technique of CPR

For CPR, any adult is considered who is more than 8-year-old. A child is in ages 1–8. An infant is less than 1-year-old.

When to Start CPR?

Cardiopulmonary resuscitation should be started immediately when a person is recognized in cardiac arrest, because victims have a good surviving if CPR started within first 4 minutes. They receive advanced cardiac life support (ACLS) within the next 4 minutes.

Performance Guidance for CPR

The techniques and principles of CPR are similar whether a rescuer is performing one rescuer CPR, two rescuers CPR, infant CPR or relief of an obstructed airway.

Performance Procedure

Cardiopulmonary resuscitation consist of four main parts **(Table 8.3)**:
- Chest compression (circulation)
- Airway
- Breathing
- Defibrillation

Defibrillation

Principles of Early Defibrillation

Early defibrillation is critical for victims of sudden cardiac arrest for the following reasons:
- The most common initial rhythm in witnessed sudden cardiac arrest is ventricular fibrillation (VF). When VF is present, the heart quivers and does not pump blood.

Table 8.3: Procedure of cardiopulmonary resuscitation.

Skill	Action
Check for response of the victim after ensuring that the scene is safe, the rescuer should check for a response by tapping the victim on the shoulder and loudly ask the victim "**Are you alright**" (OK)	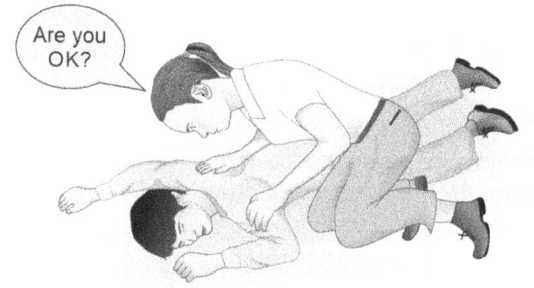 Determine unresponsiveness
Check for no breathing or no normal breathing (i.e., only gasping) Only gasping, it is a sign that the body is not receiving the oxygen it needs, it most often occurs when a person is actively dying.	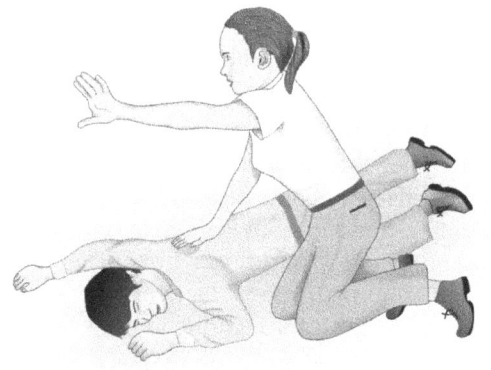 Call for help
Call for help If the victim does not respond to attempts of arousal, callout in the hope that someone will hear who can assist or activate emergency response system (**emergency medical service**)	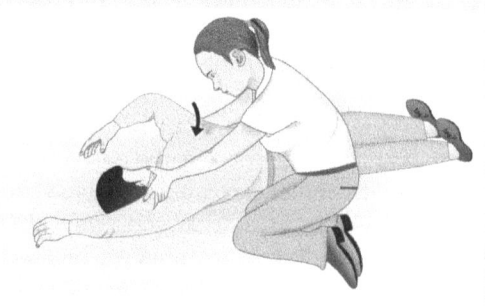 Position the victim

Contd...

Contd...

Skill	Action
Check for the pulse • Locate the carotid pulse • While maintaining head tilt/chin lift with one hand over the forehead • Locate the victims Adam apple with 2 or 3 fingers of the opposite hand • Slide your finger down into the grove lateral to the trachea (between the trachea and the sternocleidomastoid muscle) • Feel for carotid pulse, at the side nearest to the rescuer (this should take 5–10 seconds), the pulse must probed gently, avoiding the compression of the artery • If breathing is absent but pulse is present provide rescue breathing (1 breath every 5 seconds, about 12 breaths/minute) • If pulse is not present, announce cardiac arrest and commence external chest compressions	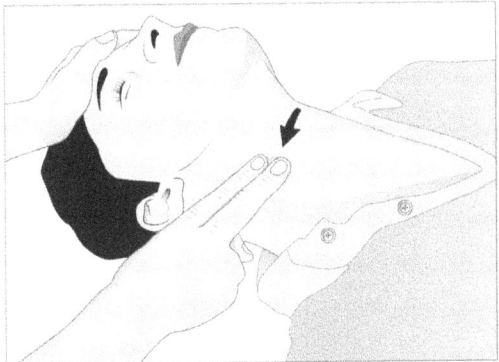 Locate the carotid pulse
Chest compression technique • Initiate compression within 10 seconds of identifying cardiac arrest • Position yourself at the victim side • Make sure the victim is lying on his back on a firm, flat surface if the victim is lying face down, carefully roll him on to his back • Move or remove all clothing covering the victim chest. You need to be able to see the skin • Put the heel of one hand on the center of the victim bare chest between the nipples • Put the heel of your other hand on top of the first hand • Straighten your arm and position your shoulders directly over your hands • Push hard and fast, press down 4–5 cm with each compression for each chest compression, make sure you push straight down on the victim breast bone At the end of each compression, make sure you allow the chest to recoil or re-expands completely. Full chest recoil allows more blood to refill the heart between chest compressions. Incomplete chest recoil will reduce the blood flow created by chest compression	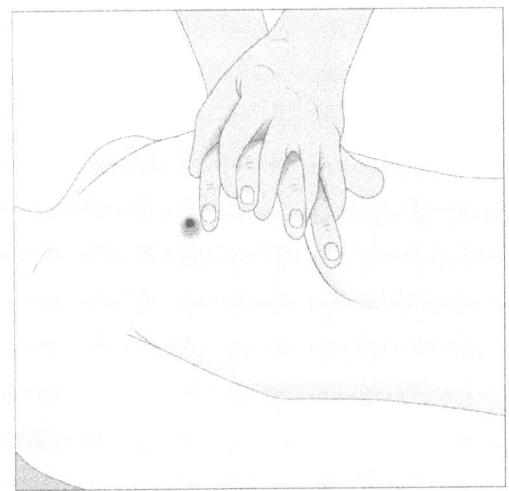 Chest compression
• Deliver compression in a smooth fashion at a rate of 100 compressions/minute • Opening the airway and giving breath • Position yourself at the victim side so that you are ready to open the airway • Begin giving breaths to the victim • Place one hand on the victim forehead and push with your palm to tilt the head back • Place the fingers of the other hand under the bony part of the lower jaw near the chin • Lift the jaw to bring the chin forward	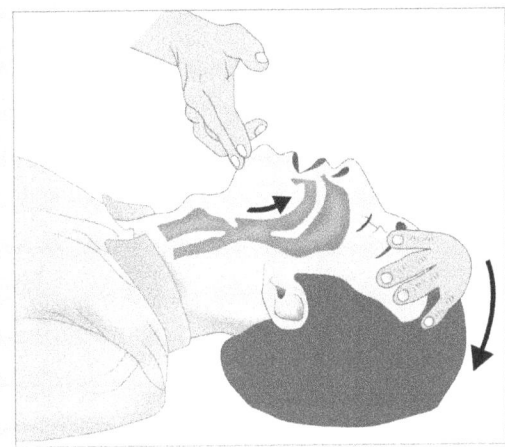 Open the airway

Contd...

Contd...

Skill	Action
Assess the breathing	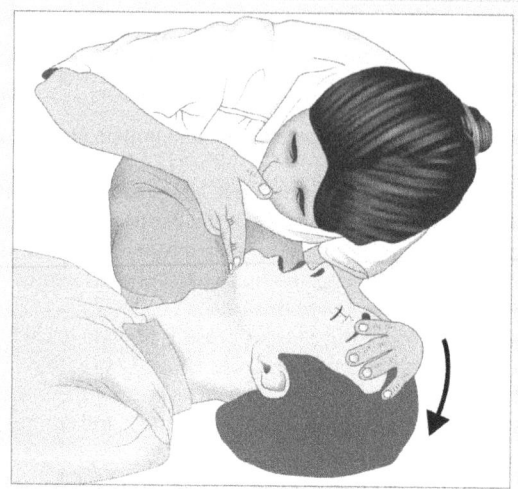 Assessing breathing
Mouth to mouth breathing • Mouth to mouth breathing is a quick, effective way to provide oxygen to the victim • Hold the victim airway open with a head tilt-chin lift • Pinch the nose closed with your thumb and index finger (using the hand on the forehead) • Take a regular (not deep) breath and seal your lips around the victim mouth creating an airtight seal. • Give first breath (blow for 1 second). Watch for the chest to rise as you give the breath • If the chest does not rise, repeat the head tilt-chin lift • Give a second breath (blow for 1 second). Watch for the chest to rise	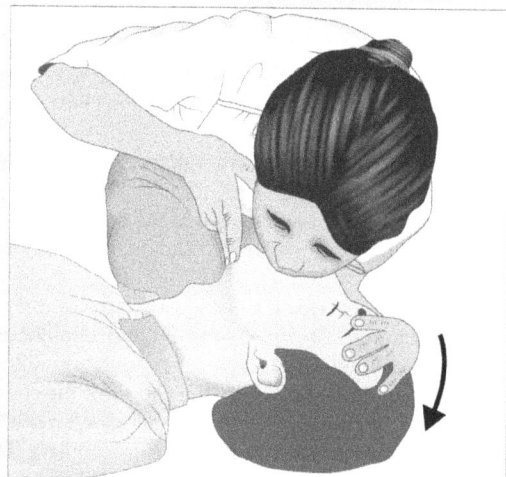 Initiate rescue breathing
If you give breaths too quickly or with too much force, air is likely to enter the stomach rather than the lungs. This can cause gastric inflation To prevent gastric inflation: • Take 1 second to deliver each breath • Deliver enough air to make the victim chest rise **Mouth ventilation** To use a mask, the lone rescuers are at the victim side. This position is ideal when performing 1 rescuer CPR because you can give breaths and perform chest compressions when positioned at the victim side. The lone rescuer will hold the mask against the victim's face and open the airway with a head tilt-chin lift. **Seal the mask against the face** • Using your hand that is closer to the top of the victim's head, place the index finger and thumb along the border of the mask • Place the thumb of your other hand along the lower margin of the mask • Place the remaining fingers of your hand closer to the victim's neck along the bony margin of the jaw. Perform a head tilt-chin lift to open the airway • Deliver air over 1 second to make the victims chest rise	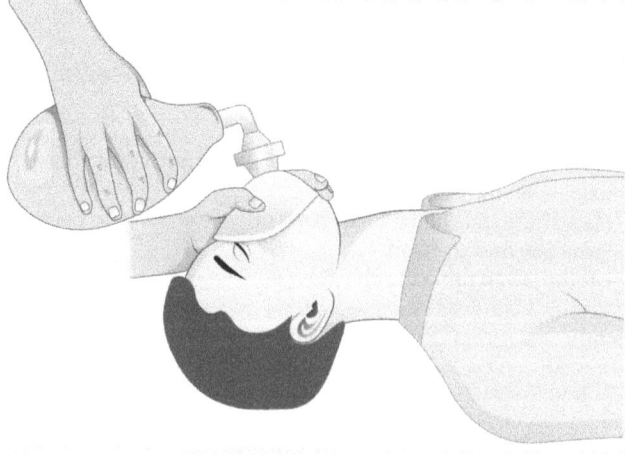 Mask Ventilation

Contd...

Contd...

Skill	Action

Compression ventilation ratio
- **One rescuer:** It should use a universal compression ventilation ratio of 30 compressions to 2 breaths when giving CPR to victim of all ages (except neonates)
- **Two rescuers:** It should use a compression-ventilation ratio of 15 compression to 2 breaths when giving CPR to children and infants
- Rescuer should make every effort to deliver breaths efficiently. This will minimize interruptions in chest compression. When you give chest compressions, it is important to press deeply at a rate of about 100 compressions per minute and allow the chest to recoil completely

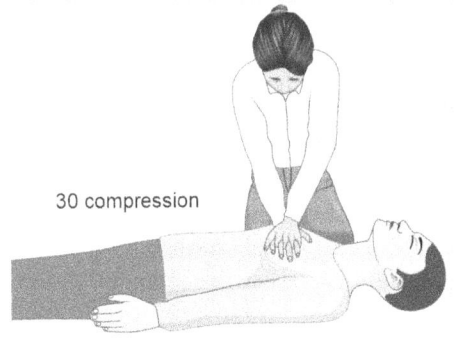
30 compression

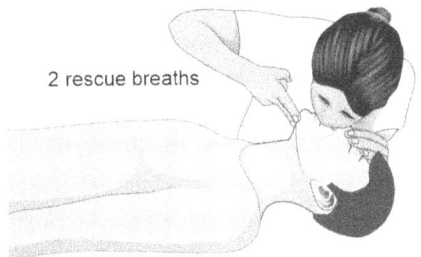
2 rescue breaths

Compression with rescuer

Open airway and check for breathing
To assess breathing you must look, listen and feel for breathing, this evaluation procedure should take at least 5 seconds but no more than 10 seconds. If the healthcare provider does not detect adequate breathing within 10 seconds, the rescuer should give 2 breaths.
Follow this step to look, listen, and feel for breath
- Open the victim airway with a head tilt-chin lift maneuver
- Place your ear near the victim mouth and nose
- While observing the victim's chest
  - Look for the chest to rise and fall
  - Listen for air escaping during exhalation
  - Feel for the flow of air against your cheek
- If the victim is not breathing adequately give 2 breaths (1 second each) while watching for the victim chest to rise
- After giving 2 breaths, check for the pulse (carotid pulse)

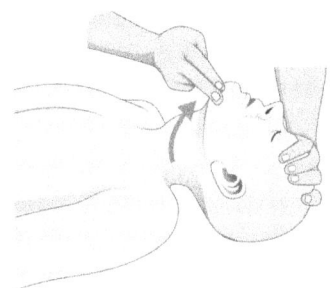
Open airways by lifting the chin slightly

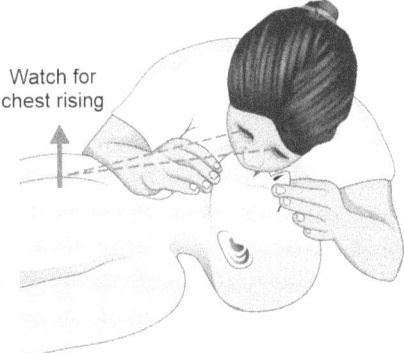
Pinch nose and give 2 rescue breaths
Open airway and check for breathing

- The most effective treatment for VF is electrical defibrillation (delivery of a shock to stop the VF).
- The probability of successful defibrillation decreases quickly overtime.
- VF deteriorates to a systole if not treated.
- The earlier defibrillation occurs, the higher the survival rate. When VF is present, CPR can provide a small amount of blood flow to the heart and brain but cannot directly restore an organized rhythm. Restoration of a perfusing rhythm requires immediate CPR and defibrillation within a few minutes of the initial arrest.
- Without by stander CPR, the chance of survival from VF cardiac arrest declines by 7-10% per minute without defibrillation. Bystander CPR improves survival from VF cardiac arrest at most defibrillation intervals.
- The use of automated external defibrillators (AEDs) increases the number of people (lay rescuers and healthcare providers) who can perform CPR and attempt defibrillation, thus shortening the time between collapse and defibrillation.

Structure and Function of Automated External Defibrillators

Automated external defibrillators are computerized devices that are attached to a pulseless victim with adhesive pads, they will recommend shock delivery only if the victim's heart rhythm is one that a shock can treat. AEDs give rescuers visual and voice prompts to guide rescuer actions.

The word "automated" actually means semiautomated, because most commercially available AEDs will "advice" the operator that a shock is needed but will not deliver a shock without an action by the rescuer (i.e., the rescuer must push the "shock" button).

A small number of fully automated AEDs are now in use, if a fully automated defibrillator detects a rhythm that a shock can treat it will deliver a shock without operator intervention.

Adhesive electrodes attach the AEDs to the patient. Most AEDs operate in the same way and have similar components.

Use AEDs only in victims, who have the following three clinical findings:
1. No response
2. No breathing
3. No pulse

The patient in cardiac arrest may demonstrate agonal gasps. Agonal gasps are not effective breathing. A victim who has agonal gasps and does not respond and has no pulse is in cardiac arrest. Remember that agonal gasps are not effective breaths.

The Universal AED: Common Steps to Operate AEDs (Table 8.4)

- Once the AED arrives, put it at the victim's side, next to the rescuer who will operate it. This position provides ready access to the AED controls and easy placement of electrode pads. It also allows a second rescuer to perform CPR from the opposite side of the victim without interfering with AED operation.
- AEDs are available in different models. There are small differences from model to model, but all AEDs operate in basically the same way.

Using an AED on a Child

For unwitnessed, out of hospital cardiac arrest in children perform 5 cycle or 2 minutes of CPR before using and attaching the AED.

For any in hospital cardiac arrest of a child or for any sudden collapse of a child out of hospital, use an AED as soon as it is available.

Choosing the AED Pads or AED Child System

Some AED systems have been designed to deliver both adult and child shock doses. If you use an AED on a child, it can deliver a child shock dose. Follow the AED instructions to select the lower (child) shock dose. You may need to turn a child key/switch or use child-size pads, or both to reduce the shock dose. You must be careful not to deliver the child shock dose for victim over 8 years of age because the smaller dose may not be effective for the larger or older victim. You need to be familiar with your AED.

If you are using an AED for a child 1-8 years of age and the AED does not have a child pads or child key or switch, you may use the adult pads and deliver the adult dose.

If an AED has optional child pads or key or a switch to enable the child dose to be delivered, it is important to select the pads and settings that are correct for the victim.

Outcomes and Actions after Shock Delivery

"Shock indicated" Message: Recurrent VF

Follow these steps after AED delivers a shock to the victim:

Immediately resume CPR beginning with chest compression. Do not delay CPR to check the patients pulse even if a displayed rhythm looks normal

After 5 cycle (about 2 minutes) of CPR, allow the AED to analyze the heart rhythm, if a shock is not advised, résumé CPR (beginning with chest compressions) for 5 more cycles (about 2 minutes)

Continue until advanced care providers take over or the victim starts to move. Advanced care providers will indicate when a pulse check or other therapies are appropriate

"No Shock Indicated" Message: Pulse and Breathing Absent

If the AED does not detect a rhythm requiring a shock, the AED will prompt you to resume CPR, beginning with chest compressions. Do not recheck to see if there is a pulse. The AED may voice prompts. Continue until advance care providers take over or the victim starts to move. Advanced care providers will indicate when a pulse check or other therapies are appropriate.

Table 8.4: Universal steps for operating an AED.

Steps	Action
Power on the AED (this activates voice prompts for guidance in all subsequent steps)	• Open the carrying case or the top of the AED • Turn the power on (some devices will power on automatically when you open the lid or case)
Attach electrode pads to the victim's bare chest	Choose correct pads (adult vs. child for size/age of victim). Use child pads or child system for children <8 years of age if available
Do not use child pads or child system for victims of 8 years and older	• Peel the backing away from the electrode pads • Quickly wipe the victim's chest if is covered with water or sweat • Attach the adhesive electrode pads to the victims bare chest • Place one electrode pad on the upper right side of the bare chest to the right of the breast bone, directly below the collar bone • Place the other pad to the left of the nipple, a few centimeters below the left arm pit • Attach the AED connecting cables to the AED box (some are preconnected)
"Clear" the victim and analyze the rhythm	• Always clear the victim during analysis. Be sure that no one is touching the victim not even the person in-charge of giving breaths • Some AEDs will tell you to push a button to allow the AED to begin analyzing the heart rhythm. Others will do that automatically. The AED may take about 5–15 seconds to analyze. • The AED then tells you if a shock is needed.
If the AED advises a shock, it will tell you to be sure to clear the victim	• Clear the victim before delivering the shock: Be sure no one is touching the victim to avoid injury to rescuers • Loudly state a "clear the patient" message, such as I am clear, you are clear, everybody clear or simply clear • Perform a visual check to ensure that no one is in contact with the victim • Press the shock button • The shock will produce a sudden contraction of the victim's muscles
	As soon as the AED gives the shock, begin CPR starting with chest compressions
	After 2 minutes of CPR, the AED will prompt you to repeat steps 3 and 4

Implantable Cardioverter Defibrillator

An implantable cardioverter defibrillator (ICD) treats dangerously fast rhythm disorders called ventricular tachycardia and ventricular fibrillation in the lower chambers of the heart. The ICD sends a shock to the heart muscle to interrupt the rhythm disorder and allow the heart to resume its normal rhythm.

An ICD corrects rapid, abnormal heart rhythms. It constantly watches the heart and delivers treatment to stop an abnormally fast rate such as VT and VF. ICDs can treat slow rhythms as well. They do this by sending tiny electrical impulses to the ventricle, the atrium, or both and it sends electrical pulses to the heart muscle through the leads. The electrical pulses slow the heart, therefore restoring a more normal rate.

Implanted Pacemakers

Victims who have a higher risk for sudden cardiac arrest may have implanted defibrillators/pacemakers that deliver shocks directly to the myocardium. You can immediately identify these devices because they create a hard lump beneath the skin of the upper chest or abdomen. The lump is half the size of a deck of cards, with a small overlying scar. If you place an AED electrode pad directly over an implanted medical device, the device may block delivery of the shock to the heart.

If you identify an implanted defibrillator/pacemaker:
❖ Place the AED electrode pad at least 2.5 cm to the side of the implanted device
❖ Follow the normal steps for operating an AED.

Occasionally, the analysis and shock cycles of implanted defibrillators and AEDs will conflict, if the implanted defibrillator is delivering shocks to the patient, the patient muscle contract in a manner like that observed after an AED shock, allow 30-60 seconds for the implanted defibrillator to complete the treatment cycle before delivering shock from the AED.

Transdermal Medication Patches

Do not place AED electrodes directly on top of a medication patch (e.g., a patch of nitroglycerin, nicotine, pain medication, hormone replacement therapy, or antihypertensive medication). The medication patch may block the transfer of energy from the electrode pad to the heart and may cause small burns to the skin.

To prevent the medication patch from blocking delivery of energy, remove the patch and wipe the area clean before attaching the AED electrode pad.

FIRST AID IN EMERGENCY

HEMORRHAGE

Hemorrhage is the loss of blood from the body, bleeding is also called hemorrhage. Blood loss can occur in almost any area of the body.

Types of Bleeding

1. **Internal bleeding:** Refers to blood loss inside the body.
2. **External bleeding:** Blood loss in outside the body is called external bleeding.

Blood loss from bleeding tissue can also be apparent when blood exits through a natural opening in the body, such as the mouth, vagina, rectum, and nose.

Causes of Hemorrhage

Hemorrhage is a common symptom. A variety of incidence or conditions can cause bleeding. Possible causes include:

Traumatic injuries:
- Abrasions
- Hematoma
- Lacerations
- Puncture wounds
- Crushing injuries
- Gunshot wounds

Condition that can cause bleeding:
- Menstrual bleeding
- Leukemia
- Platelet disorders
- Lung cancer
- Vitamin K deficiency
- Medication, such as blood thinner, aspirin, and nonsteroidal anti-inflammatory drugs (NSAIDs)

Clinical signs may begin to appear with a blood volume deficit of 15–25% of an adult with a normal circulating volume. Individual may develop shock if a loss of blood is >25% circulating blood volume. The severity of shock depends on the amount and length of time over which the blood loss occurs.

Clinical Signs of Hemorrhage

- Blood loss, if >40% is called class IV acute hemorrhage, results in increased pulse rate, more than 140, respiratory rate more than 35, decreased blood pressure, confused, lethargy.
- Blood loss, if <30–40% is called class III hemorrhage, results in increased pulse rate, more than 120, respiratory rate more than 30, decreased blood pressure, confused, and anxious.
- Blood loss, if <15% is called class I hemorrhage, which results in increased pulse rate, less than 100, respiratory rate 14–20, blood pressure will be normal, slightly anxious.
- Individual loss blood over a period of days or week tolerates their blood loss better than clients whose blood loss occurs rapidly or minute or hour.

SHOCK

Shock is a complex clinical syndrome that may occur at any time and in any place. It is life-threatening condition often requiring team action by many healthcare providers, including nurses, physicians, laboratory technician, pharmacists, and respiratory therapists.

Definition

Shock is defined as failure of the circulatory system to maintain adequate perfusion of vital organs, leading to inadequate tissue perfusion results in decreased oxygenation at the cellular level. This inadequate oxygenation results in anaerobic cellular metabolism. If not treated, cell death and organ death occurs.

Classifications of Shock

Hypovolemia Shock

Hypovolemic shock is due to inadequate circulating blood volume resulting from hemorrhage with actual blood loss. Burns with loss of plasma, proteins and fluid shifts or dehydration with a loss of fluid volume, it is the most common type of shock.

Etiology

Hemorrhage: Clinical manifestations indicative of hypovolemic shock may begin to appear a blood volume deficit of 15–25% or about 500–1,500 mL in an adult with a normal circulating volume.

Burns: Hypovolemic shock, produced by burns, occurs most often in persons with large partial thickness burns. There is a shift of plasma from the vascular space into interstitial space. The client may have cardiac dysfunction due to presence of myocardial depressant factor.

Dehydration: Shock occurs from either reduced oral fluid intake or significant losses of fluid, for example, excessive urine output, prolonged vomiting or diarrhea, exercise causing fluid loss from sweating and hot environment.

Cardiogenic Shock

Cardiogenic shock is due to inadequate pumping action of the heart because of primary cardiac muscle dysfunction or mechanical obstruction of blood flow caused by myocardial infarction (MI), vascular insufficiency due to disease or trauma, cardiac dysrhythmias or on obstructive condition, such as pericardial tamponade or pulmonary embolism (PE). Cardiogenic shock occurs in 15–20% of the all clients following MI and have at least 80% mortality rate. Cardiogenic shock after an MI, usually occurs when 40% or more of the myocardium has been damaged.

Etiology

Cardiogenic shock results primarily from an inability of heart muscle to function adequately or mechanical obstruction of blood flow to or from the heart.

Myocardial infarction: Impaired heart muscle action is most often caused by MI. The area of dead or dying tissue that occurs with infraction impairs contractility of the myocardium and the cardiac output decreases. It may occur in blunt cardiac trauma, cardiomyopathy and heart failure.

Obstructive conditions: Mechanical obstruction to blood flow causing cardiogenic shock includes a large PE, pericardial tamponade and tension pneumothorax.

Pericardial tamponade: It is an accumulation of blood or fluid in the pericardial space.

Tension pneumothorax: It is the significant amount of air in the pleural space.

Other causes: Cardiac valvular insufficiency from trauma or disease, myocardial aneurysms (previous MI), rupture of ventricle, aortic stenosis, and mitral regurgitation.

Obstructive Shock

In obstructive category, shock develops in conditions that lead to sudden obstruction of blood flow; these problems include cardiac tamponade, tension pneumothorax, and PE.

Distributive Shock

It is due to changes in blood vessels tone that increase the size of the vascular space without an increase in circulating blood volume.

Acute Allergic Reaction (Anaphylactic Shock)

Anaphylactic shock occurs as a result of an acute allergic reaction from exposure to a substance to which the client has been sensitized. Common sensitizing agents are penicillin and its derivatives, bee stings, chocolates, strawberries, peanuts, snake venom, iodine based contrast for X-ray and NSAIDs.

Spinal Cord Injury (Neurogenic Shock)

Neurogenic shock occurs from severe central nervous system (CNS) complications. As it results in low blood pressure (BP), occasionally with a slowed heart to the disruption of the autonomic pathways within the spinal cord.

Septic shock is the systemic response to infection. The process begins with the growth of various microorganisms at the site of infection.

Stages of Shock

Nonprogressive Stage

In nonprogressive stage, the body compensatory mechanism can maintain blood pressure and perfusion to the vital organs. During this time, the systemic circulation and microcirculation work together which lead to increase in lactic acid levels which reserve the entire system.

Progressive Stage

During progressive stage, supply of oxygenated blood to the tissues is reduced as vasoconstriction continues, this will lead to anaerobic metabolism, this causes decreased venous returns, and thus blood supply is progressively retained in the capillary. Decreased vascular capacity decrease the heart function result in decreased cardiac output.

Irreversible Stage

The shock state become progressively more severe, if immediately not interrupted. The shock progress to more severe, cellular ischemia and necrosis lead to organ failure and death.

Risk Factors

- Trauma
- Heart muscle injury
- Allergen
- Invasive procedure
- Exposure to pathogen

General Clinical Manifestation

- Restlessness and anxiety
- Decreased level of consciousness
- Irritability, dry mouth, and thirsty, dry mucous membranes
- Cyanosis, cold and clammy skin
- Dilated pupils, flat neck vein
- Nausea and vomiting
- Rapid thready pulse, slow capillary refilling and collapse
- Diaphoresis
- Tachycardia
- Hypotension
- Oliguria, decreased urinary volume
- Decreased oxygen saturation
- Decreased systolic BP <20 mm Hg with heart rate increased >20 beats per minute.

Diagnostic Assessment

- 12-lead electrocardiogram (ECG)
- Complete blood count (CBC)
- Arterial blood gases (ABGs) analysis
- Pulse oximetry

- Spirometry
- Central venous pressure (CVP) measurement
- Pulmonary artery or Swan–Ganz catheter measurement

Management

Medical Management (Emergency Care)

As prescribed by the concerned physician, which may include as per type of shock:
- Stop external bleeding, transfuse with fresh whole blood/packed cells, fresh frozen plasma
- Start intravenous (IV) fluids are given to correct specific problems
- Dopamine/Dobutamine infusions
- Begin to compensate for acid base imbalance. Positive end expiratory pressure may be added when the client is being mechanically ventilated
- Elevate the leg side of the bed (in modified Trendelenburg position), in lower extremities are elevated 30-45 degrees

Drug Choice

1. If one sure that it is septic shock, then use norepinephrine.
2. If it is anesthesia related or spinal shock, then use phenylephrine.
3. If it is cardiogenic shock, then use dobutamine and norepinephrine.
4. If it is anaphylactic shock, then use epinephrine.
5. If the patient is with bradycardia and hypotensive, then use the epinephrine.
6. If one do not know what is causing the shock, then use epinephrine or dopamine.
7. Maintain adequate perfusion.

Vasoconstriction

Vasoconstriction elevates the BP by constricting peripheral arterioles.

Vasodilators

Vasodilators may be helpful during shock, when vasoconstriction is severe.

Improving Oxygenation

Supplemental oxygen is administered to protect against hypoxemia. Endotracheal tube or tracheotomy may be performed to test an exhausted client during severe or prolonged shock and to correct respiratory failure (if the client not ventilated).

Assisting Circulation

Mechanical devices that assist circulation or decrease heart work load, may be used as temporary measures. For example, medical antishock trousers (MAST) and intra-aortic balloon pump.

Providing Autotransfusion

It involves collecting and transfusing blood into the same client. It is used in prevention or treatment of existing hypovolemic shock caused by hemorrhage. It is common in the treatment of chest injuries.

Evaluating Fluid Replacement

It can be evaluated by the CVP monitoring. If CVP is low, IE below 4 cm H_2O_2 mm Hg, continue the infusion of fluids or blood. When CVP is higher than normal, IE above 15 cm H_2O/mm Hg, benefit cannot be expected from the continued infusion of fluids or blood beyond maintenance amounts.

Monitoring Urinary Output

Impaired kidney function may result from inadequate renal tissue perfusion in any attempt to prevent acute renal damage, the urinary output is monitored with an indwelling catheter and diuretics (e.g., furosemide) may be given, if tubular necrosis is present peritoneal dialysis/hemodialysis may be needed until regeneration of functioning renal tubular epithelium occurs.

Preventing Gastrointestinal Bleeding

An early physiological response to shock is a decrease in splanchnic circulation. This reduces the blood supply to the stomach and bowel causing inadequate gastrointestinal tissue perfusion and delayed gastric emptying thus vomiting with aspiration of gastric contents into the lungs may occur. For this reason and for diagnostic purpose, nasogastric suction is often used during treatment of shock.

Noninvasive Management

Noninvasive management techniques can be performed rapidly and relatively easily. They require equipment and are readily observable. The first step in assessing a person in shock is a general overview, giving attention to the airway, breathing and circulation (ABC). Once the airway is patent, air exchange is adequate, a pulse is present and the cervical spine is immobilized perform a rapid, initially head to toe physical assessment, the goal is to identify major problems and gross abnormalities. The following observation should be made.

1. **Airway patency:** Noisy respirations and obstruction
2. **Breathing :** Respiration rate and efforts
3. **Respiratory pattern:** Chest wall expansion, chest wall bulges or deflates
4. **Circulation:** Pulse, BP, skin color and temperature
5. **Level of consciousness:** Orientation to place, time and person. Ability to move extremities, sensation in all extremities, pupil size and reaction to light.
6. Monitor hydration and perfusion of the skin
7. Monitor circumference of abdomen and extremities, and peripheral pulses

8. Presence of lacerations, contusion and bone deformities.
9. Doppler instrument usage
10. **Temperature monitoring (core temperature):** An indwelling flexible rectal probe connected to a continuous display monitors is more accurate and less traumatic than intermittent rectal temperature measurements. Core temperature can also be obtained if the client has a thermo dilution (Swan-Ganz) catheter in place.
11. **Cardiac monitor:** For assessment and evaluation purpose, the electrical activity of the heart needs to be continuously monitored in all clients in shock, regardless of age. Frequent ECG is must.

DROWNING

Children under 3 years of age are most vulnerable. Most infants, (<1year) who are victims, when the parent or caretaker leaves the child alone for a few minutes to answer the phone, or fetch something.

In adults, most drowning occurs in males who are intoxicated. It often happens within a few meters of the seashore, boat or dock. Suspect trouble if the swimmer's strokes become erratic and jerky or stop, or if the body sinks so that only the head shows above the water. Spinal injuries more common in diving accidents and should always be suspected.

A child or adult, who nearly drowns but has been rescued, is still in danger because fluid could build up in the lungs a few hours later. This may even lead to "secondary drowning", a fatal condition. A person who drowns dies from suffocation caused by lack of oxygen.

To Prevent Drowning

- Person who do not know how to swim should not go to deep water.
- Inform and remind children of the possible dangers of playing in deep water.
- Do not leave children playing in the water alone (such as in water basins).
- Learn how to swim.
- Do not swim alone.
- Do not swim in night.
- Place a guard or railing on open wells or ponds.
- Do not swim in waters where there are undercurrents.
- Keep children away from bodies of water and watch them carefully.

What to Check?

- Presence or absence of breathing
- Presence or absence of heart beat

First Aid for Drowning

a. If there is a presence of breathing, bring the person to shore and check the patient for any other injuries.
b. If the person does not breathe, start mouth-to-mouth breathing at once even before the person is out of the water or as soon as the water is shallow enough to allow you to stand. If you cannot blow air into the drowning person's lungs when you reached the shore, quickly put him on his side with the head lower than the body and push the belly upward to force the water out.
c. Resume mouth-to-mouth breathing.
d. If there is the presence of a heartbeat do check for any other injuries.
e. If the patient do not have a heartbeat do CPR.
f. If these step of first aid did not help the patient, bring them to the nearest hospital.

Point to Note

Make sure that you are a good swimmer before attempting to rescue a person who is drowning. If not, get help and have the drowning person brought to shallow water before giving first aid.

First Aid for Drowning Victims

If drowning in a river: First, check the scene to be sure that it is safe to attempt a rescue. Check the victim, and then send someone to get emergency help then care for the person until help arrives.

In the event of drowning, first remove the victim from the water. Check for consciousness and for breathing. If the victim is not breathing, do not waste time trying to remove water from the victim's lungs. Quickly remove any obstructions such as seaweed or excess mud from the victim's mouth, and open the airway and apply mouth-to-mouth resuscitation.

If breaths do not do in, retilt the head and attempt rescue breathing again. If air still does not go in, give children and adults abdominal thrusts using the Heimlich maneuver to clear the airway. Once the airway is clear, begin mouth-to-mouth and chest compression as necessary.

Hypothermia is the result of body temperatures falling below 35°C (95°F). The casualty will show signs of shivering and slurred speech, then confusion, irrationality, sleepiness, clumsiness, and shivering may stop. Babies may exhibit drowsiness and floppiness, and the face, hands, and feet will feel very cold.

Hypothermia victims should be gradually rewarmed by a warm bath and hot drinks. These are much preferable to a mere hot water bottle or electric blanket. If there are no other means of warmth, body heat can be used to warm the victim. The casualty should move to improve circulation, especially moving the legs, but the skin should not be rubbed.

Immediate Treatment

- Get the person out of the water. Do not try to rescue someone if it will severely endanger your life. Rather call for help, and try to reach the person from land with a pole or rope. Tie yourself to something secure on shore if you have to swim to the person.
- Do the ABCs. Check for foreign bodies in the airways, such as weed, but do not waste times by trying to drain swallowed water. If the person needs CPR, start immediately.
- Once on shore, place the person in the recovery position if there are no spinal injuries. Keep the person warm.
- If you suspect a spinal injury and CPR is not required, do not move the person to land. Keep him lying face up in the water until help arrives.
- All near-drowning victims should be observed in hospital for 24 hours.

Near drowning is the term used to describe victims who have been resuscitated and survive for at least 24 hours. If the victim dies within 24 hours of the original incident, drowning is listed as the primary cause of death. If the victim dies after the initial 24 hour period, death is attributed the "complications arising from the incident", with near drowning listed as a secondary cause of death.

INJURIES TO THE BONES, JOINTS, AND MUSCLES

Fractures

A fracture is a broken or cracked bone. The break is usually complete, but in the young, the bone can be bent without breaking completely. This is called a greenstick fracture. Correct first aid management of fractures, in both conscious and unconscious casualties, is essential, in order to reduce the amount of tissues damage, bleeding, pain and shock.

Classification of Fractures

- **Simple or closed:** Where the skin is unbroken and the cut ends of the bone do not cut open the skin and blood is lost into tissues.
- **Compound or closed:** Where the broken end of the bone protrudes through the skin. Blood loss maybe severe.
- **Complicated:** Where in addition to the fracture an important internal organ may also be injured or damaged, e.g., hip fracture with an injury to the bladder or kidney, a rib fracture with an injury to the lungs. A complicated fracture may also be simple or compound.

Causes

- **Direct force**—a blow that breaks the bone at the point of impact
- **Indirect force**—when the bone breaks at some distance from the point of impact, e.g., where a fall on an outstretched hand results in a fracture of the collar bone
- **Abnormal muscular contraction**—a sudden contraction of a muscle may result in a fracture, e.g., an elderly persons napping the knee cap after tripping and trying to prevent fall.

Effect

- Bleeding—fractures of large bones may result in considerable loss of blood, e.g., a fractured thigh results in the loss of 1 or 2 liters of blood
- Damage to surrounding tissues and blood vessels
- Pain
- Possibly shock.

First Aid Tips—Fractures

If any bone that gets broken with or without displacement of broken fragments.

Look out for indication such as:

- Very intense pain increasing on movement of affected area
- Bruising may or may not be there
- Swelling
- Injured area looks abnormal as compared to opposite side
- Difficulty in moving the injured area
- Shock
- Unconsciousness may temporarily be there.

What to do:

1. Immobilization of the affected area is required-Get Help!
2. Keep the patient still and support the injured area.
3. For arm fractures a sling can be made to support and immobilize the affected area, which can be hung around the neck using triangular bandage or cloth.
4. Splints (any long firm object) can be used for support and immobilization, but usually splinting to another part of the body is best.
5. In case of leg fractures, the patient's both legs can be tied together. Open fractures control the bleeding with sterile dressing and pressure if required.

DON'TS
1. Give massage to affected area
2. Try to straighten the broken limb
3. Move the patient without support
4. Ask the patient to move on his own
5. Move the joints above and below the fracture

Signs and Symptoms of a Fracture

- Pain at or around the site of the fracture.
- Tenderness (pain on gentle pressure) over the area. Do not press hard.
- Swelling over the area with discoloration.
- Loss of normal movements of the affected part.
- Deformity of the limb may be caused. The limb may lose its normal shape and there may be apparent shortening of the limb.

- If the fracture is close to the skin, the uneven outline of the bone can be plainly felt.
- When one end of the broken bone moves against the other, a crackling sound may be heard. This is called crepitus (grating). This should never be elicited by the person giving first aid.
- Unnatural movements may be felt at the site of the fracture. This too should never be elicited by the first-aid provider.

In addition the victim may himself say that he heard the snap of the bone. It is important to compare the injured limb with the normal limb while making an assessment.

Aims of first aid
- To prevent further damage
- To reduce pain
- To make the patient feel comfortable
- To get medical aid as soon as possible

Management
1. Fractures often occur along with other injuries. So the rescuer must assess for other injuries and decide which of them requires care on priority. Heavy bleeding is more urgent and requires higher priority care over fracture.
2. If there is no danger to life then temporary attention to the fracture is often sufficient.
3. Handle the patient very gently. Avoid all unnecessary movement.
4. Treat for shock if present.
5. If the broken ends of the bones show out, do not wash the wound or apply antiseptics to the end of the bone.
6. Do not handle the fracture unnecessarily.
7. Never attempt to reduce the fracture or to bring the bones to the normal position.
8. Stabilize and support the injured part so that no movement is possible. This stops further injury and helps to control the bleeding.
9. Immobilize the fracture area and the joints on both sides of the fracture site (above and below) by using bandages or by using splints wherever available. It is essential that the rescuer be familiar with the use of bandages and splints.

Using bandages
Usually, it is enough to use the other (uninjured) limb or the body of the victim as the splint. The upper limb can be supported by the body, and the lower limb by the other limb provided that also is not fractured. Most fractures except those of the forearm can be immobilized in this manner:
- Do not apply bandage over the area of the fracture.
- The bandaging should be firm so that there is no movement of the fractured ends but should not be too tight as blood circulation to the affected area could be reduced. If there is further swelling of the injured area, the bandage may be too tight and therefore may need to be loosened.
- Always place padding material between the ankles, knees and other hollows if they have to be tied together so that when the limbs are bound together they are comfortable and steady.
- If the patient is lying down, the bandage should be passed through the natural hollows such as the neck, the lower part of the trunk, knees, just above the ankles, etc., so that the patient's body is not jarred.
- Always tie the knots on the sound side.

Using splints
Splints are used only when necessary expertise is there.
- A splint is a rigid piece of wood or plastic material or metal applied to a fractured limb to prevent movement of the broken bone.
- Reasonably wide splints are better than narrow ones.
- Splints should be long enough so that the joints above and below the fractured bones can be made immobile.
- The splints should be well padded with cotton or cloth so as to fits snugly and softly on the injured limb.
- Splints are best applied over the clothing.
- In an emergency, splints can be improvised using a walking stick, an umbrella, a piece of wood, a book or even a firmly folded newspaper.
- Use of splints becomes obligatory only when both legs and both thigh bones are broken.

Fractures involving the back (vertebral column) require special care. In such cases, the victim should note allowed to get up. Further movement must be avoided as much as possible and emergency medical help must be sought.

Management of Fractures with Different Areas
Fracture collar bone: symptoms and signs
- Immediate pain and swelling in the area of the fracture.
- A crackling or grinding sound in the affected area when moving the shoulder.
- The shoulder sagging forward and downward.
- The patient will hold the arm immobile in an attempt to relieve the pain.
- Very rarely, patient will complain of numbness or tingling.

Management
1. DRABC
2. Control bleeding and cover all wounds
3. Check for fractures—open, closed or complicated
4. Ask the casualty not to move the injured part
5. Immobilize fractures with slings, bandages or splints to prevent movement at the joints above and below the fracture
6. Watch for signs of loss of circulation to the foot or hand
7. Move the casualty only if there is danger to you or the casualty
8. Handle gently
9. Observe casualty carefully and manage shock if necessary
10. Seek medical aid

D: Danger
Check to see if it is safe to approach the injured person.

R: Response
Check if the person is conscious or unconscious. Shake them lightly and shout to them. If they do not respond they are unconscious.

A: Airway
The airway must be protected, roll them onto their side, being aware that their neck may be injured and needs to be stabilized while they are being rolled.

B: Breathing
Once on their side check that the mouth is clear of any obstructions such as blood or vomits and make sure that they are breathing.

C: Circulation
Stop any bleeding by applying direct pressure with bandages or clothing. If possible, elevate the bleeding part above the level of the chest. Keep the injured person as still as possible by packing, clothing and equipment around them to prevent movement to the spine and any broken bones.

Fracture of upper arm
Symptoms and signs
- Pain, made worse by movement of the shoulder
- History of a fallen to the outstretched arm or elbow
- The casualty may support the arm at the elbow and incline the head toward the injured side
- The shoulder appears to be lower than the uninjured side
- Tenderness and swelling around the collarbone

Management
1. DRABC
2. Follow the general rules for fracture management
3. Support the arm on the injured side
4. Seek medical aid.

If the injury is closed to, or involves the elbow:
1. Lay the casualty down, supporting the injured area
2. Check the pulse at the wrist and the color of the hand and finger
3. Gently place the injured limb on supporting material by the side of the body. Do not bend the elbow
4. Immobilize the arm firmly to the body with broad bandages
5. Tie bandages in front on the uninjured side
6. Check the pulse
7. Seek medical aid.

If the injury is not close to the elbow:
1. Apply collar and cuff sling
2. Do not support under the elbow. Allow the elbow to hang freely
3. Places the padding between the elbow area and the chest

4. Immobilize the arm with two broad bandages (or narrow ones for a small person): One above the fracture, over the arm and surround the chest, the other below the fracture
5. Tie off the bandages in front on the uninjured side
6. Check the pulse
7. Seek medical aid.

Fracture of forearm
Symptoms and signs
- Pain
- Loss of power
- Deformity
- The casualty may support the injured forearm with the other arm

Management
If fracture is not near the elbow:
1. Immobilize the limb firmly to splint which extends from the elbow to the finger.
   Bandage:
   - Above the fracture, below the elbow
   - Below the fracture
   - At the wrist/hand
2. Apply an arm sling
3. Seek medical aid
4. Check pulse and color of finger.

If the fracture is near the elbow:
1. Immobilize the arm in the position found
2. Check the pulse
3. Seek medical aid urgently.

Fracture of the hands and the fingers
Symptoms and signs
- Pain
- Swelling
- Deformity
- Bleeding, if there is wound.

Management
Hand fractures:
1. DRABC (Danger, Response, Airway, Breathing and Circulation)
2. Place soft padding between the chest and the limb
3. Support at the arm with abroad bandage over the forearm, tied off on the uninjured side
4. Check pulse
5. Seek medical aid.

Finger or thumb fractures:
1. DRABC
2. Rest the injured hand on a well-padded splint and secure with a bandage
3. Elevate the hand for as long as possible
4. Seek medical aid.

Fracture of thigh

Symptoms and signs
- Usually a history of a fall on an outstretched hand
- Pain and swelling
- Tenderness
- Weakness of the hands and fingers
- Deformity often present.

Management
1. Rest the forearm and hand on a well-padded splint. Additional padding under the hand and wrist maybe required
2. Secure the limb to the splint by bandaging below the elbow, across the back of the hand and around the middle of the forearm
3. Elevate the limb
4. Apply a large arm sling
5. Seek medical aid.

Fracture of neck of the thigh bone

Symptoms and signs
- Severe pain at the site of the injury
- Loss of power
- Tenderness at the site of the injury
- Deformity
- Swelling
- Possibly a rotation of the foot of the injured leg
- Possible shortening of the injured leg
- Shock.

Management
1. DRABC
2. Cover open wounds
3. Place padding between legs
4. Gently bring uninjured limb to the injured limb
5. Apply a figure-of-eight bandage around the knees and tie on the uninjured side
6. Seek medical aid.

If expert assistance is likely to be delayed:
1. DRABC
2. Cover open wounds
3. Gently bring uninjured limb to the normal position
4. Place a well-padded splint between the legs
5. Place one hand under the heel and the other around the toes of the injured limb
6. Gently draw down to apply traction to the foot, while rotating the leg to a position as nearly normal as possible against the splint
7. Apply a narrow figure-of-eight bandage around the ankles and feet
8. Pass bandages under:
    i. The thighs above the fracture
    ii. The thighs below the fracture
    iii. Both knees
    iv. Between the knees and the ankles
9. Tie on the uninjured side
10. Check the circulation of both limbs (note the color and temperature of the skin and feet).

Fracture of hip

Symptoms and signs
- Pain in the area of the hip, thigh or knee when moving the limb
- Loss of power
- Tenderness over the hip
- Put ward rotation of the foot of the injured leg
- Shortening of the injured leg
- Bruising (seen later)

Management
1. DRABC
2. If the casualty has been lying on the ground for a long period of time, manage any scalds to the skin from urine and feces
3. Reassure the casualty comfortable
4. Place padding between legs and under tender spots
5. Apply a figure-of-eight bandage at the ankle and a broad bandage at the knees
6. Seek medical aid.

Fracture of kneecap

Symptoms and signs
- Pain over knee cap, aggravated by movement
- Loss of power at the knee
- Inability to straighten the leg
- Tenderness and swelling over the kneecap
- Sometimes a gap can be felt at the front of the knee
- Sometimes the displaced knee cap can be felt.

Management
1. DRABC
2. Lay the casualty on the back with head and shoulders raised
3. Raise the leg about 30 cm and support it in the most comfortable position
4. Do not attempt to straighten the knee
5. If the limb can be splinted without increasing discomfort, then
    i. Apply a pressure bandage around the knee (figure-of-eight crepe or conforming bandage)
    ii. Apply a splint along the back of the limb from buttock to beyond the heel
6. Ensure that the splint is adequately padded, particularly under the natural hollows of the knee and ankle
7. Secure the limb to the splint by a figure-of-eight bandage around the thigh, and broad bandage around the lower leg
8. Seek medical aid.

Fracture of lower leg

Symptoms and signs
- Pain
- Inability to walk

- ❖ Shortening of injured leg
- ❖ Deformity
- ❖ Swelling
- ❖ Rotation of foot of injured leg
- ❖ Protruding bone
- ❖ Bleeding.

Management
1. DRABC
2. Control bleeding and cover wounds
3. Place padding between the legs
4. Bring the uninjured limb to the injured limb
5. Steady and support the injured limb.
6. Apply a figure-of-eight bandage around the ankle and feet
7. Apply a broad bandage the knees, and tie on the uninjured side.

If expert assistance is delayed:
1. DRABC
2. Control bleeding and cover wounds
3. Lace a well-padded splint between the legs, from the thighs to the ankles
4. Pad between the thighs, knees, and ankles
5. Apply a figure-of-eight bandage around the ankles and feet
6. Apply a broad bandage around the thighs, at the knees, above and below the fracture
7. Seek medical aid.

Fracture of feet and toes

Symptoms and signs
- ❖ Pain
- ❖ Inability to walk
- ❖ Tenderness
- ❖ Swelling

Management
1. DRABC (Danger, response, airway, breathing and circulation)
2. Only remove shoes and socks if there is an open wound
3. If casualty is not wearing shoes, apply a compression bandage
4. Raise foot and rest on pillow
5. Seek medical aid.

Fracture of ankle

This fracture may be mistaken for a sprain, particularly if no deformity is present.

Symptoms and signs
- ❖ History of a twisting injury
- ❖ Pain and swelling on either or both sides of the ankle
- ❖ Inability to bear weight on the ankle tenderness, particularly over the bony prominences on either side of the ankle
- ❖ Deformity, which may be severe.

Management
If no deformity is present:
1. RICE (rest, ice, compression, elevation)
2. Avoid any weight bearing on the affected limb
3. Seek medical aid.

If deformity is present:
1. Steady and support the injured limb on pillows or a folded blanket
2. Do not apply any compression bandages around the ankle
3. Seek medical aid urgently.

FIRST AID FOR ACCIDENT

Road Traffic Accidents

If you witness an accident or are involved in an accident where someone is hurt–it is important to:
- ❖ Call the ambulance quickly and explain what has happened.
- ❖ Do not try and move the person if bones are broken–especially the back.
- ❖ Carefully move person into recovery position–ensure there is nothing blocking the person's airways if they are unconscious.
- ❖ If the person is able to move and you have access to transport. As a first aid provider, you may be required to render assistance at the scene of a road traffic accident.

If so, remember to be calm and methodical in your actions as others involved who have not had the benefit of first aid training will look to you for support and guidance.

Approaching the Scene

Consider your safety and that of bystanders and the casualty. Always take time to have a good look at the scene before you approach. Approach the scene methodically, keep away from traffic, and ask someone to accompany you as an assistant.

Examine the Scene

Give yourself time to think about your next move: Is the vehicle stable; will it roll or move? Is there spilt fuel? Is there any danger of fire? Are power poles involved? What about oncoming traffic? If a van or truck; is the load safe? Do not touch anything until you are sure that it is safe.

Control the Scene

As you move to the scene, ask bystanders to move back. Ask a responsible person to slow down or redirect any oncoming traffic. Ask someone else to make sure that bystanders (especially children) do not become involved with passing traffic. Ask bystanders not to smoke near any damaged vehicles. Unless there is someone else present with more advanced medical knowledge, you become the person in-charge of the casualties.

Assess the Scene

Initial impressions should be to assess:
- How many casualties?
- Are they walking around?
- Unconscious?
- Talking?
- Any obviously dead?
- Any trapped

After the initial quick assessment, ask the person who accompanied you to contact the ambulance service and provide information on location, number of casualties, estimated seriousness of injuries, and if road rescue is required for trapped casualties.

Attending the Casualties

Perform a quick examination of the casualties for bleeding, burns, fractures, other injuries. This will tend to confirm your initial first aid. Use any helpers to move the casualties with minor injuries (walking wounded) away from the scene to a safe place. This will give you more room to attend to the more serious cases. Always try to have a responsible person to help you attend to serious casualties–it helps to have assistance and support.

What to look for?

Always consider the effects of the accident: Side impact leads to fractured upper leg (femur) and/or lower leg. Consider a fractured pelvis. Suspect a shoulder or upper arm injury on the side of impact, and if the "B" pillar has been damaged, suspect a head injury.

- **High speed impact:** Deceleration injuries involving severe internal bleeding, multiple fractures, impacted pelvis, head and spinal injuries, and multiple lacerations. Be alert for deterioration in unconscious casualties with head injuries.
- **Rear end collisions:** Cervical spine injuries ("whiplash" effect) and facial injuries.
- **Ejection from the vehicle:** Head and spinal injuries, unconsciousness, multiple fractures, multiple lacerations to top of body and head, and internal bleeding.
- **Roll over:** This mechanism of injury provides for the complete range of damage to the human body. Drivers and passengers are usually thrown around, irrespective of their seat belt restraints, and they have no control over their movements.

  Pay particular attention to children, as they are not usually correctly restrained by seat belts designed for adults.
- **Motorcycle accidents:** Injuries commonly sustained by riders and pillion passengers are fractures of the femur, wrist and ankle fractures, head injuries, and deceleration injuries resulting in severe internal bleeding.

  Motor cyclists' helmets must not be removed unless the airway is obstructed or the casualty is not breathing. Casualties should remove their own helmets wherever possible. If a helmet has to be removed, it requires two rescuers to do so, and it should be done carefully with no movement of the neck.
- **Bicycle accidents:** Cyclists are liable to sustain multiple fractures, multiple lacerations, and head injuries. Children are susceptible to "greenstick" fractures of the arms, and wrist injuries through falling off at relatively low speed.
- **Pedestrians:** Generally, adults are struck on their side as they try to turn away from the danger. Their injuries are usually more pronounced on the side that has received the impact. Children and the elderly are more likely to be struck as they turn to face the oncoming vehicle.

Most pedestrians are "run under" rather than "run over" as they are their feet by the impact and may be thrown over the vehicle, or for some distance from the point of impact. Head and spinal injuries are common. Small children may be "run over", and be still under the vehicle when it stops.

Treatment of Casualties

Treat any casualties in accordance with the need. Do not remove any seriously injured casualties from the vehicle unless fire, fear of further collision, airway protection, control of severe bleeding, or CPR is necessary. Wait for the ambulance to arrive. Provide what treatment and reassurance you can, keep the casualties warm with blankets if available, and periodically check on the "walking wounded" who have been moved from the scene.

Remember that shock is a life-threatening condition, and is common after trauma sustained in a road traffic accident. Be ready to treat any signs and symptoms that indicate that a casualty is progressing into shock.

On arrival of the ambulance, take care of the shifting part as per the injury and on reaching to the casualty department give all the information you have and any treatment you have provided.

FIRST AID FOR BURNS AND SCALDS

Burns are wounds caused by excessive exposure of the body to heat, such as by flame, hot liquids. Of all the injuries that fire performers, accumulate burns are probably the most common. Early treatment of a burning the first few minutes after it occurs can make a huge difference in the severity of the injury.

Before giving first aid, it is necessary to evaluate the extension, involved body part, and severity of the burn. Then treat the entire burn as per the need. If in doubt, treatment should be carried out as for severe burn.

By giving immediate first aid before the arrival of medical team can help to lessen the severity of the burn. Prompt medical attention in case of serious burns can help to prevent scarring, disability, and deformity. Burns on the face, hands, feet, and genitals can be particularly serious.

Children under age 4 and adults over age 60 have a higher chance of complications and death from severe burns.

Causes

Burns can be caused by dry heat (like fire), wet heat (such as steam or hot liquids), radiation, friction, heated objects, the sun, electricity, or chemicals.

Thermal burns are the most common type. Thermal burns occur when hot metals, scalding liquids, steam, or flames come in contact with your skin. These are frequently the result of fires, automobile accidents, playing with matches, improperly stored gasoline, space heaters, and electrical malfunctions. Other causes include unsafe handling of firecrackers and kitchen accidents (such as a child climbing on top of a stove or grabbing hot iron).

Burns to your airways can be caused by inhaling smoke, steam, superheated air, or toxic fumes, often in a poorly ventilated space. In case of a fire, there is a risk for carbon monoxide poisoning. Anyone with symptoms of headache, numbness, weakness, or chest pain should be treated immediately.

Types of Burns

The first step, regardless of the type or class of burn, is to put a stop to it! Get the heat source away from the skin and extinguish any flames. Use a wet towel to put out any burning toys that may be tangled and near the skin (especially in case of child) and work to remove any hot metal from the skin as quickly as possible. Once the heat source is removed, examine (but do not touch!) the burned to assess the class of burn.

There are three levels of burns: First-degree, second-degree, and third-degree.

First-degree Burns

First-degree burn is caused by brief exposure to heat and affect only the outer/top layer of the skin. Sun burn is a type of first degree.

Signs
- Red
- Painful to touch
- Mild swelling on the skin

Treatment
- Apply cool and wet compresses, or immerse in cool, fresh water, until pain subsides.
- Cover the burn with a sterile, nonadhesive bandage or clean cloth.
- Do not apply ointments or butter to burn; these may cause infection.

First aid
- Over-the-counter pain medications may be used to help relieve pain and reduce inflammation.
- First-degree burns usually heal without further treatment. However, if a first-degree burn covers a large area of the body if the victim is an infant or elderly, seek emergency medical attention.

Second-degree (Partial Thickness) Burns

Second-degree burns caused by prolonged exposure to heat or very high temperature and involve the first two layers of skin and affect both the outer and underlying layer of skin. The skin may be intact or it may appear to be partially peeling. It may also appear moist or have a mottled appearance. Any burn with blisters is second-degree.

Signs
- Deep reddening of the skin
- Pain
- Blisters
- Glossy appearance from leaking fluid
- Possible loss of some skin.

Treatment
- Immerse in fresh, cool water, or apply cool compresses. Continue for 10–15 minutes.
- Dry with clean cloth and cover with sterile gauze and protect it from pressure and friction.
- Do not break blisters.
- Do not apply ointments or butter to burns; these may cause infection
- Elevate burned arms or legs.
- **Take steps to prevent shock:** Lay the victim flat, elevate the feet about 12 inches, and cover the victim with a coat or blanket. Do not place the victim in the shock position if a head, neck, back, or leg injury is suspected, or if it makes the victim uncomfortable.
- Further medical treatment is required. Do not attempt to treat serious burns unless you are a trained health professional.

Third-degree (Full Thickness) Burns

A third-degree burn is the most serious type of burn and is caused by prolonged exposure to very high temperature. It penetrates the entire thickness of the skin and permanently destroys deeper tissue, and causes white or blackened, charred skin that may not be painful (numb), as the pain receptors of the skin have been destroyed along with the skin.

Signs
- Loss of skin layers
- Often painless (pain may be caused by patches of first- and second-degree burns which often surround third-degree burns).
- Skin is dry and leathery
- Skin may appear charred or have patches which appear white, brown or black.

Treatment
- Cover burn light with sterile gauze or clean cloth (Do not use material that can leave Linton the burn).

- Protect the burned area from pressure and friction by elevating it.
- If the victim has stopped breathing or his/her airway is blocked, open the airway and perform rescue breathing and CPR as needed.
- If the victim is breathing, cover the burn area with a moist, cool sterile bandage or clean cloth.
- Do not apply ointments or butter to burns and be careful not to break burn blisters; these may cause infection.
- Separate the victim's fingers and toes with dry, sterile, nonadhesive bandages, to avoid adherence.
- Do not put the victim in this position if he or she is uncomfortable or if you suspect a head, neck, back or leg injury.
- Watch closely for possible breathing problems.
- Elevate burned area higher than the victim's head when possible. Keep person warm and comfortable, and watch for signs of shock.
- To prevent shock, lay the victim flat, elevate the feet 12 inches and cover the victim with a coat or blanket.
- Do not place a pillow under the victim's head if the person is lying down and there is an airway burn. This can close the airway.
- Immediate medical attention is required. Do not attempt to treat serious burns unless you are a trained health professional, but monitor vital signs frequently till arrival of the medical team.

Immediate Treatment for Burn Victims

1. "Stop, Drop, and Roll" to smother flames.
2. Remove all burned clothing. If clothing adheres to the skin, cut or tear around burned area.
3. Remove all jewelry, belts, tight clothing, etc., from over the burned areas and from around the victim's neck. This is very important; burned areas swell immediately.

First Aid Assistance for Major Burns

- Do not apply ointment, butter, ice, medications, fluffy cotton, adhesive bandages, cream or oil spray these can interfere with the healing process.
- Do not allow the burn to become contaminated, avoid coughing or breathing on the burn.
- Do not bother blistered and dead skin.
- Do not give the victim anything to ingest if he/she has a severe burn.
- Do not immerse a severe burn in cold water or apply cold compresses this can cause shock.
- Do not place a pillow under a victim's head.

Call emergency assistance immediately if:
- The victim has a severe or extensive burn
- The victim has a chemical or electrical burn
- The victim shows signs of shock are present
- Airway burn has occurred.

Remember: When in doubt, seek medical attention for a burn. Burns are complicated and these medical injuries may require very advanced care for severe cases.

Prevention

To help prevent burns:
- Install smoke alarms in your home. Check and change batteries regularly.
- Teach children about fires a safety and the hazards of matches and fireworks.
- Keep children from climbing on top of stove or grabbing hot items such as irons and oven doors.
- Turn pot handles toward the back of the stove so that children cannot grab them and they cannot be accidentally knocked over.
- Place fire extinguishers in key locations at home, work, and school.
- Remove electrical cords from floors.
- Know about and practice fire escape outs at home, work, and school.
- Set temperature of water heater at 120 degrees or less.

Health Education

In a continuing effort to increase burn awareness in the community should be initiated:
- High-risk industry employees (electrical facilities, paper mills, etc.)
- Elementary, middle, and high school students
- Nursing, occupational/physical therapies student groups
- Fire fighters, emergency medical services (EMS), paramedics and other safety/rescue personnel.

FIRST AID FOR POISONING

Poisoning may be accidental, involving everyday substances, or deliberate, as in attempted suicide. It can be caused by eating contaminated food or poisonous plants, and by misuse of drugs and alcohol.

Features of poisoning vary depending on the poison, the method of entry, and the amount taken. A conscious casualty or onlooker may report a poisoning. If the casualty is unconscious, poisoning may be deduced from external features such as a fume-filled room or a suspect container.

Medical attention is always advisable in cases of poisoning, and is essential in severe cases. Although poisoning can be fatal, most cases are treated successfully.

What is a Poison?

A poison or toxin is a substance that can cause temporary or permanent damage if taken into the body in sufficient quantity. Once introduced into the body, a poison can quickly be carried to the entire tissues via the bloodstream. Signs and symptoms vary, depending on the poison and its method of entry. Vomiting is common to many cases.

There are four ways a person can be poisoned are:
1. **Ingestion (by swallowing):** It includes foods, alcohol, medication, household and garden items and certain plants.
2. **Absorption (through the skin):** Absorbed poisons enter the body through the skin; they may come from plants, fertilizers or pesticides.
3. **Inhalation (breathing it):** Inhaled poisons may be gases, such as carbon monoxide from car exhaust, carbon dioxide from sewers, and chlorine from a pool or fumes from household products such as glue, paint, and cleaners or drugs.
4. **Injection (injected into the body):** Injected poisons enter the body through bites or stings of insects, spiders, ticks, marine life, snakes and other animals or medications injected with a hypodermic needle.

The first aid you give before getting medical help can save a victim's life. In a poisoning emergency immediate first aid is critical.

It is important to note that the absence of a warning on a package label does not necessarily mean that the product is safe.

Suspect poisoning if someone suddenly becomes sick for no apparent reason.

Suspect inhalation poisoning if the victim is found near a furnace, a car, a fire, or in an area that is not well ventilated. Symptoms of poisoning may take time to develop. However, if poisoning is suspected, do not wait for symptoms to develop before getting medical help.

Causes

Common causes include:
- Medicines (such as an aspirin overdose)
- Household detergents and cleaning products
- Carbon monoxide gas (from furnaces, gas engines, fires, space heaters)
- Household plants (eating toxic plants)
- Paints (swallowing or inhaling fumes)
- Insecticides
- Cosmetics (incorrectly used)
- Illicit drug overdose (accidental or intentional)
- Occupational chemical exposures
- Food poisoning (such as botulism)
- Animals (exposure to the toxic substances produced by some animals)

Symptoms

Symptoms vary according to the poison, but may include:
- Abdominal pain
- Bluish lips
- Chest pain
- Confusion
- Cough
- Diarrhea
- Difficulty inbreathing
- Dizziness
- Double vision
- Drowsiness
- Fever
- Headache
- Heart palpitations
- Irritability
- Loss of appetite
- Loss of bladder control
- Muscle twitching
- Nausea and vomiting
- Numbness or tingling
- Seizures
- Shortness of breath
- Skin rash or burns
- Stupor
- Unconsciousness
- Unusual breath odor
- Weakness

Always call for local poison control center or emergency medical service for help.

First Aid Management

Poisoning by Swallowing

1. Check and monitor the victim's airway, breathing and circulation. If necessary, begin rescue breathing and CPR.
2. Try to make sure that the victim has indeed been poisoned. It is not always obvious. Some signs include chemical-smelling breath, burns around the mouth, difficulty in breathing, vomiting, or unusual odors on the victim. If possible, identify the poison.
3. Only induce vomiting if the medical service is available.
4. If the victim vomits, protect the airway. If you must clear the victim's airway, wrap a cloth around your fingers before cleaning out his or her mouth and throat. If the victim has vomited a plant part, save the vomitus as it may allow identification by an expert who can then determine an antidote.
5. If the victim starts having convulsions, protect him or her from injury and give convulsion first aid.
6. Reassure the victim and keep him or her comfortable. Position the victim on his/her left side while getting or awaiting medical help. If the poison has spilled on the victim's clothes, remove the clothing and flush the skin with water.

For Inhalation Poisoning

1. Call for emergency help. Never attempt to rescue a victim without notifying the emergency services first.

2. If it is safe to do so, rescue the victim from the danger of the gas, fumes, or smoke. Hold a wet cloth over your nose and mouth. Open windows and doors to move the stored fumes.
3. Take several deep breaths offers hair, and then hold your breath as you going in.
4. Avoid lighting a match as some gases may ignite.
5. After rescuing the victim from danger, check his or her airway, breathing, and circulation. If necessary, perform rescue breathing and CPR.
6. As necessary, perform first aid for skin burns, eye injuries (eye emergencies), or convulsions.
7. If the victim vomits, protect his or her airway.
8. Even if the victim seems perfectly fine, get medical help.

Do not
- Do not give an unconscious victim anything by mouth.
- Do not induce vomiting unless you are told to do so by the doctor. A strong poison that burns on the way down the throat will also do damage on the way backup.
- Do not try to neutralize the poison with lemon juice or vinegar, or any other substance, unless you are told to do so by the doctor.
- Do not use any "cure-all" type antidote.
- Do not wait for symptoms to develop if you suspect that someone has been poisoned.

Call immediately for emergency medical assistance prevention

Prevention of poisoning is the best path for your safety and health. In addition to danger of the poison, none of the medical procedures or drugs used to treat poisoning is risk-free. Some of the antidotes for poisoning are risky in their own right, and even simple procedures such as pumping a stomach carry a certain level of risk.

Be aware of poisons in and around your home. Take steps to protect young children from toxic substances. Store all medicines, chemicals used for cleaning, cosmetics, and household chemicals out of reach of children, or in cabinets with childproof latches.

- Be familiar with plants in your home, yard, and vicinity. Keep your children informed, too. Remove any noxious plants. Never eat wild plants, mushrooms, roots, or berries unless you know what you are doing.
- Teach children about the dangers of substances that contain poison. Label all poisons.
- Do not store household chemicals in food containers, even if they are labeled. Most non-food substances are poisonous if taken in large doses.

If you are concerned that industrial poisons might be polluting nearby land or water, report your concerns to the local health department.

In the case of an emergency, try to determine what the person was exposed to and what part of the body was affected before you take action. If the person is unconscious, having trouble breathing, or having convulsions, gives needed first aid immediately. Call for your local emergency service. Remember to act fast because speed is crucial! But equally important is taking the right action. In most cases, the hazardous product's label provides you with a "First Aid Instructions" to follow in emergencies. The appropriate first aid treatment depends on the kind of poisoning that has occurred. If first aid instructions are not available, follow the general guidelines below and/or call the poison control center or emergency medical service.

FIRST AID FOR FOOD POISONING AND POISONOUS PLANTS

Food poisoning may be caused by eating food that is contaminated, either by bacteria or by toxins produced by bacteria present in the food at sometime.

Bacterial food poisoning is often caused by the *Salmonella* group of bacteria. Symptoms may develop within a few hours, or be delayed for a day or so.

Toxic food poisoning is often caused by toxins produced by the bacterial group *Staphylococcus*. Symptoms usually develop rapidly, sometimes within 2–6 hours of consumption.

Prevention of Food Poisoning

In order to prevent food poisoning: Ensure that frozen meat and poultry are fully defrosted before cooking; cook meat, poultry and eggs thoroughly to destroy any dangerous bacteria; do not keep food lukewarm for long periods (bacteria multiply); ensure hands are clean before preparing food (wear protective gloves if hands have wounds).

In cases of food poisoning, the casualty may suffer from: nausea and vomiting; cramping abdominal pains; diarrhea (sometimes bloodstained), headache, fever, shock and collapse.

Treatment of Food Poisoning

- Help the casualty toiled own and rest
- Contact a medical practitioner
- Give the casualty plenty to drink, and a bowl in case of vomiting
- If the casualty's condition worsens, contact the emergency service.

Poisonous Plants

Poisonous plants can cause serious illness if eaten. These include a few varieties of mushrooms, seeds, bulbs, rhizomes and berries.

Treatment of Ingestion of Poisonous Plants

- Check and clear the airway.
- If the casualty is unconscious, check breathing and pulse, and be prepared to resuscitate if necessary. Place the casualty in there cover position. The casualty may vomit.

Do not attempt to induce vomiting:
- ❖ Assess the need to contact a medical practitioner or the emergency service. If in doubt, always contact the emergency service.
- ❖ Try to identify the plant, and which part of it has been ingested. Keep samples of the plant, and any vomited material, to show the medical practitioner, or to send to hospital with the casualty.

Poison in Eye

If poison splashes into an eye, remove contact lenses if necessary, hold the eyelid open and wash quickly and gently with clean running water from the top or a gentle stream from a hose for at least 15 minutes. Eye damage can occur in a few minutes with some types of toxic chemicals. If possible, have someone else contact the emergency service for you while the victim is being treated. Do not use eye drops or chemicals or drugs in the wash water.

Poison on Skin

Call for emergency service, if a toxic chemical splashes on the skin. Drench area with water and remove contaminated clothing. Wash skin and hair thoroughly with soap and water. Later, discord contaminated clothing or thoroughly washes it separately from other laundry.

Suspect inhalation poisoning if the victim is found near a furnace, a car, a fire, or in an area that is not well ventilated.

Symptoms of poisoning may take time to develop. However, if poisoning is suspected, do not wait for symptoms to develop before getting medical help.

FIRST AID FOR BLEEDING

Bleeding is the loss of blood from the body. **Hemorrhage** is the medical term for bleeding. In common usage, a hemorrhage means particularly severe bleeding; although technically it means escape of blood to extravascular space. The complete loss of blood is referred to as exsanguination. Children are put more in danger by bleeding as they have less blood to lose. The average adult human will biomedical danger after 1 liter (2 pints) and could die of hypovolemic shock if more blood is lost.

The human body generates blood at a rate of about 2 liters (2 quarts) per week. The technique of blood transfusion is used to replace severe quantities of lost blood.

Causes, Prevalence and Risk Factors

Hemorrhage generally becomes dangerous, or even fatal, when it causes hypovolemia (low blood volume) or hypotension (low blood pressure). In these scenarios various mechanisms come into play to maintain the body's homeostasis. These include the "retro-stress-relaxation" mechanism of cardiac muscle, the baroreceptor reflex and renal and endocrine responses such as the renin-angiotensin-aldosterone effect.

Death from hemorrhage can generally occur surprisingly quickly. This is because of "negative feedback". An example of this is "cardiac repression", when poor heart contraction depletes blood flow to the heart, causing even poorer heart contraction. This kind of effect causes death occurs more quickly than expected.

Types of Bleeding

- ❖ **Minor traumatic bleeding:** Bleeding from small and superficial wounds; the loss of blood is not dangerous and the bleeding will stop spontaneously; the main risk is the wound itself (dysfunction of the organs involved and infection).
- ❖ **Severe traumatic bleeding:** The flow of blood can soak a paper or cloth handkerchief in a few seconds; in such a situation, the bleeding will caused within a few minutes.
- ❖ **Externalized bleeding:** The blood flow through a natural orifice, such as the nose, the ears, the mouth (spitting and vomiting blood), the vagina (except for the natural menstruation), the urethra and the anus; the blood comes from the interior of the body and reveals a hidden trauma or a disease.
- ❖ **Internal bleeding:** The blood flows inside the body; it cannot be seen, but can be suspected by shock symptoms.

Further, bleeding can be categorized by the type of the damaged blood vessel:
- ❖ **Arterial bleeding** occurs from arteries, the major blood vessels which carry oxygen-rich blood from the heart throughout the body. This type of bleeding is characterized by spurts with each beat of the heart, is bright red in color (although blood darkens when it meets the air) and is usually severe and hard to control. Arterial bleeding requires immediate attention.
- ❖ **Venous bleeding** occurs from veins, vessels which return the blood to the heart. Venous bleeding is characterized by a steady flow and the blood is dark, almost maroon in shade. Venous bleeding is easier to control than arterial bleeding.
- ❖ **Capillary bleeding** occurs from capillaries, the smallest of our body's blood vessels. It is usually slow, oozing in nature and this type of bleeding usually has a higher risk of infection than other types of bleeding. It is much easier to control than other types of bleeding.

Hemorrhage in the Brain

Internal bleeding can occur in any part of the brain. Blood may accumulate in the brain tissues itself, or in the space between the brain and the membranes covering it. The bleeding may be isolated to part of one hemisphere (lobar intracerebral hemorrhage) or it may occur in other brain structures, such as the thalamus, basal ganglia, pons, or cerebellum (deep intracerebral hemorrhage).

An intracerebral hemorrhage can be caused by a traumatic brain injury or abnormalities of the blood vessels (aneurysm or angioma). When it is not caused by one of these conditions, it is most commonly associated with high blood pressure (hypertensive intracerebral hemorrhage). In some cases, no cause can be found. Blood irritates the brain tissues, causing swelling (cerebral edema). It can collect into a mass called a hematoma. Either swelling or a hematoma will increase pressure on brain tissues and can rapidly destroy them. Symptoms vary depending on the location of the bleed and the amount of brain tissue affected. The symptoms usually develop suddenly, without warning, often during activity. They may occasionally develop a stepwise, episodic manner or they may get progressively worse.

Minor Traumatic Bleeding

The minor traumatic bleeding stops spontaneously, the loss of blood is not dangerous in itself. But the wound can still endanger the life of the casualty.

Severe Traumatic Bleeding

The general management:
- **Protect:** Remove the cause of wound so nobody else gets hurt, or lead the casualty away and mark out the dangerous area; when the casualty cannot walk, do not move him unless the danger is deadly and real;
- Stop the bleeding;
- Leave the casualty in the position he feels comfortable;
- Ask someone to call for help, or do it yourself if you are alone; describe the general state of the casualty (check for breathing or not).
- Follow the instructions given by the EMS.

Immediate management: A major technique of first aid is to control bleeding through direct pressure with the hand (possibly protected by a plastic bag, a glove or other material); it can be replaced when necessary by the application of a bandage over the wound. If the casualty is conscious and alert, he can press on the wound himself for a short time (e.g., the time needed for a bystander to get protection for the hands, something to make bandage).

When the direct pressure is not possible (e.g., there is a foreign body inside the wound, or a broken bone comes outside, or the wound is too large for the hand), then it is possible to compress the artery against bone, between the wound and the heart.

In extreme cases of an injured limb, a tourniquet may be used. If medical care is delayed (after a few hours), the injured limb must generally be amputated afterward, just below the level the tourniquet is applied; this is "losing a limb to save a life". This risk is very low in the urban environment of a developed country but must be taken into account in wilderness or in countries that do not have organized prehospital medical services. Some first aid instruction no longer teaches the use of the tourniquet because the risk may be greater than the benefit; some other considers that saving a life is above the rest. However, this should always be the last choice.

Severe Bleeding

To stop serious bleeding, follow these steps:
1. Lay the affected person down. If possible, the person's head should be slightly lower than the trunk of his or her body or the legs should be elevated. This position increases blood flow to the brain. Elevate the site of bleeding, if possible to reduce the blood flow.
2. Do not attempt to clean the wound.
3. Apply steady, firm pressure directly to the wound using a sterile bandage, a clean cloth, or your hand. Maintain pressure until the bleeding stops, then wrap the wound with a tight dressing and secure it with adhesive tape. Most bleeding can be controlled this way. Call for emergency help immediately.
4. If the bleeding continues and seeps through the bandage, add more absorbent material. Do not remove the first bandage.
5. If the bleeding does not stop, apply pressure to the major artery that delivers blood to the area of the injury.
6. When the bleeding has stopped, immobilize the injured portion of the body. You can use another part of the body, such as a leg or torso, to immobilize the area. Leave the bandages in place and take the person for immediate medical attention or call for emergency service.

Externalized Bleeding

The only minor situation is a spontaneous nosebleed, or a nosebleed caused by a slight trauma (such as a child putting his finger in the nose). Just sit down, slightly tilt your head forward, and pinch the bridge of your nose. Do not blow your nose! Keep doing this for about 10 minutes, which is the time the clot forms correctly (a shorter compression is not efficient). Consult a doctor when the bleeding does not stop or starts again.

Any other situation (including nosebleed due to a severe nose trauma or to a head trauma) must be considered as an emergency: place the person in a comfortable situation (lying or seated), call for help and follow the instructions.

Internal Bleeding

Internal bleeding, often more serious than external bleeding, is usually the result of crush injuries, fractures, or a burst peptic ulcer. Blood lost internally can pool in connected tissues and cause a build-up of pressure on vital organ, a hemorrhage inside the skull, for example, can lead to compression of the brain. Both internal and external bleeding can reduce blood pressure and cause shock.

Internal bleeding should be suspected if the person has pale, clammy skin, and a rapid, feeble pulse. (Note that the pulse may be slow if bleeding inside the skull has occurred.) Breathing may become shallow, with air hunger (yawning), restlessness, and thirst. Coughing or vomiting blood is another sign. There may also pain and swelling at the site of bleeding, or bruising under the skin.

First, encourage the person to rest quietly with legs raised, unless recourse there is a chest injury, in which case he or she should sit propped up. Keep the person warm observe the patient closely until help arrives. There is nothing else you can do, unless you have special training.

Risk of Blood Contamination

Concerning the direct exposure of the first-aider's skin to the blood: the skin is water tight, so if the skin is not wounded (skin disease or very recent wound), there is no risk of contamination by a disease of the casualty. Before any further activity (especially eating, drinking, touching the eyes, the mouth or the nose), the hand must be carefully and softly washed with clear water, then bathed 5 minutes in diluted sodium hypochlorite.

However, to avoid any risk, it is highly recommended to protect the hands, e.g., by a plastic bag or a cloth, before pressing the wound. If there is nothing to protect the hands, examine your hand to be sure it is not wounded, or use a distant compression of the artery pressure point with your hand if you know the anatomic references, or tourniquet.

In case of blood exposure, even on safe skin, the first-aider should go to the emergency service, where on antiretroviral therapy will be started just in case.

FIRST AID FOR AN INSECT BITE

Insect bites and stings are common and, although bothersome, seldom have serious consequences. The severity of an insect bite varies from person to person. The type of reaction which occurs after an insect bite depends so the species of insect, the age of the person and whether or not the person has been exposed to the insect before.

Insects not only bite, but also cause irritation to the skin. Most reactions to insect bites depend on a reaction to the saliva or venom. Insect bites can be single or multiple, depending on the feeding habits of the insect concerned. For example, fleas may produce multiple bites while a mosquito may bite only once.

Most reactions because a stinging sensation, redness, mild swelling, and some annoying itching confined to the sting site that disappear within a day or so. For some, especially in children, the swelling and redness may extend beyond the sting site, be more pronounced, and last 2-3 days.

A few people are allergic to insect bites and will experience itchy bumps, itching and swelling in other areas of the body. There might be tightness in the chest, difficulty breathing and swelling of the face and tongue. Only a small percentage of people develop an anaphylactic reaction which may be life-threatening. Mosquito, bedbugs and flea bites are the most common insect bites. In certain areas, some mosquitoes can transmit malaria. Bee and wasp stings are common during summer but not usually dangerous unless the person is allergic to these insects or if they are stung in the mouth or throat. These stings cause a painful red bump or swelling. Ticks are parasites that embed their heads in the skin to feed on the blood of mammals. They range in color from brown to grey and are usually found in the veld and on domestic animals. Tick bites are more common during spring and summer. They seldom lead to serious problems but some ticks may transmit organisms which could lead to illnesses, such a stick bite fever.

Home Treatment

- Itching can be relieved with an ice cube or cold compresses, a baking soda paste or bath, a meat tenderizer-water solution or soothing lotions such as calamine, Prep or witch hazel. 1% hydrocortisone cream is also effective.
- Take an oral antihistamine, such as Phenergan, to reduce fever and itching. Give paracetamol for pain.
- Remove a bee stinger by gently scraping the skin with the blunt edge of a knife, a credit card or with your fingernail. Try to do so within 30 seconds to avoid receiving more venom. Do not grasp the stinger as this could release more venom. If the stinger is below the skin surface, leave it alone and see a doctor. Do not rub the skin.
- Wash the bite area with soap and water.
- If you are severely allergic to bee or wasp stings, ask your doctor about an emergency kit containing an adrenaline syringe (Epipen), and try to avoid being outdoors. Wear a Medic Alert tag. An ice cube will also reduce blood flow.
- If you've been outdoors, check your whole body for ticks, especially hairy areas, skin clefts and crevices. If a tick is found, remove it immediately. Do not use bare fingers to remove the tick, but clutch it with fine-tipped tweezers as close to the skin as possible and pull it out in a straight line-do not jerk or twist it. Make sure that the head is also removed. If the head remains behind, it could cause a small necrotic ulcer. Do not squeeze or crush the tick. Save the tick in a container in case you develop a tick-borne illness and tests need to be done. Wash your hands and the bite site. Apply an antiseptic cream.

Get help immediately if:

- You have a severe allergic reaction to an insect bite. Follow steps for allergic reactions. Do not wait for the reaction to occur if you have a history of previous severe reaction to the insect's bite. Get to a hospital.

You've been stung on your face or neck. It may cause rapid swelling which could obstruct the airway.

Call for help if:
 There are signs of infection.
 There are multiple bites causing swelling around the eyes.
 You develop urticaria (hives).
 If you have developed an allergy to an insect bite. Allergy desensitization treatment is highly effective.
 The whole tick could not be removed.
 You develop flu-like symptoms.

Management for Insect Bites

1. Examine the stings it closely, looking for the stinger that may still be in the skin.
2. If a stinger is visible and accessible, attempt to remove it by carefully scraping it and the attached poisons from the skin. Do not use tweezers, fingers or anything that might squeeze more poison into the body.
3. To reduce the irritation at the site of the sting, apply rubbing alcohol or a paste of baking soda and water. Ice can also be used. Never use alcohol near the eyes.
4. If the sting is in the mouth, give the person a mouthwash of one teaspoonful of baking soda in a glass of water, or a piece of ice to suck on. Monitor the casualty for swelling or difficulty breathing. If symptoms occur, get medical help.

Signs of an Allergic Reaction to Insect Bite

A person suffering an allergic reaction to an insect bite or sting may display some or all of these symptoms:

1. General itching—a rash may develop around the bite, spreading over the body.
2. A bump on the skin—may is white, pink, reddish or blotchy.
3. Generalized swelling—especially of the airway.
4. Weakness and headache.
5. Fever.
6. Breathing difficulties.
7. Anxiety.
8. Abdominal cramps and vomiting.

Prevention

 Use insect repellents, such as coils and sprays, containing 10% DEET to prevent mosquito and flea bites.
 Sleep under mosquito net with a fan next to you and wear protective clothing after dusk.
 Make sure that the household pets are free of fleas by regular use of anti-flea preparations. If fleas are obviously infesting the house then fumigation may be needed.
 Stay out of the "territory" of stinging insects by using nests. If you encounter any flying stinging insects, stay calm and move away slowly. Do not wait at it; rather, gently brush it aside.

 Many insects are attracted by flower smells, so avoid perfume when outdoors. Wear white clothing if you are visiting an area where bees are common. Wear closed-toe shoes outdoors and do not go barefoot.
 Keep food covered when eating or drinking outdoors. Remember that stinging insects crawl into open cool drink cans.

Foreign Bodies

A foreign body is anything inside of the body that is not meant to be there, such as dirt, glass, viruses and so on. Only the most superficial foreign bodies should be removed from the eyes by non-physicians. If medical care is not readily available, the eye should be irrigated with lukewarm water, or a moist piece of cotton can be used to brush out the foreign body. A little bit of mineral oil instilled into the eye will relive most of the irritation. Avoid rubbing eye and avoid trying to scrape out a foreign body with any hard object.

Foreign bodies in the eye can be classified as:
 Free floating on the surface of the eye
 Adherent to or embedded on the conjunctiva or corneal part of the eye
 Penetrating the eye ball.

If a foreign body is on or in the eye, it is essential to take a look at the surface of the eye and under the eyelids, where possible, to determine the location of the foreign body and the action to be taken. Never use a matchstick, splinter probe or any other sharp object to attempt any treatment.

Free Floating Foreign Bodies

 Flush the eye with disposable eye wash or clean running water.
 If flushing does not remove the foreign body, a trained first aid person may make one attempt to remove it from the white of the eye, with well-moistened surgical spears on an applicator stick.
 If the foreign body cannot be removed, pad the eye lightly and arrange prompt medical assessment.

Adherent or Embedded Foreign Bodies

 Arrange for prompt medical assessment.
 Do not attempt to remove.

Penetrating Foreign Bodies

If a person reports being struck in the eye while grinding, sanding, chipping or hammering metal and no foreign body is seen, always suspect a penetrating foreign body and arrange for prompt medical assessment.

If a penetrating eye injury is obvious:
 Assist the injured person to rest in the most comfortable position.
 Arrange urgent medical assessment.

Nose

If one can get the patient to sneeze, the foreign body will often be extruded. This can be accomplished by having him inhale some pepper through his nostrils or by tickling the opposite nostril.

Ears

Foreign bodies in the ear should not be attacked by lay people as damage may result to this delicate structure. The best first aid is to place some olive oil, mineral oil, or castor oil into the ear and let it stay there for few minutes. This will usually bring out the foreign body. No great harm will result if foreign body remaining in the ear until medical attention is obtained.

Splinters

Only those splinters that can be grasped firmly by a protruding end and can be gently withdrawn should be attacked by laymen. Soft splinter or broken off splinters should be treated by physicians. If a piece of foreign body is allowed to remain in the skin, it will usually become infected. If medical care is not available, warm soaks for a period of a few days will often bring a splinter to a position where it can be withdrawn with a pair of tweezers.

Stab Wounds (Knives, Shrapnel, or Other Weapons)

Protruding objects of this type should usually be left in place until medical care can be obtained. Removal by nonphysicians may result in severe hemorrhage. The best first aid is to place a sterile dressing over the area and transport the patient to the nearest hospital.

What Should be Done About Pieces of Clothing or Dirt that Have Gotten into on Abrasion or Laceration?

Thorough washing with soap and water will usually dislodge such foreign bodies. This should be done as soon as possible after the injury. The injured area should then be covered with a clean dressing, and medical attention should be obtained.

Transportation of the Injured

The two-person arm carry, can be used in some cases to move an injured person. However, it should not be used to carry a person who has serious wounds or broken bones. Other two-person carry, which can be used in emergencies. Two rescuers position themselves beside the casualty, on the same side, one at the level of the chest and the other at the thighs. The rescuers interlock their adjacent arms as shown, while they support the victim at the shoulders and knees. In unison, they lift the victim and roll his or her front toward theirs. This carry must not be used to move seriously injured persons.

Once the casualty has been rescued from the immediate danger slow down and do not rush. From this point on, handle and transport the casualty with every regard for the injuries that have been sustained. Casualties should not be moved before the type and extent of injuries are evaluated and the required emergency medical treatment is given (The exception to this occurs, of course, when the situation dictates immediate movement for safety purposes. For example, it may be necessary to remove a casualty from a burning vehicle; the situation dictates that the urgency of casualty movement outweighs the need to administer emergency medical treatment). In the excitement and confusion that almost always accompany an accident, rescuers are likely to feel rushed, wanting to do everything rapidly? Speed is essential in treating many injuries and in getting the casualty to a medical treatment facility. However, it is not reasonable to let yourself feel so hurried that you become careless and transport the victim in a way that will aggravate the injuries.

Emergency Vehicles, Equipment, and Supplies

In most peacetime emergency situations, some form of ambulance will be available to transport the victim to a medical treatment facility. Ambulances vary in size and shape from the old "gray ghost" to modern van and modular units. Although there are many differences in design and storage capacity, most ambulances are equipped to meet the same basic emergency requirements. They contain equipment and supplies for emergency airway care, artificial ventilation, suction, oxygenation, hemorrhage control, fracture.

COMMUNITY EMERGENCIES

COMMUNITY EMERGENCIES AND COMMUNITY RESOURCES

Introduction

Community emergencies is storm to pandemic to fires in these situation emergency preparedness is essential for keeping you and others safe. Self-reliance is vital when a large scale disaster effects on entire community since emergency services can become overwhelmed.

Role of Community in Emergency

In case of any disaster community itself acts as a first responder before the external help reaches to victim, so if the capacity building of community is done, community will be ready to face the disaster and it will reduces the work load on external agencies coming to help.

Emergency Action Plan
- Assemble a disaster
- Consider situation
- Determine the correct action
- Create rally point
- Verify safe route for every one
- Drill
- Keep reviewing

Communication and Coordination

A key to effective hazard management is effective communication, this is especially true for hazards like tsunamis and flash floods, since inundation arrives times may be measured in just minutes such a short fused events require an immediate careful systemic appropriate response.
- Warning reception
- Warning point and community emergency operation enters each needs redundant pathway to receive things and respond quickly

Community Disaster Planning

Preparedness plan should list the, responsibilities during emergencies and contact number and address for the for the emergency response focal. The team members at each operational level and people in change of:
- Activities response services
- Community with headqutres
- Approach that seek to actively engage at role communities in the identification, analysis, implementation, monitoring and evaluation of disaster risk in order to reduce their vulnerability and enhance their capacity.

Community Disaster Preparedness Plan

1. Assemble a disaster supply kit
2. Locate safe place for each type of disaster
3. Determine the best evacuation route
4. Become trained in first aid and CPR
5. Show each family member how and where to keep utilities (water, gas, electricity)

Emergency Kit Include

- Contact information for important people and care provider
- A list of medicine ,dosage, instruction
- Styles and serial number of all medical and assistive devices
- Need to know the information for first responder and other who might need to help health care providers.

Community Emergency Response Team

Community emergency response team (CERT) have been developed around the country to assist professional. Emergency management personnel first responders is responding to disaster and emergencies. The federal emergency management agency under its citizen corps program has established minimum training standards. However each community uses its CERT Voluntaries as it deems most appropriate and providers' additional training as it applicable, while many committees including same with airport have established CERT into airport emergency response plan.

Community Disaster Response Team (CDRT)

The CDRT is designed to complement and strengthen the existing role of the district emergency organization by helping to increase its capacity. The Red Cross trains and equip community disaster response team in each community to enable them to carryout emergency first response when disaster occurs.

Role of Community in Emergency

In case of any disaster community it act a first responder before the external help reaches to victim. So if the capacity building of community is done, community will be ready to face disaster and it will reduce the work load on external agencies coming to help.

Community Resources

Fire protection and suppression systems (fire sprinklers, fire extinguishers fire pumps and water supplies extinguisher for computer rooms and special hazards).

What are the Community Emergencies

Communities are becoming vulnerable to the hazards that cause disaster. Disasters are not conformed to one community or society they can occur anywhere at any time. Events that occur are increasing frequently. There are many types of disaster with destructive impact.

TYPES OF DISASTER

It includes fire explosion, floods, earthquakes, famines, etc.

Fire Explosion

Fire explosions are reactions, and conversions, respectively, of solids, liquids, or gases comprising the release of high levels of energy that are triggered by an ignition or self-ignition of the substance system. This causes a strong increase in temperature which results in fire. Different fires have different hazards and risks. Use the wrong type of fire extinguisher could do more harm than good.

Types of Fire

1. Fire involving solid materials such as wood, paper, or textiles
2. Fire involving flammable liquids such as petrol, diesel, or oil, etc.
3. Fires involving gases
4. Fire involving metals
5. Fire involving electrical apparatus

Causes of Fire

Oxygen, heat, and fuel frequently referred to as the *fire triangle* and fourth one is chemical reaction. The important things to remember is take any of these four things away, you will not have a fire or fire will be extinguished.

Fire Extinguishment Principle

1. Cooling of flame
2. Reduction of flame by cooling of the liquid, dilution of the liquid or blanketing of the liquid
3. Reduction of oxygen
4. Interference with combustion reaction

Types of Fire Extinguisher

The different types of fire extinguishers include specialist dry powder, standard dry powder, foam, water spray, water mist, water spray, wet chemical and carbon dioxide. There is no single fire extinguisher that can be used on all classes of fire.

Prevention and Safety Tips

However you can take safety, install smoke alarm on every level of your home, inside bedrooms and outside sleeping areas, test smoke alarm every month, talk with all family members about a fire occurs in your home get outstay out, and call for help.

Most common cause of house fires, and some tips to take precautions:

1. Cooking equipment
2. Heating equipment
3. Smoking in bed rooms
4. Electrical equipment
5. Candles
6. Curious children
7. Faulty wiring
8. Barbecues

Prevention

How can fire and explosion be prevented?

1. Fire resistance protective clothing
2. Routine checking and supervision
3. Items to be worked on removed to safe area
4. Remove or protect combustible or flammable materials
5. Prevent suppress and control sparks
6. Prevent, suppress and control heat.

Fire Protection and Emergency Plans

Fire protection plans

1. Where there are fire hazards at any place responsible person must ensure that their health and safety documents include a fire protection plan must take into account
2. Likely source of fire, taking into account the presence of ignition sources and oxygen
3. Precaution to be taken to protect against, to detect and combat the outbreak and spread of fire
4. Avoiding or controlling the source of ignition
5. Minimize the amount of flammable materials
6. Detecting fires and giving warning in the event of fire
7. Minimizing the spread of fire, smoke, fumes or toxic gases
8. The actions to be taken on discovery of a fire

Floods

Floods are the most frequent type of natural disaster and occurs when an overflow of water submerges land that is usually dry, floods are often caused by heavy rainfall, rapid snowmelt or a storm surge from a tropical cyclone or tsunami in coastal areas. Floods can cause widespread devastation, resulting in loss of life and damages to personal property and critical public health infrastructure.

Types of Floods

There are three common types of floods:

1. Flash floods are caused by rapid and excessive rainfall that raises water heights quickly, and rivers, streams, channels or roads may be overtaken.
2. River floods are caused when consistent rain or snow melt forces a river to exceed capacity.
3. Coastal floods are caused by storm surges associated with tropical cyclones and tsunami.

Floods are also increasing in frequency and intensity, and the frequency of extreme precipitation is expected to continue to increase due to climate change.

The World Health Organization (WHO) Health Advisory provides guidelines to countries on adapting all existing preparedness and response plans and procedures for cyclone, tropical storms, tornadoes, floods earthquakes and potential outbreak of other diseases to their COVID-19 Strategic Preparedness and Response Plan. It also provides advice on how to test the required capacities through simulation as and when necessary to ensure the strategic objectives of pandemic response.

WHO advises governments and partners to consider the following aspects of preparedness:

Coordination mechanisms:

Multisectorial disasters risk management COVID-19 preparedness and response should be well-coordinated, this includes collaboration at national and local level for planning and implementation of priority actions through the engagement of all key factors.

Scenario based planning:
Countries need to build potential scenarios that describe how the impact can affect preparedness and response for other hazards in various part of the country.

Adaptation of National and Local Plan to Repurpose the Available Resources

National and local disasters management plans and hazard specific contingency plan will need to be linked to ensure to optimal measures and capacities are in place.

Early Warning and Risk Communication

Public communication of early warnings for cyclones, tropical storms, tornadoes, floods, earthquakes should include risk communication messages should be adopted accordingly to inform all stakeholders mitigation, prevention, preparedness and response in order to reduce the morbidity and mortality from all potential hazards.

Earthquakes

Any sudden shaking of the ground caused by the passage of seismic waves through earth's rocks. Seismic waves are produced when some form of energy stored in earth's crust is suddenly released, usually when masses of rock straining against one another suddenly fracture and slip.

Types of Earthquakes

There are four different types of earthquakes—tectonic, volcanic, collapse and explosion. A tectonic earthquake is one that occurs when the earth's crust breaks due to geological forces on rocks and adjoining plates that cause physical and chemical changes.

Many earthquakes are followed several hours or even days later, by further tremors, usually of progressively decreasing intensity. To reduce the destructive effect of earthquakes a number of precautions are essential.

Precaution to be Taken During and After an Earthquake

If you are indoors when earthquake hits:
1. Drop down and take cover under a desk or table
2. Stay inside until the shaking stops and it is safe to exit
3. Pick a safe place where things will not fall on you
4. Wait in your safe place until the shaking stops, then check to see if you are hurt. It will be better able to help others if you take care of yourself first, then check the people around you
5. Stay away from book cases and other furniture that can fall on you
6. Stay away from windows and light fixtures
7. If you are in bed-hold on and stay there
8. Inspect your home
9. Check yourself and others for injuries
10. Stay out of damaged buildings
11. Be careful around broken glasses and debris
12. Keep away from the stairs, which might collapse suddenly
13. People who are outside should stay there keeping away from building to avoid collapsing walls and away from electrical cables
14. Anyone in vehicle should park it, keeping away from bridges and buildings.

Stay indoor until the shaking stops and you are sure it is safe to exit. More injuries happen when people move during the shaking of earthquakes, after shake has stopped, if you go outside, move quickly away from the building.

After Earthquakes

Earthquakes can cause a lot more damage after the first shock. They are often followed by aftershocks, causing even more damage to already weakened buildings and roads. Land especially hills, can also be damaged by earthquakes and result in devastating landslides and mudslides.

Stay Calm. Help Others If You are Able

- Stay prepared for after shocks
- Listen to the radio or television for information from authorities
- Check your home for structural damage and other hazards
- Do not light matches or turn on light switches until you are sure that there are no gas leaks or flammable liquids spilled
- Look for structural damage
- Obey the authorities instructions
- Give first aid to the injured and alert the emergency services
- Make sure water is safe to drink

Famines

The word *famine* is defined by images of mass starvation, where whole communities are literally starving, famine severe and prolonged hunger in a substantial proportion of the population of a region country resulting in widespread acute malnutrition and death by starvation and disease. Famines usually last for a limited time, ranging from a few months to a few years. They cannot continue indefinitely, if for no other reason than that the affected population would eventually be decimated.

Crop failures caused by natural disaster including poor weather, insect, and plant disease, crop destruction due to warfare, and enforced starvation as a political tool are some causative factors of famine.

Historical Responses to Famine

The British government wrote the first modern codification of responses to famine during its occupation of India. The highly detailed Indian Famine Code of 1883 classified situation of food scarcity according to a scale of intensity and it laid out series of steps that in the event of a famine. The code continues to influence, contemporary policies, such as food for work program and what the code called gratuitous relief for those unable to work.

What Need to Be Done?

Averting future famines and building long-term food security require a paradigm shift, a strategy that goes beyond proverbial relief and development dilemma, in short, local communities must develop food system with high level resilience. In the meantime, traditional approaches to managing the famine must be deployed. Set of strategies as follows:

1. Humanitarian aid
2. Rebuild communities
3. Strengthen local food system resilience
4. Economic strategies

Development assistance should aim to foster economic diversification and otherwise expand employment opportunities. This will help ensure food security, especially when combined with investments and long-term agriculture research.

Index

Page numbers followed by *b* refer to box, *f* refer to figure, and *t* refer to table.

A

Abdomen 38
   physical examination of 207
Abdominal binders 243
Abdominal examination 137
Abdominal surgery, previous 137
Abrasion 85, 274
Absorption 220, 268
Accident
   and emergency department, preparation of 37
   bicycle 265
   first aid 264
   motorcycle 265
   road traffic 264
   scene 237, 239
   victim 237
Accidental injury, action after 178
Accountability, framework for 57
Acid-base imbalance 193
Acoustic nerve 132
Acquired immunity 172
Activated partial thromboplastin time 153, 154
Activities 76, 77
   follow-up 100, 143, 231*t*
Actual pressure sores, assessment of 93
Acute pain 200, 200*t*
   signs of 200*t*
Adequate fluid balance 185
Adhesive type 198
Administer medication 209
Administering enema 100, 101
   steps of 101*t*
Administering injections 218
Administering medications, safety in 209
Administering oxygen, indications for 187
Administrating meter dose inhaler, steps of 227
Administrating small volume nebulizer, steps of 227
Admission
   procedure 35, 36
   records 52, 55
   sheet 52
   types of 35
Admitting clients, first step in 35
Admitting department 21
Adolescent 46
Adrenocorticotropic hormone stimulation test 155
Advanced cardiac life support 249
Advanced nursing practice 3
Agent
   biological 171
   causative 171
   change 5
   chemical 171
   mechanical 171

   nutritional 171
   physical 171
   social 171
Air-borne spread 173
Airway 250
   breathing and circulation 239
   clearance 184
   open 251, 253
   patency 258
Alanine transaminase 153
Albumin 153
Alcohol 72
Alkaline phosphates 153
Allergic reaction 185, 219
   acute 257
Allergy, history of 210
Ambiguous statement 61
Ambulance bag, equipment in 37
Ambulation 74, 74*t*
Ammonia dermatitis 85
Anaphylactic shock 257
Anaphylaxis 219
Anchor final bandage with tape strips 247*f*
Anemia 93
Animal starch 110
Ankle, fracture of 264
Antibody 172
Anticipation 44
Antigen 172
Antivitamin factors 112
Anuria 202
Anxiety factors, common 28
Apical pulse assessment 145
Apnea 185
Arm grasp, through 79
Arterial blood 155
   gas, common investigation 156
   pressure, physiology of 148
Arterial puncture 155
Asepsis, concept of 175
Aspirate transaminase 153
Assisting patient, suggestion for 115
Athlete's foot 91
Attending casualties 265
Attitudes 45
Audit 52
Auditory canal purposes, external 226
Auscultation 126, 127, 135
Automated external defibrillators
   child system 254
   structure and function of 254
Autopsy 121, 122
Autotransfusion 258
Awareness, level of 30
Axillae examination 136
Axillary temperature, procedure of taking 143*t*

B

Balance scale 116
Balanced diet 112
Balanced traction 199
Bandages 241
   elastic 241
   flannel 241
   gauze 241
   general purposes of 241
   muslin 241
   plastic adhesive 241
   position of 198
   spica 242
   types of 241
   using 261
Bandaging 239, 247
   recurrent 247*f*
Basal metabolic rate 138
Baseline vital signs 38
Basic cardiac life support 248
   indications for 249
Basic first aid kit 239
Basic food group guides 113
Basic guidelines 78, 78*t*
Basic hospital diet 114
Basic human needs 25, 26
Bathing patient 86
Bed 30
   amputation 84
   and bed making 81
   bath 86
      procedure 87, 87*t*
   cardiac 84
   divided 84
   fracture 84
   kinds of 84
   making, clinical guidelines for 81
   occupied 82
   postanesthetic 84
   postoperative 84
   recovery 84
   sores 92
   stump 84
   unoccupied 81
Bedpans 98
   disinfection of 178
   types of 98
Bedridden patient, shampooing hair of 88
Bedtime rituals, supporting 72
Behavior 129
   change 33
   wellness 23
   illness 23, 27
Bilirubin 153

Index

Biomedical waste
  categories of 182t
  disposal of 182t
  management 182
Bleeding
  arterial 270
  capillary 270
  cause of 256
  external 256
  externalized 270, 271
  internal 256, 270, 271
  minor traumatic 270, 271
  severe 271
  source of 186
  stop serious 271
  times 154
  types of 256, 270
  venous 270
Blood 156
  contamination, risk of 272
  dispraises 219
  fasting 154
  glucose 154
  level of glucose, measure of 154
  lipids 153
  specimen, nursing protocol for 152
  urea nitrogen test 154
  volume 148
Blood pressure 148
  assessing 148, 149
  assessment, sources of error in 149t
  digital monitor 151
  factors affecting 148
  measurement, indication of 150
  measuring 150
  procedure of measuring 150t
Blood vessel
  superficial 92
  type of damaged 270
Bloodstream 174
Bodily sensation 200
Body
  alignment 198
  cells, increased temperature of 138
  elimination deviation, care of 202
  heat 93
    production, factors affecting 138
  images, change of 27, 33
  lice 88
  mechanics 73
  movements and gestures 42
  repositioning 94
  structure 129
Body temperature 137
  alterations in 138, 189
  assessment of 139
  care of 189
  factors affecting 138, 189
  kinds of 138
  measurement 139t
Bone
  conduction test 132
  injuries to 260
Bowel elimination
  alteration in 205
  common problems in 96
  role of nurse in 207

Bradypnea 185
Brain
  death 120
  hemorrhage in 270
Breast
  binder 243, 243f
  examination of 136
  female 136
  male 137
Breath sounds
  adventitious 135
  normal 135
Breathing 250, 258, 268
  abilities, assessment of 186
  absent 254
  assess 252
  assessing 252
  check for 253
  initiate rescue 252
  mouth-to-mouth 252
  pattern 185
Brevity 55
Buccal route 213
Build trust 51
Burn 256
  first-degree 266
  second-degree 266
  third-degree 266
  types of 266
  victims, treatment for 267

C

Caffeine 72
Calcitonin 155
Calcium 192
  high 115
Canning 112
Cap principles 176
Capillary blood 152
Carbohydrate 110, 114, 115
Cardiac arrest 248
Cardiac massage, external 248
Cardiac monitor 259
Cardiac output 143, 148
Cardiogenic shock 256
Cardiopulmonary resuscitation 248
  guidance for 250
  parts of 250
  procedure of 250t
  technique of 249
  training 249
Cardiovascular system, effect on 219
Care, continuity of 57
Caregiver 4
  role 122
Carotid arteries 134
Carotid pulse 251
Cast
  care of 199
  types of 199
Casualties, treatment of 265
Catheter, presence of long-term 105, 203
CD4 cell count 153
Cellulose 110
Celsius to fahrenheit, convert
  from 140
Census record 53

Central cyanosis 186
  assessment of 186
Central Sterile Supply Department, purposes
  of 21
Cereal grains 110
Cervical scrape 159
  procedure of 159t
Changing position procedure 80, 80t
Chest 38, 134
  anterior 135
  compression 250, 251
    technique 251
  infection 174
Cheyne-Stokes respiration 185
Child-birth process 177
Chloride 193
Cholesterol 111, 113, 248
  high 248
Circulation 198, 258
Circulatory system 249
Cleaning 179
Cleansing baths 86
  types of 86
Client advocate 5
Client goals 62, 63
  establishing 62
Client records, types of 52
Client to nursing unit, admission
  of 35
  procedure of 36t
Client's health
  problems 60
  values and beliefs 62
Client's priorities 62
Client's pulse, assessing 144
Clinical record 53
Clinical waste 177
Clostridium difficile, case of 173
Clothing
  pieces of 274
  removal of 38
Clustering data 60
Code of conduct, elements of 13
Code of ethics 13, 18
Coma 193
Comatose patient, initial assessment
  of 194
Coombs test 154
Communication 40, 44, 51, 184, 275
  approaches 48
  barriers to effective 43
  difficulties 46
  forms of 41
  health team members 50
  kinds of 40
  levels of 40
  measures to improve 184
  model 42
  modes of 41
  nonverbal 41
  process 40
    basic elements of 41
    factors influencing 44
  verbal 41, 44
  with child and adolescent 46
  with hearing impaired client 47
  with mute client 47

Communicator 4
Community disaster
   planning 275
      preparedness plan 275
      response team 275
Community emergency
      274, 275
   response team 275
   role of 274, 275
Community resources 275
Complete blood count 153
Compression ventilation
      ratio 253
Consciousness 131
   level of 128, 258
Constant fever 139, 189
Contact lenses 90
Convection 138
Converting metric units 221
Coordination mechanisms 276
Copper diet, restricted 115
Core temperature 259
Corn 91
   starch 86
Correct grasp technique 79, 79t
Cough 186
Counter traction 198
Crab lice 88
Crimean war 11
Critical decision point 130
Critical thinking
   attitude for 56
   competencies 56
   in nursing, levels of 56
Crohn's disease 115
Cross-infection 173
   safety for preventing 32
Cuff 149
Culture and sensitivity 153
Customary English system 221
Cyanosis 186

D

Daily living, activities of 94
Daily nursing care record 53
Dandruff 88
Danger 262
Data
   collection, method of 59
   identification 167
   processing 59
   types of 58
Dead body, care of 123, 123t
Death 121
   biological 120, 248
   care after 121
   circulatory 120
   clinical 120, 248
   declaration certification 121
   sign of impending 120
   types 120
Decoding 42
Deep penetrating necrosis 92
Defensiveness 44
Defibrillation 250
Deformity, prevention of 198
Dehumanization 28

Dehydration 256
   causes of 190, 191t
   symptoms of 190, 191t
   treatment of 190, 191t
Depression 91
Developing illness, risk factors
      for 27
Dextrin 110
Diabetic diet 114
Diagnostic process, steps of 59
Diagnostic testing, phases of 151
Diaper rash 85
Diarrhea 96, 205
   causes 96
   severe 115
   symptoms 96
Diastolic pressure 149
Diet 72, 220
   in health and disease 110
   planning and serving 115
   type of 112
Dietary guidelines 113
Dietary services, types of 20
Digital thermometer, using 141
Dignity 13
Direct antiglobulin test 154
Disaster, types of 275
Discharge against medical
      advice 39
Discharge procedure 35, 39, 39t
Disease 105, 203
Disinfection 179
Disposable gloves 142
Disposable injection units 218
Distress, acute 130
Distributive shock 257
Diurnal variations 138
Doctor's examination 38
Documentation 247
   methods of 54
   systems of 54
Domestic services 21
Domestic waste 177
Dominating emotion 44
Dorsalis pedis pulse 144f
Drowning 259
Drug 222
   classification of 222
   data 210
   effects of 219
   in other forms, application of 227t
   interactions 219
   into body cavity, insertion of 225
   measurement, system of 221
   parenteral administration of 213
   storage and maintenance of 218
   tolerance 219
   tropical 227t
   use 222, 223
Drug administration
   buccal routes 213
   oral route 211
   rights of 210t
   routes of 211
   sublingual route 213
Drying hand after scrubbing 175f
Dumping syndrome diet 115

Dying
   care of 3
   patient Bill of Rights 121
Dyspnea 185
   managing 123
Dysuria 104, 202

E

Eagerness 44
Ear 132, 274
   canal 133f
   care of 90
   drops
      instillation of 226, 226t, 227t
      irrigation of 226
   irrigation 226t
   swab 159
      collection of 160, 160t
Early defibrillation, principles of 250
Early life and education 10
Earthquake 277
   after 277
   precaution during and after 277
   types of 277
Eat foods
   with adequate starch 114
   with fiber 114
Edema 132
Education 45
   for women 10
Educational opportunities 3
Ejection from vehicle 265
Elasticated tubular bandage,
      application of 244, 245t
Elasticity 148
Elbow grasp 79
Electrical hazards, prevention of 31
Electrical safety 31
Electrolyte
   balance 190
   imbalance 190
Emancipation of women 10
Emergency
   action plan 275
   aid 239
   cardiac care 248
   care 194, 258
   concept of 239
   department, admission of patient to 37
   kit 275
   medical assistance prevention 269
   personnel, complete information to 238
   plans 276
   transportation 238
   vehicles 238
      equipment, and supplies 274
Emotion 33, 46
   assessment of 166
   physiological effects of 34
   types of 34
   ways of expressing 34
Emotional change 27, 33
Emotional response
   common 34, 34t
   patterns 34
Emotional state 30
Emotional wellness 25

Enema
    prepackaged 101
    types of solutions for 100
Enuresis 104, 202
Environment 17, 24, 45, 72, 138, 173
    manipulation of 95
Environmental conditions 220
Environmental distractions, reducing 72
Environmental health 25
Environmental hygiene 85
Environmental safety 29
Enzyme-linked immunosorbent assay 153
Epidural injection 232
Epinephrine 138
Equipment 119
    care of 218
    collecting stool specimen 99
    disinfection of 178
    position 77
    required 116, 117
Erythema 85
Erythrocyte sedimentation rate 153
Essential fatty acids 111, 112
    deficiency of 112
Ethical implications 152
Euthanasia 122
Examine scene 264
Examine victim 238
Excessive dryness 85
Excretion 221
Exercise 138, 148
    general guidelines for 95
Extraocular movement 132
Eye 132
    care of 90
    contact 41
    glasses 90
    injury, penetrating 273
    poison in 270
    shields 176
    structure, external 132
    swab 160

F
Face mask principles 176
Facial expression 41, 129
Facilitating bowel elimination 206
    equipment 206
    procedures 206
Facilitating urine elimination 203
    equipment 203
    procedures 203
    types 203
Fahrenheit to celsius, convert
        from 140
Family roles, change in 27, 33
Famines 277
Fat 111, 113, 114
    controlled, low cholesterol diet 115
    diet, restricted 114
    functions of 112
    high 114
    modification in 114
    requirements 112
    sources 111
Fecal impaction 96, 205
    causes 96
    symptoms 96

Fecal incontinence 96, 206
    causes 96, 206
Feces
    characteristics of 97, 97t, 204t
    inspecting 207
Feeding, artificial method of 117, 117t
Feet
    and toes, fracture of 264
    care of 90, 91
Fever 138
    clinical signs of 139, 189
    common types of 138, 189
    remittent 138, 189
Fiber 110
    diet, high 116
Figure-of-eight
    bandaging 247f
    turns 242
Finger 262
    clubbing of 186
Fingertips over trachea, placement
        of 134f
Fire
    causes of 276
    explosion 275
    extinguisher, types of 276
    extinguishment principle 276
    protection 276
    types of 276
First aid 236, 237, 239, 267
    administrant 237
    before victim transported 239
    bleeding 270
    burns 265
    drowning victims 259
    emergency 256
    equipment and materials 238
    food poisoning 269
    general principles of 237
    insect bite 272
    kit 239
        preparation of 239
    major burns 267
    management 268
    poisoning 267
    poisonous plants 269
    procedures in 239
    rules of 239
    scalds 265
    techniques in 239
    tips, fractures 260
Fissures 91
Flatulence 97, 206
    causes 97
Floods 276
    types of 276
Fluid
    and electrolytes imbalance,
        care of 190
    balance record 53
    intake 105, 184, 203
        promoting 105, 205
    replacement, evaluating 258
    volume
        disturbances in 190
        measures to maintain 184
Folate level 154
Folic acid 154

Food poisoning
    prevention of 269
    treatment of 269
Food, variety of 112
Foot problems callus, common 91
Forearm, fracture of 262
Foreign bodies 273
    adherent 273
    embedded 273
    free floating 273
    penetrating 273
Formulating nursing diagnoses 60
Fracture 260
    causes 260
    closed 260
    complicated 260
    compound 260
    management of 261
    pan 98
    signs of 260
    symptoms of 260
Fracture collar bone 261
    signs 261
    symptoms 261
Freezing 112
Friction 92
Fructose 110
Fruit 110
    sugar 110

G
Galactose 110
Gargle, direct application of 224
Gargling procedure 225, 225t
Gastrointestinal bleeding, preventing 258
Gastrointestinal system, effects on 219
General hospitals 19
General physical examination,
        equipment and supplies for 128t
General survey 128
    observations 129t
Genetic differences 220
Genitalia
    female, support for external 243f
    male, support for eternal 243f
Glass waste 177
Gloves 176
    principles of changing 176
Glucose 156
    tolerance test 155
Gluten-free diet 115
Glycogen 110
Goggles 176
Good nutrition 95
    status, clinical signs of 113
Good record report, characteristics of 55
Gown
    principles 176
    use of 179
Groin, spica for 242f
Gums 133

H
Hair
    and scalp 132
        problems 88
    care of 88
    shampooing, contraindications for 89

Index

Hallux valgus 91
Hammer toe 91
Hand
  and fingers, fracture of 262
  washing 175, 178
Hazards 182
Head 38, 132
  and neck 132
  lice 88
Health 23
  and disease 23
  and sickness 96
  determinants of 24
  dimensions of 25
  education 267
  illness continuum 26
  maintenance 3
  related research 19
  restoration 3
  risks 60
  services available 24
Health assessment 125, 126
  process of 126
Health personnel 58
  education 19
Health problem
  and risks 60
  urgency of 62
Health promotion 3, 19
  implications 48
Healthcare
  agencies, types of 18
  teams 23
Heart 135
  attack 248
  murmur 136
Heart sound
  first 136
  fourth 136
  second 136
  third 136
Heat injury 246
Heat loss 138
Height measuring scale 116
Help, call for 250
Hematocrit 154
Hemoglobin 153
Hemoptysis 186
Hemorrhage 256, 270
  causes of 256
  clinical signs of 256
Heparin lock 230
  administration of 230t
Heparin medication, administration of 231t
Heredity 24
Hesitancy 104, 202
Hierarchy 25
Hip, fracture of 263
Home care considerations 106
Hormones 138
Hospice care 22
Hospital 18
  acquired infection, source of 173
  admission 35
  classification of 19
  diet for therapeutic purpose, modification of 114

discharge 35
  from 39
functions of 19
health services departments 19
language, lack of understanding of 28
unit and preparation of unit, admission to 35
waste, types of 182
Hospital-acquired infection 172, 173, 181
  common 174
  potential for 174
Hospitalization, effect of 28
House fires, cause of 276
Household system 221
Housekeeping department 21
Hydration, altered 86
Hygiene 93
Hygienic activities 86
Hygienic needs 85
Hypercalcemia 192
Hyperkalemia 191, 192t
Hyperlipoproteinemia, dietary management of 115
Hypermagnesemia 192t
Hypernatremia 190
Hyperphosphatemia 192t
Hyperpnea 185
Hypertonic dehydration 190
Hypertonic overhydration 190
Hypertonic solution 100
Hyperventilation 185
Hypocalcemia 192, 192t
Hypokalemia 191, 191t
Hypomagnesemia 192t
Hyponatremia 190, 191t
Hypophosphatemia 192t
Hypothermia 139
  clinical signs of 140
  physiologic process of 139
  risk for 140
  victims 259
Hypotonic dehydration 190
Hypotonic overhydration 190
Hypovolemia 190
  shock 256

I

Ideal weight, maintain 113
Idiosyncratic reaction 219
Illness 23, 27, 71, 172
  and nursing implications 34, 34t
  causes for developing 27
  effect of 28, 33
  impact of 28
  types
    acute 27
    chronic 27
Illness-wellness continuum 26, 26t
Immobility 86
  prevent problems of 94
Immune response 173
Immunity
  active 172
  passive 172
Immunization 173, 177
Implantable cardioverter defibrillator 255
Industrial revolution 10
Infected linen, disinfection of 178

Infected materials, protection against 177
Infection
  chain of 170, 171
  control 170
  during injection, preventing 213
  elements of 171
  factors increasing 172
  mode of spreading of 170
  nature of 170
  prodromal stage of 172
  severity of 172
  stages of 171
  types of 170, 171
Inflammation
  causes of 173
  stages of 173
  types of 173
Inflammatory response 173
Inflatable bladder 149
Ingestion 268
Ingrown toenails 91
Inhalation 218, 227, 268
  poisoning 268
Inhaler, guidelines for using 227
Injection
  intra-arterial 232
  intradermal 217
  intramuscular 216
  intraosseous 232
  intraperitoneal 232
  intrapleural 232
  intrathecal 232
  types of 213
Injury
  accidental inoculation of 178
  types 238
Ink, use of 54
Inner oral mucosa, inspection of 133f
Insect bite
  management for 273
  signs of allergic reaction to 273
Insects, safety from 32
Insomnia, type of 72
Insulin
  administration 228, 228t
  mixing 229
    procedure for 229t
  types of 228
Integumentary system 131
Intellectual health 25
Intermittent fever 138, 189
Interview
  questions 104, 203
  technique 125
Intestinal obstruction, partial 115
Invasive method 188
Iodine uptake test 155
Iron diet, high 115
Irritation and discomfort, freedom from 71
Isolation 179
  precautions 178
    essentials of 178
Isometric exercise 94
Isotonic dehydration 190
Isotonic exercise 94
Isotonic overhydration 190

Index

J
Job satisfaction 57
Joint
   injuries to 260
   stiffness 247
Jugular veins, external 134

K
Kaiserswerth training 10
Kardex and nursing care plan 52
Ketogenic diet 114
Ketones 156
Kneecap, fracture of 263

L
Laceration 274
Lactose 110
Lactose-free diet 115
Language 45
Laundry department 21
Leader 5
Left against medical advice 39
Leg muscles, lift with 76
Legal documentation 52
Legal implication 152
Legible document 54
Lesions, structural 193
Lethargy 44
Lice 88
Life, respect for 17
Lifting and moving techniques 76, 77t
Limbs 38
Linen 177
   categories of 177
Lip 133
Lipid profile 153
Lipoprotein 153, 248
   profile 153
Liquid
   direct application of 224
   fecal seepage 96
Listening, active 51
Liver function test 153
Love and belonging needs 26
Low carbohydrate diet 114
Low kilocaloric diet 114
Lower leg, fracture of 263
Lower lip 133f
Lung
   assessment 135
   inspect 135

M
Magnesium 192
Maintenance department 21
Making occupied bed, procedure for 83t
Malformed infant, conflict related to 17
Maltose 110
Management functions 44
Manometer 149
Mask
   use of 179
   ventilation 252
Maslow's hierarchy of needs 25
Maturity, degree of 112
Maxillary sinus 133
   palpation of 133f

Meal service, consideration in 115
Mechanical department 21
Mechanical devices 86
Mechanical diet 115
Medical asepsis 178
   practices 178, 178t
Medical department 19
Medical education, changes in 9
Medical history sheet 52
Medical records 21, 58
   source-oriented 52
Medical technology, development of 9
Medical treatment plan 62
Medical waste, types of 182
Medication
   action, types of 221
   administration of 209
      errors in 211
   delivery 210
   dose calculation formula 221
   errors 211
   forms of 211, 211t
   mixing 228
   orders 209
   prescription 209
   purpose of 209
   record 53
   routes of administration of 211
   storing of 218
Medicine 6
   cabinet and drugs, care of 218
Medicolegal issues 40
Memory 131
Mental status and speech 131
Messages, interpretation of 44
Metabolic acidosis 193
Metabolic alkalosis 193
Metabolic disorders 193
Metabolism 220
Meticulous hygiene 95
Metric system 221
Microorganisms 31
Minerals 115
Minute volume 186
Mobility 93
   status 30
Modern medicine and hospitals 9
Moisture 92, 131
Mood assessment 166
Mortuary, placing body in 122
Motion exercises, active range of 94
Mouth 133
   ventilation 252
Movement exercise, passive 73, 73t
Moving patients and equipment,
   safety in 32
Muscle
   activity 138
   deltoid 217
   dorsogluteal 217
   injuries to 260
   vastus lateralis 216
   ventrogluteal 217
Muscular contraction, abnormal 260
Musculoskeletal problems 94
Mute client 47
Myocardial infarction 257

N
Nails 132
   care of 90, 91
Narrative charting 53
Nasal cannula 188, 188t
Nasal swab 162
   procedure of collecting 162t
Nasogastric intubation 117, 118
   procedure of 118t
Nasogastric tubefeeding 119
   procedure of 119t
Natural immunity 172
Neck 134
   of thigh bone, fracture of 263
Needle 217
   sticks injuries, prevention of 223
Nervous systems, effects on 219
Neurogenic shock 257
No breathing, check for 250
Noises 31
Noninvasive management 258
Nonprofessional health service
   departments 21
Norepinephrine 138
Normal sleep, factors affecting 71
Nose 133, 274
   care of 90
Nosocomial infection 173
Nurse
   and client 62
   and coworkers 16
   and people 17
   and practice 16
   and profession 17
   assesses skin 131f
   functions of 4
   implication for 16, 17
   initial assessment of 38
   knowledge base for 209
   professional conduct for 18
   responsibility 85, 218
   role 197
      and responsibilities of 13, 38
Nurse-patient relationship 50
   characteristics of 50
   steps of 50
Nursing
   actions, types of 65
   alert 226, 229, 230
   and medicine 6
   brotherhoods 9
   competencies, specialty 3
   concept 1
   dark period of 10
   department 19
   diagnoses 59, 183
      format 60
   diagnostic statement 61, 61t
   ethics in 13
   historical prospective of 56
   history of 5
   holistic 23
   implementation 123
   important dates in 232-233
   in ancient times 5
   management 194
   nature of 3

practice 3
responsibilities 152
scope of 3
sisterhoods 9
skills, basic 40
standards 152
Nursing care
evaluating quality of 66
modern approaches to 23
of patient 29
of unconscious patient 195t
Nursing intervention
for patients with fever 139, 190
monitor 190
schedule 72
Nursing process 56
steps in 57
Nursing profession 1, 12, 12f
development of 5
Nursing role 152
assess, guidelines for 151
Nursing service department 21
functions of 22
Nursing strategies
developing alternative 64t
generating alternative 64
guidelines for implementing 66
time needed for 62
Nursing unit 22
functions of 22
safety guidelines in 29
types of 22
Nutrition 93, 112
ideal 112
in illness, factors affecting 112
Nutritional needs 109
Nutritional status 131, 172
alteration in 85
assessing 116
procedure to assess 116t

O

Obesity 113
Observation skills, accurate 126
Observation technique 125
Obstructive conditions 257
Obstructive shock 257
Occult blood, stool for 156
Occupational health 25
Occupied bed, making 83
Odors 127t
Oil retention 100
Olfaction 126, 127
Olfactory nerve 133
Oliguria 202
Operating theater 20
Oral cavity, care of 90
Oral drug administration 211t
Oral mucosa, inflammation of 90
Oral nutrition 117
Oral temperature, procedure of taking 141t
Organisms, mode of entry of 174
Organizing data 59
Ostomy, management of 104, 203
Outpatient department 20
Overweight 113

Oxygen 189
administration, method of 187
inhalation 186
mask 187, 188t
safety 31
tent 188
therapy 187, 187t
Oxygenation, factors affecting 186
Oxyhood 188

P

Pacemakers, implanted 255
Padding 245
Pads and slings, supporting 198
Pain
can affect sleep 71
care of 199
chest 186
chronic 200, 200t
clinical manifestations of 200
factors influence responses to 201b
management 123
general strategies for 201
nursing diagnosis patient with 201
patient with 200
psychogenic 200
referred 200
types of 200
Palpation 126, 135, 136
method 151, 151t
Paramedical departments 20
Parasomnias 73
Parathormone 155
Parathyroid hormone 155
Parenteral administration 213
Parotitis 90
Patent airway, maintaining 184
Patient
admission of 35
basic needs of 70
care 19
education 136, 184, 245
information 32
property and valuables 38
with pressure sores, assessing 93
with traction, general nursing care of 198
Pedestrians 265
Pediculosis 88
capitis 88
corporis 88
pubis 88
Penile swab 162
Perceptual alterations 30
Percussion, types of 127
Performance procedure 250
Pericardial tamponade 257
Perineal care 90, 91
Periodontal disease 90
Peripheral cyanosis 186
Peripheral pulse assessment 145
Personal hygiene 85, 129
Personal information 17
Personal space 45
Personnel department 21
pH 156
direct measurement of 156
Pharynx 133

Phenylalanine diet, restricted 115
Phosphate 192
Phosphorus diet, high 115
Physical assessment 126, 183, 185
anus 207
rectum 207
Physical barriers 43
Physical examination 126, 129, 183, 203
techniques of 126
Physical health 25
Physical injuries, risk for 30
Physical restraints, kinds of 84
Physician's order 52
Physician's role 210
Placing hand over groove 146f
Planning 61, 184, 201
care 52
nursing strategies 64
types of 61
Plant sources 110
Plantar warts 91
Plaque 90
Plaster rolls 245
Plaster splint material, prepare 246
Plastic apron 176
Poison 267
Poisonous plants 269
treatment of ingestion of 269
Polymerase chain reaction 153
Polyunsaturated fats 111
Polyuria 202
Posture, movement, and position, assess 130
Potassium 190
permanganate 86
Potential pressure sore sites 93
Practice nursing, entry to 3
Preadolescent 46
Prehistoric medicine 5
Prepare patient properly 152
Pressure 92
Pressure areas
assessing 93
care of 92
Pressure sore 93, 246
categories of 92
causes of 92
formation of 92, 93
infection of 92
preventing 95
Prevention tips 276
Privacy 14
lack of 28
PRN order 210
Profession, criteria of 12
Professional growth 57
Professional health service departments 19
Professional nursing
emergence of 9
essential components of 1
Professional practice, scope of 14
Progress records, types of 53
Protective clothing 175
Protective towels, equipment and solutions 226
Protein 114, 156
diet
high 115
restricted 115

high 114
    modification in 115
    total 153
Psychogenic causes 193
Psychological assessment 166
Psychological factors 220
Psychological preparation 131
Psychological stress 72
Public distance 45
Pulmonary diseases 185
Pulse 143, 254
    characteristics of 145
    check for 251
    oximetry 156
    physiological basis of 143
    rate 145
        factors affecting 144
    rhythm 145
    sites 144
    technique 145
    volume 145
Purchasing department 21
Pyrexia 189

Q
Quality clients care 57

R
Radial pulse assessment, procedure of 146t
Radiation 138
Radioactive iodine uptake 155
Range of motion 73
    exercises, passive 94
    types 73
Readable document 54
Reagent strip testing 156
Reagent tablet testing 156
Record 50
    and reports 58
    and reports, special 52
    keeping form, common 52
    purposes of 50
Recording and reporting 51, 76, 158
Rectal clinical thermometer 142
Rectal suppository, insertion of 225
Rectal swab 163
Rectal temperature, procedure of taking 142t
Rectum 225
    medicated packing in 225
    procedure of collecting specimen from 163t
Reef knot 244
Regimentation 28
Rehabilitation
    center 22
    process 22
Relapsing fever 138, 189
Relaxation 105, 205
Relieve discomfort, measures to 184
Report 50
    and records, purposes of 51
    kinds of 55
    written 55
Research 5, 52

Reservoir 171
Residue diet, restricted 115
Respiration 145
    assessing 146, 147
    characteristics of 146
    physiological basis for 145
    procedure of assessing 147t
    resting 147f
Respiratory acidosis 193
Respiratory alkalosis 193
Respiratory arrest 249
    causes of 249
Respiratory condition 71
Respiratory diseases
    signs of 185
    symptoms of 185
Respiratory droplet 173
Respiratory pattern 258
Respiratory rate 186
Response, check for 250
Rest 71
    and sleep, promoting 72
    importance of 71
Restraints 84
    hazards of 85
    indication for 85
    principles of 85
    use 85
Resuscitation 248
Retention 104, 203
Rheumatoid factor 154
Rights of drug administration 209
Rinne air condition 132
Rinne test 133f
Rocking motion, use of 78
Rocking movements, use 76
Roll over 265
Roller bandage
    basic terms for 242
    removing 243
Routine and terminal cleaning 178
Rubber tubing 149

S
Safe bedside unit 29
Safe environment, creating 72
Safety alert 189
Safety and security needs 26
Safety devices 84
Safety knowledge 29
Safety measures, use 152
Safety precautions 33
Safety tips 276
Saline water baths 86
Saline, physiologic normal 100
Sample recording 54
Saturated fats 111
Scalp, scaling of 88
Schilling test 154
School-age child 46
Scultetus binder 244f
Seal mask against face 252
Self awareness, lack of 51
Self-concept, change in 27, 33
Self-esteem 26, 46
    disturbance in 61
Semantics 44

Semen 163
    specimen
        collection of 164
        procedure of collecting 164t
Sensation, altered 86
Sensory alterations 30
Sensory perception 129
Septic shock 257
Serum
    creatinine 154
    electrolytes 153
    free triiodothyronine 155
    values 154
Service
    opportunities 4
    type of 19
Shampooing hair of bedridden patient, procedure of 89t
Sharp disposal bin 176
Shock 256
    classifications of 256
    delivery 254
    stages of 257
Shoes 176
Sick among primitive people, care of 5
Sickle cell test 154
Sickness and sin 6
Side effect 219
Silence, maintain 51
Sinus 133
Size and bed capacity 19
Skeletal traction 199
Skills, implementing 66
Skin 131
    and mucous membrane
        application to 224
        care of 85
    excretions on 86
    folds, measure 116
    poison on 270
    puncture 152
    secretions on 86
    traction 197, 199
Sleep 30, 71
    apnea 73
    disorders, common 72
Slipper pan 98
SOAP format 53
Soap suds solution 100
SOAPIE 53
Social distance 45
Social health 25
Social service departments 21
Sociocultural background 45
Sociocultural conditions 24
Socioeconomic conditions 24
Sociopsychological barriers 43
Sodium 190
    bicarbonate 86
    diets, restricted 115
Soil variation and climate 112
Sorbitol 110
Sores, grading scale of 93b
Speaker's message 44
Special hospitals 19
Special nursing care 199

Specimen
    collection of 151
        protocols for 152
    from penis, collection of 163, 163t
    from rectum, collection of 163
    from throat swab, collection of 164
    from vagina, collection of 165
    transport 152
Speech 129, 131
Sphygmomanometer 148
Spillage 177
Spinal accessory nerve 134
Spinal cord injury 257
Spiral bandaging 247f
Spiral reverse turn 242
Spiral turn 242
Spiritual health 25
Spiritual problems 122
Splint 85, 239, 244
    application of 246
    rolls, prefabricated 245
    types of 85
    using 261
Splinters 274
Sputum production 186
Staff monitoring operations, developing 5
Staff's poor technique and discipline 173
Starch 110
State orders 210
Statement 18
Statistics 52
Sterile
    clean container 165t
    technique 180
Sterilization 179
Stimulants 72
Stimulating test 155
Stimulus 200
Stockinet 245
Stoke volume 143
Stomatitis 90
Stool specimen, collecting 99, 99t, 160, 161, 161t
Store specimens 152
Stress 105, 138, 148, 203
Subcutaneous injection 216
Sublingual route 213
Substance, unit of concentration of 221
Sucrose 110
Sugar 154
Superficial pressure sores, development of 92
Surgical asepsis 180
    concept of 175
    general principles of 180
    practices 180t
    principles of 181, 181t
Susceptible host 171
Swabbing throat, direct application of 224
Swallowing 268
    poisoning by 268
Swan-Ganz catheter 259
Sweets 110
Syringes, types of 217
Systematic nursing education 57
Systolic pressure 149

T
Tachypnea 185
Tap water 100
T-binder 243
    double 243f
    single 243f
Teeth 133
    and oral cavity, care of 90
Temperature 131
    axillary 142
    core 138
    monitoring 259
    oral 141
    rectal 142
    scales 140
    surface 138
Tension pneumothorax 257
Terminal illness 120, 122
    health model 123, 123t
Terminally ill 123
    and dying patient, care of 120
Termination phase 51
Theology 6
Therapeutic baths 86
    types of 86
Therapeutic communication 49t
    technique 43
Therapeutic diet, prescription of 114
Therapeutic effect 219
Therapeutic environment 30
Therapeutic nurse-patient relationship 51
Therapeutic nursing care 183
Therapeutic nutrition 114
    purposes of 114
Therapeutic relationship 50
Thermodilution catheter 259
Thermometer
    placement of 142f, 144f
    step except 141
    types of 140
Thigh, fracture of 263
Thoracic reference line, posterior 134
Throat
    gargling 225
    paining 224t
    swab 164
        procedure of collecting 164t
Thromboplastin, partial 153
Thumb
    fractures 262
    spica 243f
        steps for 242
Thyrocalcitonin 155
Thyroid 134
    gland, palpation of 134f
    stimulating hormone test 155
Thyrotrophin 155
Thyroxin output 138
Tidal volume 186
Tissue 92
    paper 142
Toilet
    chair 98
    utensils 98

Tongue 133
    inflammation of 90
Tooth decay, measures to prevent 90
Touch 42
Toxic effect 219
Toxin 172
Toxoid 172
Trachea 134
Traction
    care of 197
    classification of 197
    purposes of 197
    types of 199
Traditional patient record 52
Transdermal medication patches 255
Transfer from bed to chair and vice versa 80, 81
    procedure 81t
Transfer procedure 35
Transient circulatory disturbance 92
Transmission of disease, mode of 174
Transporting patients, safety in 32
Trauma 137
Traumatic bleeding, severe 270, 271
Traumatic injuries 256
Triangular arm slings 244
    method 244
Trustworthy 16
Tube feeding 115
Turgor 132
Typhoid fever 115

U
Ulcerative colitis 115
Unconscious patient, care of 193, 194
Unconsciousness 193
    clinical manifestation of 194
Underweight 113
Unit after discharge, care of 40
Universal precaution 181
    elements of 182
    part of 176
Unoccupied bed
    making 82
        procedure of 82t
Unpleasant odors 91
Upper airway infections, prevent 185
Upper arm, fracture of 262
Upper respiratory airway infection 183
Uric acid 154
Urinals, disinfection of 178
Urinary catheterization 108
    procedure of 108t
Urinary diversion, management of 104, 203
Urinary elimination 103
    assessing 104, 203
    common alterations in 103, 202
    factors influencing 104, 203
    problems 104
Urinary incontinence 104, 202
Urinary output, monitoring 258
Urinary retention 104, 203
Urinary system, effect on 219
Urinary tract infection 174
Urine 164
    accidental leakage of 104
    analysis 156
    chemical properties of 157t

collection of 165
description of 104, 203
examination of 105, 204
procedure of collecting 165t
production, altered 103, 202
specimen, collecting random 107
    procedure of 107t
stream, difficulty in starting 104
tests 156

V

Vagina 225
    procedure of collecting specimen from 165t
Vaginal cream 225
Vaginal swab 165
Validating data 59
Valve, control 149
Vaporization 138
Venereal disease research laboratory 155
Venipuncture 152
Venous blood 152
Venous circulation, altered 86
Vials and ampoules, types of 218

Victim
    comfortable 237
    lying down 237
    warm 238
Visitors information 32
Visual acuity 132
Vital signs 129, 137
    assess 137
    guidelines for taking 137, 140
Vitamin 112, 115
    diet, high 115
    in food, quality of 112
Vocal fremitus 135
Voice, tone of 42
Voiding habits 105, 204
Voiding pattern 104, 203

W

Waste
    collection of 177
    segregation 182
    transportation of 177
Water and electrolyte balance 193

Webber lateralization 132
Weight-bearing activity 94
Wellness 23
Western blot 153
Wheezing 186
White blood cells 154
Wing tipped cannula insertion 231, 231t
Working as a team 15
Wound
    care of 239
    collection of specimen from 166
    dressing of 239, 240t
    infection 174
    procedure of collecting specimen from 166t
    stab 274
    swab 165
Wrist grasp
    double 79
    single 79
Writing nursing care plan 64
    guidelines for 65
Writing nursing orders 64
Writing progress notes, formats for 53

EU GSPR Authorised Reprsentative
Logos Europe, 9 rue Nicolas Poussin
1700, La Rochelle, France
Phone: +33 (0) 6 67 93 73 78
E-mail: contact@logoseurope.eu

www.ingramcontent.com/pod-product-compliance
Ingram Content Group UK Ltd.
Pitfield, Milton Keynes, MK11 3LW, UK
UKHW050458150426
5217IPUK00025B/1738